Type 1 Diabetes
IN ADULTS

Type 1 Diabetes
IN ADULTS
PRINCIPLES AND PRACTICE

Edited by

Serge Jabbour
Thomas Jefferson University, Philadelphia, Pennsylvania, USA

Elizabeth A. Stephens
Providence Portland Medical Center, Portland, Oregon, USA

Associate Editors

Irl B. Hirsch
University of Washington, Seattle, Washington, USA

Satish Garg
University of Colorado Health Sciences Center, Denver, Colorado, USA

Barry J. Goldstein
Thomas Jefferson University, Philadelphia, Pennsylvania, USA

Matthew C. Riddle
Oregon Health & Science University, Portland, Oregon, USA

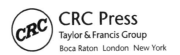

CRC Press
Taylor & Francis Group
Boca Raton London New York

CRC Press is an imprint of the
Taylor & Francis Group, an **informa** business

CRC Press
Taylor & Francis Group
6000 Broken Sound Parkway NW, Suite 300
Boca Raton, FL 33487-2742

First issued in paperback 2019

© 2008 by Taylor & Francis Group, LLC
CRC Press is an imprint of Taylor & Francis Group, an Informa business

No claim to original U.S. Government works

ISBN-13: 978-0-8493-2622-6 (hbk)
ISBN-13: 978-0-367-38827-0 (pbk)

A CIP record for this book is available from the British Library.

Library of Congress Cataloging-in-Publication Data available on application

**Visit the Taylor & Francis Web site at
http://www.taylorandfrancis.com**

**and the CRC Press Web site at
http://www.crcpress.com**

Preface

At a time of dramatic increases in the prevalence of obesity, it is appropriate that type 2 diabetes has received a great deal of attention by the endocrinology community. Clearly, the management of insulin resistance and cardiovascular risk is a critical issue. However, it is equally important to acknowledge and address type 1 diabetes, whose prevalence is also increasing and whose management remains complex. Currently it is estimated that 10–15% of those with diabetes have type 1, and often the diagnosis is challenging since many of those previously thought to have type 2 diabetes actually have late-onset type 1 diabetes (also termed latent autoimmune diabetes in adults, or LADA). Over the last decade the tools for the management of type 1 diabetes have also evolved and so there is an opportunity to more closely replicate normal physiologic insulin secretion with either basal–bolus insulin therapy or continuous subcutaneous insulin infusions. Besides insulin, there are now some added therapies such as pramlintide. While these advancements allow us to better manage our patients with type 1 diabetes, they also add complexity. An updated text to address the concepts behind the care of the person with type 1 diabetes is warranted to review these issues for endocrinologists and primary care providers with an interest in diabetes.

To achieve this goal, we have divided our textbook into four separate sections:

- In the first section, we review the pathogenesis of type 1 diabetes, including polyglandular autoimmunity, and expand our understanding of LADA.
- In the second section, we discuss in detail the management of type 1 diabetes, including blood glucose monitoring; diabetes education, nutrition, and special situations; insulin; and pramlintide therapies.
- In the third section, we review the complications of diabetes: Hyperglycemia and tissue damage, including data from DCCT/EDIC, retinopathy, nephropathy, neuropathy, and hypoglycemia.
- In the fourth and last section, we discuss special settings and situations such as pregnancy, psychology, including depression and eating disorders, and pancreas and islet transplantation.

We would like to acknowledge the mentoring of our senior editors, Dr. Irl Hirsch, Dr. Satish Garg, Dr. Barry J. Goldstein, and Dr. Matthew Riddle.

We hope you find this text to be informative and practical in your day-to-day management of type 1 diabetes patients and all the complex issues that arise in their care.

Serge Jabbour
Elizabeth A. Stephens

Contents

v

Contributors

Jo Ann Ahern   Animas Corporation, West Chester, Pennsylvania, U.S.A.

T. S. Bailey   Advanced Metabolic Care & Research, Escondido, California, U.S.A.

B. A. Boyer   Institute for Graduate Clinical Psychology, Widener University, Chester, Pennsylvania, U.S.A.

V. J. Briscoe   Vanderbilt School of Medicine, Division of Diabetes, Endocrinology and Metabolism, Vanderbilt University, Nashville, Tennessee, U.S.A.

J. M. Cropsey   Wills Eye Institute, Philadelphia, Pennsylvania, U.S.A.

S. N. Davis   Vanderbilt School of Medicine, Division of Diabetes, Endocrinology and Metabolism, Vanderbilt University, Nashville, Tennessee, U.S.A.

J. L. Edwards   Department of Neurology, University of Michigan, Ann Arbor, Michigan, U.S.A.

E. L. Feldman   Department of Neurology, University of Michigan, Ann Arbor, Michigan, U.S.A.

M. S. Fineman   Wills Eye Institute, Philadelphia, Pennsylvania, U.S.A.

K. W. Hickey   Georgetown University Hospital, Washington, DC, U.S.A.

K. K. Hood   Section on Behavioral and Mental Health Research, Section on Genetics and Epidemiology, Joslin Diabetes Center, Harvard Medical School, Boston, Massachusetts, U.S.A.

A. M. Jacobson   Section on Behavioral and Mental Health Research, Joslin Diabetes Center, Harvard Medical School, Boston, Massachusetts, U.S.A.

H. A. Keenan   Section on Vascular Cell Biology, Joslin Diabetes Center, Harvard Medical School, Boston, Massachusetts, U.S.A.

D. Lehman   Institute for Graduate Clinical Psychology, Widener University, Chester, Pennsylvania, U.S.A.

A. A. Little   Department of Neurology, University of Michigan, Ann Arbor, Michigan, U.S.A.

M. F. Magee   MedStar Diabetes & Research Institutes at Washington Hospital Center and Georgetown University School of Medicine, Washington, DC, U.S.A.

L. F. Meneghini   Diabetes Research Institute, University of Miami Leonard M. Miller School of Medicine, Miami, Florida, U.S.A.

M. Miodovnik   Washington Hospital Center, Washington, DC, U.S.A.

V. Myers   Pennington Biomedical Research Center, Louisiana State University, Louisiana, U.S.A.

R. G. Naik   Bombay Hospital and Medical Research Center, Mumbai, India

C. M. Nassar   MedStar Diabetes & Research Institutes at Washington Hospital Center, Washington, DC, U.S.A.

J. P. Palmer   DVA Puget Sound Health Care System, University of Washington, Seattle, Washington, U.S.A.

J. J. Reyes-Castano   MedStar Diabetes & Research Institutes at Washington Hospital Center, Washington, DC, U.S.A.

R. Paul Robertson   Pacific Northwest Research Institute, University of Washington, Seattle, Washington, U.S.A.

J. G. Umans   Medstar Research Institute, Hyattsville, Maryland, U.S.A.

Y. Woredekal   SUNY Downstate Medical Center, Brooklyn, New York, U.S.A.

C. H. Wysham   Washington State University, Spokane, Washington, U.S.A.

1

Pathophysiology of Type 1 Diabetes

L. F. Meneghini
Diabetes Research Institute, University of Miami Leonard M. Miller School of Medicine, Miami, Florida, U.S.A.

INTRODUCTION AND BACKGROUND

Type 1 diabetes mellitus (T1DM) is characterized by defects in beta-cell function that eventually result in absolute insulin deficiency, requiring insulin replacement therapies to ensure survival and limit the complications of hyperglycemia. Type 1A or autoimmune diabetes, which accounts for 85% to 90% of T1DM, is characterized by the presence of autoantibodies to several islet cell molecules, including insulin, GAD, and IA-2, as well as by infiltration of the islets and destruction of beta cells by mononuclear cells (insulitis). Although the presence of insulitis requires a tissue specimen for diagnosis, autoantibodies on the other hand can be measured from serum and are detectable years prior to the onset of hyperglycemia. Along with genetic screening and assessment of stimulated insulin secretion, autoantibodies can also be used to predict the development of T1DM in at-risk populations.

Although there is a 10- to 15-fold increase in the lifetime risk of developing the disease for first-degree relatives of subjects with T1DM compared to the general population, over 85% of patients who develop autoimmune diabetes do so in the absence of a positive family history. Several genetic factors that increase the risk of developing autoimmune diabetes have been identified; the best characterized and studied are the DR3/DR4 alleles in the MHC (HLA) complex. It is still unclear what triggers the initial immunologic attack on the beta cell, but a combination of both genetic and environmental factors is likely to be involved. Once autoantibodies are detectable in the serum, many of these patients will go on to develop insulitis and beta-cell destruction eventually leading to metabolic instability, hyperglycemia, and possibly ketoacidosis. The mechanisms underlying the progression of the autoimmune attack on the beta cells have been extensively assessed in the rodent model, but unfortunately remain incompletely understood in humans, where access to injured tissue (pancreatic islet cells) and other factors have limited our ability to better address the pathology of diabetes. In this chapter, we will review the natural history and the development of the metabolic abnormalities that characterize the progression of autoimmune diabetes and try to link these clinical observations to possible pathogenetic factors. We will conclude by describing the relationship of T1DM to other autoimmune syndromes that share similar genetic predisposition.

Table 1 HLA Haplotypes and Risk of Type 1 Diabetes (86)

	HLA		
Risk	HLA DRB1	HLA DQA1	HLA DQB1
High risk	0401, 0402, 0405	0301	0302
	0301	0501	0201
Moderate risk	0801	0401	0402
	0101	0101	0501
	0901	0301	0303
Weak or moderate	0401	0301	0301
Protection	0403	0301	0302
	0701	0201	0201
	1101	0501	0301
Strong protection	1501	0102	0602
	1401	0101	0503
	0701	0201	0303

HLA DR3, DQB1*0201 = DR3-DQ2; HLA DR4, DQB1*0302 = DR4-DQ8; HLA DR2, DQB1*0602 = DR2.

GENETIC PREDISPOSITION

Several factors can be used to predict the risk of T1DM. In many subjects who are diagnosed with the disease, specific genetic elements have been implicated. For example, the heterozygous HLA DR3-DQ2/DR4-DQ8 genotype is so far the highest risk genotype identified for the development of T1DM diabetes (Table 1). This combination occurs in less than 3% of the general population and in approximately 30% of patients with autoimmune diabetes. Moreover, about 90% of subjects with autoimmune diabetes carry either DR3 or DR4 allele. Individuals with the high-risk DR3/DR4 genotype have an increased lifetime risk of developing T1DM of approximately 6%, which is 20 times higher compared to individuals without it (1). Other genetic factors as well as environmental factors are thought to contribute to disease risk, given that the genetic susceptibility from HLA alleles predicts only about 50% of diabetes cases (2).

Genetic testing has been used in the attempt to identify individuals (particularly children) at-risk for T1DM, with the purpose of developing effective strategies for early disease screening and prevention studies. The diabetes autoimmunity study in the young (DAISY) longitudinally assessed the development of disease in both first-degree relatives (children) of patients with T1DM as well as a cohort of newborns from the general population identified through HLA screening, and risk classified based on HLA-DR/DQ genotyping (3). The high-risk genotype (DR3-DQ2/DR4-DQ8), which was present in 2% of newborns, correctly identified almost half of the children who went on to develop diabetes. Of the studied population, 8.2% of children were found to be positive for one or more autoantibodies (GAD, IA-2, IAA), although in 62% of the cases the antibody test was considered either falsely or only transiently positive. This transient positivity may reflect subjects in whom the autoimmune process was somehow attenuated or perhaps aborted. While in this study, the HLA-DR3/DR4-DQ8 genotype was most predictive of progression to diabetes, the presence of more than one antibody and a higher autoantibody titer also identified children who went on to develop the condition. The Finnish type 1 diabetes prediction and prevention (DIPP) screened almost 32,000 neonates from the general population for the high-risk HLA-DQB1 alleles and offered follow-up immunologic testing only to the 15%

of infants who screened positive (4). Their strategy, which cost approximately $245 per child (5), was able to identify 75% of children who went on to develop T1DM at an early age, and was clearly more cost-effective than a purely immunologic screening approach. In the Bart's-Oxford study, the highest risk genotype (HLA DR3/DR4) conferred a 5.1% absolute risk of diabetes by age 15 years (compared to 0.3% in the general population of the study) and had an overall 23% sensitivity for detecting disease (6). Presently, the use of HLA screening of the general population to identify high-risk individuals, followed by immunologic and possibly metabolic testing in subjects positive for HLA DR3/DR4, could represent a feasible strategy to identify a significant proportion of subjects without a family history of T1DM who may in the future develop the disease.

Familial transmission of autoimmune diabetes appears to be in part determined by the relationship an individual has to the proband with the disease. For example, offsprings of fathers with diabetes carry a substantially higher risk of disease (6–9%) than do offsprings of diabetic mothers (1.3–4%) (7), while if both parents have T1DM the risk increases to approximately 30% (8–10). In fraternal (dizygotic) twins the concordance rate is 5%, whereas the risk is substantially higher in identical (monozygotic) twins (30–50%). When nonidentical siblings share the same high-risk genotype (DR3/DR4), the risk of T1DM in the unaffected proband jumps to 20%, while in monozygotic twins it increases to 70% (11). Interestingly, a higher risk of diabetes concordance is seen in siblings of subjects who develop diabetes at an earlier age (12,13).

On the other hand, the HLA DQB1*0602 allele, associated with HLA-DR2, appears to confer protection against the disease and is present in approximately 20% of Caucasians and less than 1% of children with diabetes (14). The protective effect of DQB1*0602 is seen even in subjects with evidence of pancreatic autoimmunity (positive ICA or GAD antibodies) as well as in the presence of high-risk DR3 and DR4 alleles (15). In these subjects, progression to diabetes, or even loss of first-phase insulin release (FPIR), is unusual.

While genetic screening for T1DM has focused on MHC-linked genes located on chromosome 6p21.31, also known as the IDDM1 locus, other loci outside of the MHC (HLA) region may also contribute to disease susceptibility. These loci, termed IDDM2 through IDDM18, include genes that are sometimes associated with other autoimmune diseases such as rheumatoid arthritis, lupus and Graves', while others appear diabetes-specific. For example, the IDDM2 locus on chromosome 11p15 appears to correspond with a variable number of tandem repeats (VNTR) (16), which regulates the levels of insulin gene expression in the thymus—a mechanism that has profound effects on self-tolerance to insulin (17).

NATURAL HISTORY

In many cases of T1DM, however, genetic risk alone does not appear to be sufficient to initiate the autoimmune attack. Environmental factors, such as viruses, early dietary exposure to milk proteins, vaccinations, and other factors are thought to possibly "trigger" an autoimmune event in genetically susceptible individuals (18–23). Autoantibodies become detectable in the blood of subjects who eventually experience insulitis and beta-cell injury. The presence of multiple antibodies as well as their respective titers has been used to predict the risk of developing hyperglycemia (24). This autoimmune assault appears to occur months to years before the onset of hyperglycemia. Subjects who will go on to develop diabetes usually transition through loss of FPIR, followed by glucose intolerance and eventually frank hyperglycemia, and often ketoacidosis (25). Currently, the use of autoantibody numbers and titers, along with the loss of first-phase insulin secretion following an intravenous glucose tolerance test (IVGTT) are the most accurate methods for predicting the future T1DM risk. Although T1DM does occur in adults, the peak incidence for the disease is between the age of 11 to 15 years.

A number of studies have evaluated the changes over time in the metabolic status of antibody-positive subjects prior to the diagnosis of diabetes (hyperglycemia). Much of our understanding of the natural history of T1DM is gleaned from these trials. The largest of these studies is the diabetes prevention trial in T1DM (DPT-1), which screened 84,228 first- and second-degree relatives of patients with T1DM for islet cell antibodies (ICA) (26). Those that had ICA titers of 10 JDF (Juvenile Diabetes Foundation) units or higher (3.7% of those screened) were further evaluated to (i) exclude the presence of the protective haplotype HLA-DQA1*0102,DQB1*0602 (DR2), (ii) confirm ICA positivity, and (iii) test for insulin antibodies. Additionally, they underwent testing of FPIR by IVGTT and oral glucose tolerance test (OGTT). These assessments were then used to quantify their future risk of developing T1DM. Subjects with a low FPIR on IVGTT (< 10% for siblings, offsprings, second-degree relatives, or < 1% for parents, compared to a standardized mean for a nondiabetic population), or impaired glucose tolerance on OGTT were estimated to have a 50% risk of developing diabetes within the next 5 years ($n = 339$). They were randomized to either close observation (control group) or intervention consisting of daily low-dose subcutaneous insulin injections, plus a yearly IV insulin infusion. Subjects with positive insulin autoantibodies, but no detectable metabolic instability were considered to have a 25% to 50% 5-year risk of developing the disease and were offered inclusion in the oral insulin trial. OGTTs were done every 6 months in order to detect the primary endpoint of diagnosis of diabetes, and subjects were followed for a median of 3.7 years. Although insulin treatment did not prevent progression to hyperglycemia in the DPT-1, the data from this trial have significantly contributed to our understanding of the natural progression of disease and potential screening tools to identify high-risk individuals.

Progression to diabetes appears to be marked by gradual deterioration in glycemic control, but variable secretion of insulin, depending on age at diagnosis. From observations of the DPT-1 cohorts, it appears that with the development of autoantibodies, plasma glucose levels begin to gradually rise for up to 2 years prior to the onset of diabetes, with a more marked increase in glycemia in 6 months preceding diagnosis (25). The rise in glycemia in this cohort of the DPT-1 was accompanied by a fall in stimulated C-peptide (adjusted for glucose levels), but a relatively fair preservation and in many cases even an increase in basal C-peptide levels, possibly reflecting the development of some insulin resistance (27). At diagnosis of diabetes in the DPT-1, levels of C-peptide tended to be higher than what has been observed in clinical practice (28), probably due to more timely screening and earlier detection of the metabolic abnormality. In most individuals, glucose intolerance by OGTT was detectable prior to progressing to full-blown hyperglycemia.

Insulin secretion increases in adolescence, probably in response to the reduction in insulin sensitivity brought on by puberty-related hormonal changes (29). Insulin resistance in this group appears to peak at Tanner stage 3, returns to prepubertal levels by Tanner stage 5 (30), and is probably related to changes in growth hormone (31) and adrenal steroid levels (29). Investigators have reported that insulin secretion in children at-risk for T1DM increases both before and during puberty, probably reflecting an expansion in beta-cell mass, and then decreases or remains stable during the adult years (32). While in high-risk adults, a relative decrease in insulin secretion over time predicted the development of T1DM, this was not the case for high-risk children and adolescents. Others have also documented that stimulated C-peptide secretion increases in at-risk subjects who do not progress to T1DM compared to no such change in progressors (33). It has been postulated that progression

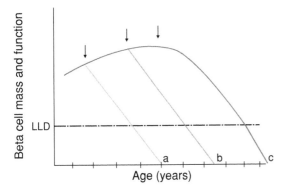

Figure 1   Model of change in beta-cell function in type 1 diabetes. The lines represented by a, b, and c illustrate the fall in beta-cell function in individuals of increasing age (32). *Abbreviation*: LLD, lower limit of detection (C-peptide of 0.03 pmol/ml).

to T1DM in children may be characterized initially by a failure to increase expected insulin secretory capacity with age, eventually followed by loss of FPIR and metabolic tolerance (34).

Another recent observation is the greater beta-cell mass estimated to be present at diagnosis of T1DM, compared to historical reports. Previous studies of beta-cell mass at diagnosis of T1DM reported values between 10% (pathologic anatomy) to 33% (stimulated C-peptide) of normal (35,36), while more recent assessments estimate the functional residual capacity to be over 50% (37). Greater beta-cell mass is associated with both older age at diagnosis and more aggressive glycemic control following the onset of hyperglycemia, although the prolongation in beta-cell function from the latter appears to be temporary (38,39). A number of researchers have documented better preservation of residual beta-cell function in adults when compared to children (40,34), substantiated by the fact that a higher percentage of subjects diagnosed at an older age have detectable C-peptide levels. Presumably, adults have had time to fully mature their beta-cell mass, while children and adolescents are still "building up" beta-cell volume. Rate of change in beta-cell function (as a surrogate marker for beta-cell mass) following the diagnosis of diabetes has been reported to be similar in children and adults in certain studies (32,37,41), although these differences have not been found consistently. Some postulate that while loss of secretory function following diagnosis may or may not be different between children and adults, the initially greater beta-cell mass in those with older onset disease translates into higher percentage of subjects with detectable C-peptide levels later on (Fig. 1).

LINK BETWEEN GENETICS AND IMMUNOLOGY

To better understand the association between HLA genes and autoimmune diabetes, and specifically the IDDM1 locus, it is important to realize that approximately 40% of the functional genes that have been identified in the class II section of the HLA locus encode for proteins that are involved in the immune response. The MHC is classified into three major sections termed class I, II, and III. Class I and II genes encode for an alpha (α) and beta (β) heterodimers that form the cleft or pocket on antigen-presenting cells (APC), where antigen is bound and presented to T lymphocytes. The amino acid sequences in these pockets are variable (polymorphic), especially for class II molecules, giving them the ability to bind to a wide variety of different peptide antigens. APCs such as macrophages, dendritic cells, activated T cells and B cells, use HLA class II molecules to bind peptides derived from extracellular proteins and specifically present them to T-helper lymphocytes (also termed CD4+ T cells, since CD4 is a molecule that is expressed on their surface) (42). When the presentation of MHC-bound antigen by the APC to the T-cell receptor (TCR) occurs in the presence of the appropriate coreceptors (i.e., CD4) and costimulatory molecules (i.e., CD80/86 with CD28; CD40 with CD154) (43), the T helper cells become activated and subsequently elicit an immune response through the release of inflammatory cytokines, the recruitment of cytotoxic killer cells (CD8+ T cells), and the production of antibody by activated B cells (also known as plasma cells). HLA class I molecules on the other hand are found on all nucleated cells of the body, bind intracellular peptides (such as small pieces of viral peptides from infected cells) and present them to cytotoxic T cells, also known as CD8+ T lymphocytes. Activated CD8+ T cells are capable of exerting direct cytotoxic effects on their target cells. T cells, whether they are T-helper (CD4+) or cytotoxic (CD8+) cells, are MHC-restricted, meaning that they can only be activated when antigen is presented to them specifically bound to either HLA class II (for CD4+ T cells) or HLA class I (for CD8+ T cells) molecules.

Disruption in the mechanisms of antigen presentation can result in either immune deficiency or autoimmunity, depending on the specific abnormalities present. For example, it has been observed that the amino acid at position 57 on the HLA-DQ beta chain is associated with either risk for or protection from autoimmune diabetes (44). Specifically, when aspartic acid (Asp57β) is present at position HLA-DQA1*0102/DQB1*0602 (DR2), then the risk of developing autoimmune disease is low. On the other hand, lack of aspartic acid at this position is observed for HLA DQB1 molecules associated with diabetes risk, such as HLA-DQB1*0201 (DR3-DQ2) and HLA-DQB1*0302 (DR4-DQ8). Variations in the MHC class II molecules have been linked not only to diabetes, but also to various other chronic autoimmune conditions, such as multiple sclerosis, celiac disease, rheumatoid arthritis, and narcolepsy. Although not entirely clear at this time, it appears that the polymorphisms encountered in the beta chain of HLA class II molecules expressed by APCs may influence presentation of autoantigens to T cells. Antigen presentation is not only important for the induction of a normal immune response, but it is also critical for the induction of immune tolerance, which is both centrally and peripherally mediated.

TOLERANCE MECHANISMS

Central (based in the thymus) and peripheral (based in lymph nodes and the circulation) tolerance mechanisms are essential in ensuring that mature lymphocytes can differentiate between pathogens and self-antigen. Disruption of these tolerance mechanisms can lead to autoimmunity to various organs and cells, and result in chronic autoimmune disease.

Although not fully elucidated, mechanisms of central tolerance are beginning to emerge. Thymocytes derived from bone marrow precursors will enter the thymus as immature T cells, which do not yet have the surface markers, CD4 and CD8 molecules, that specifically distinguish them. Within the thymus, a number of processes lead to the transformation of these cells into differentiated lymphocytes that are either CD4+ or CD8+. As lymphocytes mature, they undergo specific selection so as to eliminate (through clonal deletion) T cells that have a greater affinity for self-antigens, and positively select lymphocytes that have weak affinity for self-antigens (45) (Fig. 2). Those cells that escape this

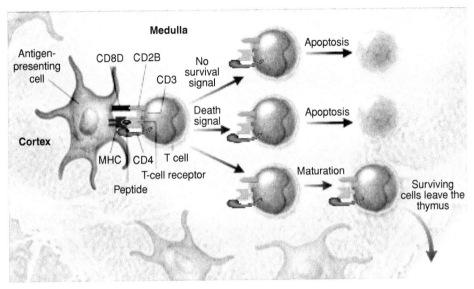

Figure 2 Central mechanisms in the induction of tolerance (87).

central tolerance mechanism are then subject to regulation through peripheral tolerance mechanisms.

The MHC–antigen complex is an essential component of the thymic selection (or deletion) of lymphocytes and their eventual maturation into CD4+ or CD8+ T cells. Both the expression of coreceptors, CD4 and CD8, and costimulatory molecules such as CD80/86 and CD40L, appear to be important in the selection of regulatory T cells and the deletion of potentially autoreactive lymphocytes. Another important mechanism in the determination of central tolerance is the expression and presentation of autoantigens in the thymic cortex and medulla. Animal studies have clearly shown that specialized cells, called medullary thymic epithelial cells (mTECs) and dendritic cells (46) are able to transcribe and express proteins usually found in peripheral tissues, such as insulin, thyroglobulin, and myelin basic protein (47–49), which have been associated with autoimmune T1DM, thyroiditis and multiple sclerosis, respectively. The qualitative and quantitative expression of these proteins by mTECs appear to, in part, determine the presence or absence of peripheral immunological reactivity to them. For example, higher levels of expression of insulin in the thymus, mediated by the INS-IDDM2 allele have been shown to be associated with protection against T1DM (17,50). The autoimmune regulator (AIRE) gene found on chromosome 21q22.3 (51) produces proteins, which are found predominantly in the thymus as well as in lymph nodes, pancreas, and adrenal cortex, and have been shown to bind DNA and variably activate the transcription of some of the peripheral tissue-specific proteins expressed by mTECs (52,53). Loss of the AIRE transcription factor results in autoimmunity to some of the organs and cells whose thymic expression by mTECs appears to be regulated through the AIRE gene (54).

GENETIC SYNDROMES

The autoimmune polyendocrinopathy-candidiasis-ectodermal-dystrophy (APECED) syndrome, also known as autoimmune polyendocrinopathy syndrome type 1 (APS1), is an autosomal recessive disease characterized by a classic triad of chronic mucocutaneous candidiasis, hypoparathyroidism, and adrenal cortical failure. Mutations in the AIRE gene

Table 2 Major Clinical Features
of the IPEX Syndrome (63)

Watery/bloody diarrhea
Failure to thrive
Type 1 diabetes mellitus
Hypothyroidism
Eczema
Hemolytic anemia
Thrombocytopenia
Lymphadenopathy
Hepatospenomegaly
Recurrent infections

are thought to be responsible for this syndrome, which is found in greatest frequency among Iranian Jews, Sardinians, and Finns (55). Although T1DM is relatively uncommon in APS Type1 (approximately 1% of affected probands), a publication on a series of Finnish patients with APECED reported a 12-fold higher prevalence of diabetes compared to the general population (56). The association between diabetes and both autoimmune adrenal insufficiency and thyroiditis is considerably greater in patients with APS type 2, also known as Schmidt syndrome (57), or Carpenter syndrome, so called when all the three conditions are present (58). Autoimmune diabetes is present in 20% to 50% of subjects with the APS type 2, and usually presents at an earlier age than either Addison's disease or thyroid disorders (59,60). As with classical type 1A diabetes, and similar to what is seen in other isolated autoimmune disorders, there is clear evidence of both humoral and cellular autoimmunity as manifested by the presence of organ-specific autoantibodies and CD8+ predominant lymphocytic infiltration (60). Addison's disease was also found to be linked to HLA DR3 and DR4 haplotypes, both independently of its association with T1DM (HLA DR3/DBQ1*0201), and in the presence of ICA (HLA DR4/DBQ1*0302) (61). Because a family history of APS type 2 is rare, it may be prudent to periodically screen patients who develop autoimmune organ damage for autoantibodies to other conditions, or at the very least to closely monitor for signs and symptoms of other autoimmune diseases.

The immunodysregulation, polyendocrinopathy, enteropathy, X-linked (IPEX) syndrome is a rare, autosomal dominant X-linked condition affecting male children usually in the neonatal period, characterized by early onset T1DM and severe enteropathy as well as by autoimmune skin disease, hypothyroidism, and variable other autoimmune manifestations (Table 2) (62–65). In the majority of cases, the condition is linked to mutations in the human *FOXP3* gene (66), which is thought to be an essential player in the regulation of T-cell activation. Mutations in this gene result in deficiencies of T regulatory cells (CD4+CD25+ T-cells), which are essential in controlling the activity of antigen-stimulated T cells. The relationship and similarities among these three autoimmune syndromes is illustrated in Table 3 and Figure 3.

AUTOIMMUNITY AND TYPE 1 DIABETES

Studies of subjects with T1DM have shown an increased frequency of antibodies directed against the beta cell (77%) as well as an increased frequency of thyroid (22%) and celiac antibodies (5–7%) (67–69). Anti-adrenal (1–2%) antibodies are less commonly detected (70), and usually result in low frequency of Addison's disease (0.8%) (71). The risk for an

Table 3 Features of the Autoimmune Polyendocrine Syndromes (62)

Feature	Autoimmune polyendocrine syndrome type I	Autoimmune polyendocrinesyndrome type II	X-linked polyendocrinopathy, immune dysfunction, and diarrhea
Prevalence	Rare	Common	Very rare
Time of onset	Infancy	Infancy through adulthood	Neonatal period
Gene and inheritance	*AIRE* (on chromosome 21, recessive)	Polygenic	*FOXP3*, X-linked
HLA genotype	Diabetes (risk decreased with HLA-DQ6)	HLA-DQ2 and HLA-DQ8; HLA-DRB1*0404	No association
Immunodeficiency	Asplenism, susceptibility to candidiasis	None	Overwhelming autoimmunity loss of regulatory T cells
Association with diabetes	Yes (in 18%)	Yes (in 20%)	Yes (in majority)
Common phenotype	Candidiasis, hypoparathyroidism, Addison's disease	Addison's disease, type 1A diabetes, chronic thyroiditis	Neonatal diabetes, malabsorption

autoimmune condition appears to extend to first-degree relatives of patients with T1DM, who may benefit from periodic screening for diabetes as well as thyroid disease (72).

Screening recommendations for subjects with T1DM should take into account the rates of positive antibodies and associated clinical disease, as well as the age of the patients. For example, even though up to one-fifth of patients with autoimmune diabetes will develop anti-peroxidase or anti-thyroglobulin antibodies, only 2% to 5% of patients with T1DM develop autoimmune thyroid dysfunction, predominantly hypothyroidism. The greatest risk

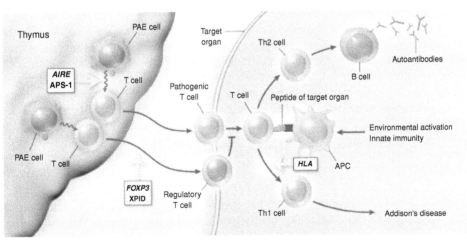

Figure 3 Pathogenic model of autoimmune polyendocrine syndrome disorders (62). *Abbreviations*: XPID, IPEX; PAE cell, peripheral antigen-expressing cell; APC, antigen-presenting cell; Th2 cell, type 2 helper T cell; Th1 cell, type 1 helper T cell.

is found in females and patients with a longer duration of disease (73,71). Interestingly, linkage analysis studies in subjects with both T1DM and autoimmune thyroid disease have revealed a significant contribution from HLA-DR3, but not from HLA-DR4 (74,75). In children and adolescents, subclinical hypothyroidism may present with only subtle findings, such as an increased frequency of hypoglycemic episodes, or a decrease in growth rate (76,77) Currently, most experts would recommend screening patients with T1DM for thyroid dysfunction at diagnosis, and periodically thereafter (every 1–2 years), even in the absence of clear symptomatology, and possibly more frequently if thyroid antibodies are positive. Screening can be done with a TSH level, and a free T4 level is obtained when abnormal TSH levels are registered. Persistently elevated TSH values should be evaluated and thyroid hormone replacement considered, with the goal of maintaining TSH levels ideally between 1 to 2 mIU/L.

The prevalence of celiac disease in the United States is reported to range between 1:133 in low-risk groups (78) with prevalence rates approaching 5–7% in patients with T1DM (69,79). The greatest risk is seen in females, those with a younger age of diabetes diagnosis and those with thyroid disease (80). Celiac disease is an autoimmune condition characterized by inflammation of the intestinal mucosa resulting in thickening of the villous crypts and villous hypertrophy, and flattening of the mucosa. The classic features of celiac disease include villous atrophy resulting in symptoms of malabsorption, such as diarrhea, weight loss, fatty stools, abdominal discomfort, all of which respond, within a few months to a gluten-free diet (81). The malabsorption associated with these pathologic changes can lead to iron deficiency resulting in anemia, vitamin D, and calcium deficiencies leading to osteoporosis and osteopenia, and vitamin B deficiency manifested through neuropsychiatric complications such as depression, anxiety, and seizures (82). Celiac disease is often asymptomatic, at least in the early stages, and may only be subtly manifested by unexpected glycemic variability, growth failure, and/or anemia. Screening for celiac disease should be carried out periodically in children (83,84), and upon suspicious findings in adults with autoimmune diabetes. This can be done by sampling serum for tissue transglutaminase antibodies (preferred) or anti-endomysial antibodies (68). Patients found positive on screening should consider undergoing a confirmatory small bowel biopsy. If disease is confirmed, the patient should be referred for nutritional counseling and placed on a gluten-free diet. Gluten, which appears to be the trigger for autoimmunity is a protein found in all forms of wheat and other grains such as rye and barley.

Screening for gastric (pernicious anemia) or adrenal (Addison's disease) autoimmunity is not usually performed on a routine basis, since the prevalence of clinically significant organ damage is relatively low. If clinical findings arise, then testing for autoimmunity with anti-parietal antibodies (and intrinsic factor antibodies) and anti-adrenal antibodies (steroid 21-hydroxylase antibodies) would be warranted (85,70). The presence of autoimmunity should be followed up by appropriate clinical evaluations and confirmation of end-organ dysfunction.

SUMMARY

Type 1A diabetes is characterized by the loss of insulin secretion due to autoimmune destruction of pancreatic beta cells, often presenting with diabetic ketoacidosis, and usually requiring insulin replacement for survival. Genetic, environmental, and possibly other unknown factors contribute to disease susceptibility. The DR3/DR4 alleles in the MHC (HLA) complex have clearly been implicated in disease risk. Mechanisms of both central and peripheral tolerance appear to play a role in the development of autoimmunity and may in part explain the association of diabetes to other polyendocrine syndromes. Patients with T1DM should undergo periodic screening to assess for the onset of thyroid dysfunction or celiac disease.

ACKNOWLEDGEMENT

I am indebted to Arleen Barreiros for the invaluable assistance in getting this manuscript to print, and to Dr. Alberto Pugliese for thoughtfully and patiently mentoring me through this project.

REFERENCES

1. Tisch R, McDevitt H. Insulin-dependent diabetes mellitus. Cell 1996;85:291–297.
2. Nerup J, Platz P, Anderson AA, et al. HLA antigens and diabetes mellitus. Lancet 1974;12: 864–866.
3. Barker JM, Barriga KJ, Yu L, et al. Prediction of autoantibody positivity and progression to type 1 diabetes: Diabetes autoimmunity study in the young (DAISY). J Clin Endocrinol Metab 2004;89(8):3896–3902.
4. Kupila A, Muona P, Simell T, et al. Feasibility of genetic and immunological prediction of type I diabetes in a population-based birth cohort. Diabetologia 2001;44(3):290–297.
5. Hahl J, Simell T, Honen J, et al. Costs of predicting IDDM. Diabetologia 1998;41:79–85.
6. Lambert AP, Gillespie KM, Thompson G, et al. Absolute risk of childhood-onset type 1 diabetes defined by human leukocyte antigen class II genotype: A population-based study in the United Kingdom. J Clin Endocrinol Metab 2004;89(8):4037–4043.
7. Redondo MJ, Eisenbarth GS. Genetic control of autoimmunity in type I diabetes and associated disorders. Diabetologia 2002;45(5):605–622.
8. Spielman RS, Bair MI, Clerget-Darpoux F. Genetic analysis of IDDM: Summary of GAW5 IDDM results. Genet Epidelmiol 1989;6:43–58.
9. Thomson G, Robinson WP, Kuhner MK, et al. Genetic heterogeneity, modes of inheritance and risk estimates for a joint study of caucasians with insulin-dependent diabetes mellitus. Am J Hum Genet 1988;43:799–816.
10. Johnston C, Pyke DA, Cudworth AG, et al. HLA-DR typing in identical twins with insulin-dependent diabetes: Differences between concordant and discordant pairs. BMJ 1983;286: 253–255.
11. Redondo MJ, Rewers M, Yu L, et al. Genetic determination of islet autoimmunity in monozygotic twin, dizygotic twin, and non-twin siblings of patients with type 1 diabetes: Prospective twin study. BMJ 1999;318:698–702.
12. Redondo MJ, Yu L, Hawa M, et al. Heterogeneity of type I diabetes: Analysis of monozygotic twins in Great Britain and the United States. Diabetologia 2001;44(3):354–362.
13. Eisenbarth GS, Ziegler AG, Colman PA. Pathogenesis of insulin-dependent (type I) diabetes mellitus. In: Kahn CR & Weir GC, eds. Joslin's Diabetes Mellitus, 13th edn. Philadelphia, PA: Lea & Febiger, 1994, pp. 216–239.
14. Baisch JM, Weeks T, Giles R, et al. Analysis of HLA-DQ genotypes and susceptibility in insulin-dependent diabetes mellitus. N Engl J Med 1990;322(26):1836–1841.
15. Pugliese A, Gianani R, Moromisato R, et al. HLA-DQB1*0602 is associated with dominant protection from diabetes even among islet cell antibody-positive first-degree relatives of patients with IDDM. Diabetes 1995;44(6):608–613.
16. Bennett ST, Lucasen AM, Gough SCL, et al. Susceptibility to human type I diabetes at IDDM2 is determined by tandem repeat variation at the insulin gene minisatellite locus. Nat Genet 1995;9:284–292.

17. Pugliese A, Zeller M, Fernandez A, et al. The insulin gene is transcribed in the human thymus and transcription levels correlate with allelic variation at the INS VNTR-IDDM2 susceptibility locus for type 1 diabetes. Nat Genet 1997;15:293–297.

18. King ML, Shaikh A, Bidwell D, et al. Coxsackie B-virus specific IgM responses in children with insulin-dependent diabetes mellitus. Lancet 1983;1:1397–1399.

19. Hviid A, Stellfeld M, Wohlfahrt J, et al. Childhood vaccination and type 1 diabetes. N Engl J Med 2004;350:1398–1404.

20. Hyoty H, Taylor KW. The role of viruses in human diabetes. Diabetologia 2002;45:1353–1361.

21. Norris JM, Barriga K, Klingensmith G, et al. Timing of initial cereal exposure in infancy and risk of islet autoimmunity. JAMA 2003;290:1713–1720.

22. Parslow RC, McKinney PA, Law GR, et al. Incidence of childhood diabetes mellitus in York-shire, northern England, is associated with nitrate in drinking water: An ecological analysis. Diabetologia 1997;40:550–556.

23. Virtanen SM, Saukkonen T, Savilahti E, et al. Diet, cow's milk protein antibodies and the risk of IDDM in Finnish children. Diabetologia 1994;37:381–387.

24. Bingley PJ, Bonifacio E, Williams AJK, et al. Prediction of IDDM in the general population: Strategies based on combination of autoantibody markers. Diabetes 1997;46 (11):1701–1710.

25. Sosenko JM, Palmer JP, Greenbaum CJ, et al. for the DPT-1 Study Group. Patterns of metabolic progression to type 1 diabetes in the Diabetes Prevention Trial-Type 1. Diabetes Care 2006;29:643–649.

26. Diabetes Prevention Trial Type 1 Study Group. Effects of insulin in relatives of patients with type 1 diabetes mellitus. N Engl J Med 2002;346(22):1685–1691.

27. Fourlanos S, Maremdran P, Byrnes GB, et al. Insulin resistance is a risk factor for progression to type 1 diabetes. Diabetologia 2004;47:1661–1667.

28. Komulainen J, Knip M, Lounamaa R, et al. for the Childhood Diabetes in Finland Study Group. Poor beta-cell function after the clinical manifestation of type 1 diabetes in children initially positive for islet cell specific autoantibodies. Diabet Med 1997;14:532–537.

29. Goran MI, Gower BA. Longitudinal study on pubertal insulin resistance. Diabetes 2001;50(11):2444–2450.

30. Moran A, Jacobs DR Jr, Steinberger J, et al. Insulin resistance during puberty: Results from clamp studies in 357 children. Diabetes 1999;48:2039–2044.

31. Caprio S, Plewe G, Diamond MP, et al. Increased insulin secretion in puberty: A compensatory response to reductions in insulin sensitivity. J Pediatr 1989;114:963–967.

32. Tsai EB, Sherry NA, Palmer JP, et al. The rise and fall of insulin secretion in type 1 diabetes mellitus. Diabetologia 2006;49:261–270.

33. Schatz D, Cuthberton D, Atkinson M, et al. Preservation of C-peptide secretion in subjects at high risk of developing type 1 diabetes mellitus—a new surrogate measure of non-progression? Pediatr Diabetes 2004;5:72–79.

34. Sherry NA, Tsai EB, Herold KC. Natural history of beta-cell function in type 1 diabetes. Diabetes 2005;54(Suppl 2):S32–S39.

35. Gepts W. Pathologic anatomy of the pancreas in juvenile diabetes mellitus. Diabetes 1965;14: 619–633.

36. Faber OK, Binder C. B-cell function and blood glucose control in insulin dependent diabetics within the first month of insulin treatment. Diabetologia 1977;13:263–268.

37. Steele C, Hagopian WA, Gitelman S, et al. Insulin secretion in type 1 diabetes. Diabetes 2004;53(2):426–433.

38. Madsbad S, Krarup T, Faber OK, et al. The transient effect of strict glycaemic control on B cell function in newly diagnosed type 1 (insulin-dependent) diabetic patients. Diabetologia 1982;22:16–20.

39. Diabetes Control and Complications Trial Research Group. Effect of intensive therapy on residual beta-cell function in patients with type 1 diabetes in the Diabetes Control and Complications Trial: A randomized, controlled trial. Ann Intern Med 1998;128:517–523.

40. Karjalainen J, Salmela P, Ilonen J, et al. A comparison of childhood and adult type I diabetes mellitus. N Engl J Med 1989;320:881–886.

41. Snorgaard O, Lassen LH, Binder C. Homogeneity in pattern of decline of beta-cell function in IDDM. Prospective study of 204 consecutive cases followed for 7.4 yr. Diabetes Care 1992;15(8):1009–1013.
42. McDevitt HO. Characteristics of autoimmunity in type 1 diabetes and type 1.5 overlap with type 2 diabetes. Diabetes 2005;54(Suppl 2):S4–S10.
43. Bromley SK, Burack WR, Johnson KG, et al. The immunological synapse. Annu Rev Immunol 2001;19:375–396.
44. Todd JA, Bell JI, McDevitt HO. HLA-DQ β gene contributes to susceptibility and resistance to insulin-dependent diabetes mellitus. Nature 1987;329:599–604.
45. Palmer E. Negative selection: Clearing out the bad apples from the T-cell repertoire. Nat Rev 2003;3:383–391.
46. Garcia CA, Kamalaveni RP, Diez J, et al. Dendritic cells in human thymus and periphery display a proinsulin epitope in a transcription-dependent, capture-independent fashion. J Immunol 2005;175:2111–2122.
47. Derbinski J, Schulte A, Kyewski B, et al. Promiscuous gene expression in medullary thymic epithelial cells mirrors the peripheral self. Nature Immunol 2001;2:1032–1039.
48. Heath VL, Moore NC, Parnell SM, et al. Intrathymic expression of genes involved in organ specific autoimmune disease. J Autoimmun 1998;11:309–318.
49. Klein L, Klugmann M, Nave KA, et al. Shaping of the autoreactive T-cell repertoire by a splice variant of self protein expressed in thymic epithelial cells. Nature Med 2000;6:56–61.
50. Vafiadis P, Bennett ST, Todd JA, et al. Insulin expression in human thymus is modulated by INS VNTR alleles at the IDDM2 locus. Nat Genet 1997;15:289–292.
51. Scott HS, Heino M, Peterson P, et al. Common mutations in autoimmune polyendocrinopathy-candidiasis-ectodermal dystrophy patients of different origins. Mol Endocrinol 1998;12:1112.
52. Kumar PG, Laloraya M, Wang CY, et al. The autoimmune regulator (AIRE) is a DNA-binding protein. J Biol Chem 2001;276:41357–41364.
53. Bjorses P, Halonen M, Palvimo JJ, et al. Mutations in the AIRE gene: Effects on subcellular location and transactivation function of the autoimmune polyendocrinopathy-candidiasis-ectodermal dystrophy protein. Am J Hum Genet 2000;66:378–392.
54. Anderson MS. Projection of an immunological self shadow within the thymus by the aire protein. Science 2002;298:1395–1401.
55. Perheentupa J. Autoimmune polyendocrinopathy-cadidiasis-ectodermal dystrophy. J Clin Endocrinol Metab 2006;91:2843–2850.
56. Ahonen P, Myllarniemi S, Sipila I, et al. Clinical variation of autoimmune polyendocrinopathy-candidiasis-ectodermal dystrophy (APECED) in a series of 68 patients. N Engl J Med 1990;322:1829–1836.
57. Schmidt MB. Eine biglandulare Erkrankung (Nebennieren und Schilddruse) bei Morbus Addisonii. Verh Dtsch Ges Pathol 1926;21:212–221.
58. Carpenter CCJ, Solomon N, Silverberg SG, et al. Schnidt's syndrome (thyroid and adrenal insufficiency): A review of the literature and a report of fifteen new cases including ten instances of coexistent diabetes mellitus. Medicine 1964;43:153–180.
59. Neufeld M, Maclaren NK, Blizzard RM. Two types of autoimmune Addison's disease associated with different polyglandular autoimmune (PGA) syndromes. Medicine 1981;60:1653–1660.
60. Betterle C, Lazzarotto F, Presotto F. Autoimmune polyglandular syndrome type 2: The tip of an iceberg? Clin Exp Immunol 2004;137:225–233.
61. Maclaren N, Riley W. Inherited susceptibility to autoimmune Addison's disease is linked to human leukocyte antigens DR3 and/or DR4, except when associated with type 1 autoimmune polyglandular syndrome. J Clin Endocr Metab 1986;62:455–459.
62. Eisenbarth GS, Gottlieb PA. Autoimmune polyendocrine syndromes. N Engl J Med 2004;350:2068–2079.
63. Gambineri E, Torgerson TR, Ochs HD. Immune dysregulation, polyendocrinopathy, enteropathy, and X-linked inheritance (IPEX), a syndrome of systemic autoimmunity caused by mutations of FOXP3, a critical regulator of T-cell homeostasis. Curr Opin Rheumatol 2003;15:430–435.

64. Wildin RS, Smyk-Pearson S, Filipovich AH. Clinical and molecular features of the immunedysregulation, polyendocrinopathy, enteropathy, X linked (IPEX) syndrome. J Med Genet 2002;39:537–545.
65. Wildin RS, Freitas A. IPEX and FOXP3: Clinical and research perspectives. J Autoimmun 2005;25:56–62.
66. Bennett CL, Christie J, Ramsdell F, et al. The immune dysregulation, polyendocrinopathy, enteropathy, X-linked syndrome (IPEX) is caused by mutations of FOXP3. Nat Genet 2001;27: 20–21.
67. De Block CEM, De Leeuw IH, Vertommen JJF, et al. Beta-cell, thyroid, gastric, adrenal and celiac autoimmunity and HLA-DQ types in type 1 diabetes. Clin Exp Immunol 2001;126:236–241.
68. Holmes GK. Screening for celiac disease in type 1 diabetes. Arch Dis Child 2002;87:495–498.
69. Maki M, Mustalahti K, Kokkonen J, et al. Prevalence of celiac disease among children in Finland. N Engl J Med 2003;348:2517–2524.
70. Peterson P, Salmi H, Hyoty H, et al. Steroid 21-hydroxylase autoantibodies in insulin-dependent diabetes mellitus. Childhood diabetes in Finland (DiMe) study group. Clin Immunol Immunopathol 1997;82(1):37–42.
71. Leong KS, Wallymahmed M, Wilding J, et al. Clinical presentation of thyroid dysfunction and Addison's disease in young adults with type 1 diabetes. Postgrad Med J 1999;75:467–470.
72. Jaeger C, Hatziagelaki E, Petzoldt R, et al. Comparative analysis of organ-specific autoantibodies and celiac disease-associated antibodies in type 1 diabetic patients, their first-degree relatives, and healthy control subjects. Diabetes Care 2001;24:27–32.
73. Kordonouri O, Hartmann R, Deiss D, et al. Natural course of autoimmune thyroiditis in type 1 diabetes: Association with gender, age, diabetes duration, and puberty. Arch Dis Child 2005;90(4):411–414.
74. Levin L, Ban Y, Concepcion E, et al. Analysis of HLA genes in families with autoimmune diabetes and thyroiditis. Hum Immunol 2004;65:640–647.
75. Sumnik Z, Drevinek P, Snajderova M, et al. HLA-DQ polymorphisms modify the risk of thyroid autoimmunity in children with type 1 diabetes mellitus. J Pediatr Endocrinol Metab 2003;16: 851–858.
76. Mohn A, Di Michele S, Di Luzio R, et al. The effect of subclinical hypothyroidism on metabolic control in children and adolescents with Type 1 diabetes mellitus. Diabet Med 2002;19: 70–73.
77. Chase HP, Garg SK, Cockerham RS, et al. Thyroid hormone replacement and growth of children with subclinical hypothyroidism and diabetes. Diabet Med 1990;7:299–303.
78. Fasano A, Berti I, Gerarduzzi T, et al. Prevalence of celiac disease in at-risk and not-at-risk groups in the United States: A large multicenter study. Arch Intern Med 2003;163:286–292.
79. Rewers M, Liu E, Simmons J, et al. Celiac disease associated with type 1 diabetes. Endocrinol Metab Clin North Am 2004;33:197–214.
80. Cerutti F, Bruno G, Chiarelli F, et al. Younger age at onset and sex predict celiac disease in children and adolescents with type 1 diabetes: An Italian multicenter study. Diabetes Care 2004;27(6):1294–1298.
81. Ubin CE, Brandborg LL, Phleps PC, et al. Studies of celiac disease: The apparent identical and specific nature of the duodenal and proximal jejunal lesion in celiac disease and idiopathic sprue. Gastroenterology 1960;38:28.
82. Addolorato G, Stefanini GF, Capristo E, et al. Anxiety and depression in adult untreated celiac subjects and in patients affected by inflammatory disease: A personality "trait" or a reactive illness? Hepatogastroenterology 1996;43:1513.
83. Freemark M, Levitsky LL. Screening for celiac disease in children with type 1 diabetes: Two views of the controversy. Diabetes Care 2003;26(6):1932–1939.
84. Silverstein J, Klingensmith G, Copeland K, et al. Care of children and adolescents with type 1 diabetes: A statement of the American Diabetes Association. Diabetes Care 2005;28(1): 186–212.

85. Carmel R. Reassessment of the relative prevalences of antibodies to gastric parietal cell and to intrinsic factor in patients with pernicious anaemia: Influence of patient age and race. Clin Exp Immunol 1992;89(1):74–77.
86. Atkinson MA, Eisenbarth GS. Type 1 diabetes: New perspectives on disease pathogenesis and treatment. Lancet 2001;358:221–229.
87. Kamradt T, Mitchison NA. Tolerance and autoimmunity. N Engl J Med 2001;344(9):655–664.

2

Latent Autoimmune Diabetes in Adults

R. G. Naik
Bombay Hospital and Medical Research Center, Mumbai, India

J. P. Palmer
DVA Puget Sound Health Care System, University of Washington, Seattle, Washington, U.S.A.

INTRODUCTION

A very large amount of clinical and basic research supports our current understanding that there are two major types of diabetes, termed type 1 diabetes and type 2 diabetes. The underlying pathophysiologic disease processes for these are usually thought to be markedly different. The disease process in classical type 1 patients is believed to be autoimmune in nature, whereas the disease process in classical type 2 is not autoimmune (1–3). In 1974, two separate groups of investigators discovered that islet cell antibodies (ICAs) were common in the sera of patients with type 1 diabetes, and this provided strong evidence that the β-cell lesion of type 1 diabetes was autoimmune in nature (4,5); autoimmune β-cell destruction leads to insulin deficiency; and circulating autoantibodies, such as autoantibodies to islet cell cytoplasm and/or to glutamic acid decarboxylase 65 (GAD65; GADA) and/or to the intracytoplasmatic domain of the tyrosine phosphatase-like protein IA-2 (IA-2A), are markers of this process. However, in clinical practice, the diagnosis of type 1 and type 2 diabetes is made phenotypically using variables such as age at onset, apparent abruptness of onset of hyperglycemia, presence of ketosis, degree of obesity (especially central and intra-abdominal), prevalence of other autoimmune diseases, and apparent need for insulin replacement. This clinical distinction is recognized to be imperfect (6,7). Our ability to distinguish the type 1 versus the type 2 disease process also has limitations due to genetic (8), immunologic (9), and functional complexity (10). There are no reliable markers for type 2 diabetes and therefore the absence of markers or manifestations of type 1 diabetes is frequently taken as indicating type 2 diabetes.

Before the recent exponential increase in childhood obesity, type 1 diabetes has been the most common diabetes seen in Caucasian children of European descent, and the disease process in these patients is almost always autoimmune. The diabetes that occurs in obese children is frequently phenotypically type 2, but we and others have found a surprisingly high frequency of islet autoantibodies in these children, which suggests a combination of the type 1 and type 2 diabetes disease processes in some of these children (11–13).

In contrast, in adults over the age of 40 in these same populations, both clinical type 1 and type 2 diabetes occur (2,14). The type 2 diabetes is thought to be common in the older age group, but the prevalence of the type 1 diabetes is unknown. Epidemiologic studies have suggested that the incidence rate of type 1 diabetes peaks twice: once close to puberty and again around 40 years of age (15), and it has been suggested that the overall incidence rate of type 1 diabetes is approximately equivalent above and below the age of 20 (16). This relatively high incidence rate of type 1 diabetes in adults is often not appreciated, probably because of the more than 10-fold greater frequency of type 2 diabetes in this age group.

Soon after the demonstration of ICAs in type 1 diabetes, in a study by Irvine et al. it was stated that ~ 11% of patients with type 2 diabetes were also positive for ICAs (17); compared to ICA⁻ type 2 diabetic patients, this ICA⁺ subset of type 2 diabetic patients tended to fail sulfonylurea therapy and needed insulin treatment earlier (17). Subsequently, several other investigators have also identified a similar subset of phenotypic type 2 diabetic patients who are positive for the antibodies commonly found in type 1 diabetes; this subset has been variously termed—latent autoimmune diabetes in adults (LADA), type 1.5 diabetes, slowly progressive IDDM, latent type 1 diabetes, youth-onset diabetes of maturity, latent-onset type 1 diabetes, "double" diabetes, and antibody-positive non–insulin-dependent diabetes (14,18–20). Although the different names have caused some confusion, the finding of this subset of phenotypic type 2 diabetic patients by many different investigators rather than just one or two groups confirms their existence as an important subset of diabetes. It is believed by many that the autoimmune β-cell destructive process proceeds more slowly in LADA than in classical childhood-onset type 1 diabetes, or the destruction may stop at a "moderate" stage (6). But some patients may have more rapid progression to complete or severe β-cell deficiency than others. In this review we will try to summarize the current state of knowledge regarding LADA, emphasizing the similarities and differences between LADA and classical type 1 diabetes. Some of the concepts expressed in this chapter have also been included in prior publications from our group (3,14,20,21).

DEMOGRAPHIC AND CLINICAL CHARACTERISTICS

Epidemiological data demonstrate that LADA accounts for 2% to 12% of all cases of diabetes (22,23). A prospective observation on the natural history of the ICA⁺ type 2 diabetes patients in Japan found that the characteristic findings in this country of "slowly progressive insulin dependent diabetes" included a late-onset, a family history of type 2 diabetes, a slow progression of β-cell failure over several years with persistently positive low-titer ICA, and incomplete β-cell loss (24). Similar presentations have been described in various other countries including Australia, Finland, New Zealand, the United States, Hong Kong, Korea, China, Mexico, and Sweden (25–28). The clinical onset of LADA may be less dramatic (25,29), the clinical recognition not always easy, and a type 2 diabetes phenotype not clear-cut; as many as 50% of "nonobese type 2 diabetes" may be late-onset type 1 diabetes (24). The typical patient, however, is generally > 35 years (age at onset 30–50 years), nonobese (lower body mass index, BMI), the diabetes is often initially controlled with diet, but within a short period (months to years), dietary control fails requiring oral agents, and progression to insulin dependency is more rapid than in antibody-negative, obese type 2 diabetes subjects. The eventual clinical features of these patients include weight loss, ketosis proneness, unstable blood glucose levels, and an extremely diminished C-peptide reserve (24); in retrospect, these subjects possess additional classical features of type 1 diabetes, viz., increased frequency of HLA-DR3 and -DR4 and ICA positivity (30).

A major question facing the diabetes community is whether all autoantibody-positive diabetes is due to the same pathophysiologic disease processes. Is autoimmune diabetes in adults due to the same underlying disease process as childhood type 1 diabetes or do some patients with autoimmune diabetes in adulthood have a distinct form of autoimmune diabetes compared to classical childhood type 1 diabetes? We have discussed some of these nomenclature issues in an editorial (31), and phenotypically we see at least three separate populations of autoimmune diabetes in adults: LADA, adult-onset type 1 diabetes, and obese patients with phenotypic type 2 diabetes who are antibody positive (type 1.5) (31). The Immunology of Diabetes Society has recently proposed several criteria in an attempt to standardize those patients referred to as having LADA. These criteria are patients should be ≥ 30 years of age, positive for at least one of the four antibodies commonly found in type 1 diabetic patients (ICAs and autoantibodies to GAD65, IA-2, and insulin), and are not treated with insulin within the first 6 months after diagnosis. The latter requirement is subjective and is likely to vary depending on the treating physician; it is, however, meant to distinguish LADA and type 1 diabetes occurring in patients > 30 years of age (21,32).

The role of obesity and the degree of insulin resistance in LADA is another area of controversy. Kahn et al. (33) demonstrated a curvilinear relationship between insulin resistance and insulin secretion; normal β-cells compensate for insulin resistance by secreting more insulin, and the product of insulin sensitivity and insulin secretion is normally a constant and this is termed as disposition index (34). The implication of this physiology is that patients with insulin resistance will demonstrate hyperglycemia with a lesser degree of absolute insulin deficiency compared to subjects who are insulin sensitive. Since LADA subjects span the spectrum from lean to obese, differences in insulin sensitivity could be an important variable in their physiology. Our group has recently documented that insulin sensitivity, taking into account obesity (BMI), is not different in LADA and antibody-negative type 2 diabetes (18).

HUMORAL IMMUNE RESPONSE

Antibody Positivity and Clustering

That the underlying disease processes in both LADA and classical type 1 diabetes is autoimmune is strongly supported by the presence of islet autoantibodies. However, there are differences in antibodies in LADA and type 1 diabetes; this suggests potentially important immunological differences between the two groups. All four islet autoantibodies—ICAs, GAD antibodies (GADAs), IA-2 antibodies, and insulin autoantibodies—are common in childhood type 1 diabetes; many type 1 diabetes patients are also positive for multiple autoantibodies. Thus, antibody clustering is a characteristic feature of classic childhood type 1 diabetes. In nondiabetic relatives of patients with type 1 diabetes, risk of future type 1 diabetes is directly proportional to the number of autoantibodies positive (35–37). For relatives with two or more of these autoantibodies, the risk of diabetes within 3 years was 39% (95% CI, 27–52) and the risk within 5 years was 68% (95% CI, 52–84). Relatives with three autoantibodies had a risk within 5 years that was even higher. The presence of low first-phase insulin release further increased the risk for relatives with one or two autoantibodies (36,37). ICAs and GADAs are also common in LADA, but IA-2 antibodies and insulin autoantibodies are much less commonly seen in LADA than in type 1 diabetes (20). As discussed earlier, type 1 diabetic patients are very often positive for multiple (two or more) autoantibodies, whereas single autoantibodies are more common in LADA patients (Fig. 1).

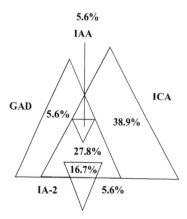

Figure 1 Clustering of autoantibodies in autoantibody-positive patients. Numbers (%) refer to the percentage of the antibody-positive patients who were positive for the respective antibodies. *Source*: Reproduced with permission from Ref. 25.

It has been shown that high GADA levels remain for up to 40 years after diagnosis of type 1 diabetes (38) in contrast to ICA, which falls after the diagnosis (39). There appears to be an ethnic difference in GADA positivity with higher frequency in Caucasian late-onset type 1 diabetes subjects than in adult-onset Asian type 1 diabetes patients suggesting that the adult-onset diabetes in the latter groups is less likely to have an autoimmune component to its pathogenesis or that different antigens (and by inference different autoantibodies) are involved (40–42).

Autoantibodies and β-Cell Function

Many studies have shown that patients positive for GADA and/or ICA have a more rapid decline in C-peptide, fail oral agents, and require insulin treatment earlier (43–48). In one study (43) the positivity rate for GADA was as high as 23.8% in nonobese and insulin-deficient patients with sulfonylurea failure, suggesting that autoimmune mechanisms may play an important role in the pathogenesis of secondary failure of sulfonylurea therapy. Another study (47) determined the prevalence of GADA and ICA in relation to β-cell function in adults newly diagnosed with diabetes mellitus. The positive predictive values for insulin deficiency of GADA and ICA were 39 and 78%, respectively. The sensitivity of both antibodies for detecting insulin deficiency was 50%. The specificity for detecting noninsulin deficiency was 85% for GADA and 97% for ICA. Positivity for both GADA and ICA gave a specificity and positive predictive value for insulin deficiency of 99% and a sensitivity of 50%. Later analysis of the United Kingdom Prospective Diabetes Study data has also shown that the presence of both ICAs and GADAs was a stronger predictor of insulin requirement than GADAs alone among patients older than 45 years of age (49).

After the diagnosis of the disease, probably in parallel with β-cell destruction (23,37,38), ICA declines in type 1 diabetic children as the duration of diabetes increases. ICA declines more rapidly than do IA-2As and GADAs (50). To clarify the relationships between islet antibodies (ICA, GADA, and IA-2A) versus the progression of β-cell dysfunction, Borg et al. followed a group of diabetic patients from their diagnosis at 21–73 years of age (51). Patients with ICA had high levels of GADA and/or IA-2 A at diagnosis and more severe β-cell dysfunction 5 years after diagnosis than those with only GADA in low concentrations. This 12-year follow-up study examined the further progression of β-cell dysfunction in relation to islet antibodies at and after diagnosis. In this prospective study of patients with adult-onset diabetes, almost all of those with GADA and/or ICA at diagnosis of diabetes had developed complete β-cell failure (undetectable fasting plasma C-peptide) 12 years after diagnosis. This was seen in patients of all ages. In this context, isolated GADA positivity was associated with a slower development of β-cell failure than positivity for multiple antibodies. Patients with isolated GADA positivity had some preserved function 5 years after diagnosis of diabetes; however, most of them (80%) had developed β-cell failure 12 years after diagnosis. Indeed, β-cell failure 12 years after diagnosis was restricted to patients who were autoantibody positive at diagnosis. Among patients antibody positive at diagnosis, the frequencies of ICA and IA-2A decreased 50% from diagnosis to 12 years after diagnosis, whereas almost all patients with GADA at diagnosis remained GADA positive during the entire study period of 12 years. This study showed that GADA measurements may be performed many years after the diagnosis of diabetes with preserved sensitivity. In addition, ICA developed many years after diagnosis in some patients who were ICA⁻ at diagnosis, and C-peptide declined more rapidly in these patients than in those who remained antibody negative. This may argue for repeated antibody measurements after diagnosis. This study very strongly argued for the importance of conducting islet antibody measurements at or near the time of diagnosis in most patients with adult-onset diabetes; islet antibody positivity very specifically identified all patients with future β-cell failure.

Antigenic Differences Between LADA and Type 1 Diabetes

Other observations also suggest antigenic differences between LADA and type 1 diabetes. The ICAs and GADAs found in LADA versus type 1 diabetes may differ. Seissler et al. demonstrated that over 90% of ICA⁺ sera from type 1 diabetic patients was also positive for GADAs or IA-2 antibodies; on the contrary this was observed in < 20% of LADA patients (52). The investigators also found that the ICA staining in ∼ 60% of type 1 diabetic patients' sera could be blocked by GAD and IA-2; however, this was seen in a much lower percentage of LADA patients, suggesting that antibodies to antigens other than GAD and IA-2 are more prevalent in LADA (52). This raises the intriguing possibility that some unidentified antigens are more commonly involved in LADA than in type 1 diabetes.

Another large study involving 569 type 2 diabetes subjects looked for possible associations of GADA epitope specificity and clinical characteristics using GAD65/67 chimeric molecules (53). Of the 11% of GADA-positive type 2 diabetic patients, ∼ 80% had antibodies directed to both middle and COOH-terminal epitopes; these patients had a lower BMI, lower basal C-peptide, and a higher frequency of insulin treatment than GADA-negative patients. The 20% of GADA-positive patients with antibodies directed solely at the mid-portion of GAD65 were phenotypically similar to GADA-negative type 2 diabetic patients (53).

Using recombinant 35 S-GAD65/67 fusion proteins, we, in collaboration with Chris Hampe and Åke Lernmark, investigated possible differences in epitope specificity of GADAs in LADA versus type 1 diabetes. More than 90% of type 1 diabetes patients' sera bound to the middle or COOH-terminal portion of GAD65; similar binding was seen in only 65% of sera from LADA patients. In contrast, the NH₂-terminal portion of GAD65 was recognized by 20% of LADA patients compared with 5% of type 1 diabetic patients (54). We have found similar results using GAD65-specific recombinant Fabs in more recent studies (55).

Epitope differences between LADA and type 1 diabetes have also been confirmed in the slowly progressive insulin-dependent diabetes (Japanese equivalent of LADA). Using

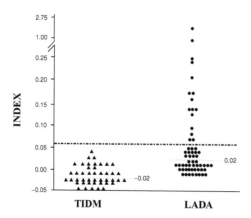

Figure 2 GADA IgG$_4$ subclass distribution in patients with type 1 diabetes ($n = 45$) and in patients with LADA ($n = 60$). Patients with an index below –0.05 are not shown in the figure. The cutoff level for negativity was fixed at 0.06 (represented by dotted line). The median index levels in each group are shown in the figure as –0.02 for type 1 diabetes and 0.02 for LADA. *Source*: Reproduced with permission from Ref. 57.

GAD65/67 chimeric molecules, unique NH$_2$-terminal linear epitopes in the GADAs of slowly progressive insulin-dependent diabetes that did not react with sera of adult-onset type 1 diabetes have been identified (56). These observations demonstrate heterogeneity of GADA epitope specificity and suggest important differences between LADA and type 1 diabetes. Differences in the GAD antibody IgG subclasses also appear to exist in type 1 diabetes versus LADA. The IgG4 subclass of GADA was more frequent in LADA than in type 1 diabetic patients, implying a greater TH2 or regulated immune response in LADA (Fig. 2) (57).

T-CELL STUDIES

Type 1 diabetes is a T-cell–mediated autoimmune disease. Over the last few years, our group has developed T-cell assays to measure reactivity to islet antigens in human type 1 diabetes; one such assay called cellular immunoblotting uses proteins from human islets separated into 18 different molecular weight regions using SDS-PAGE. An excellent sensitivity and specificity was demonstrated by this assay in a recent, National Institutes of Health–Immune Tolerance Network Workshop (58). The cellular immunoblotting assay has been used to describe the T-cell reactivity of recently diagnosed type 1 diabetic patients to multiple different molecular weight islet proteins (59), to describe the antigen spreading that occurs during the prediabetic (type 1 diabetes) period (60), and to compare T-cell responses of type 1 diabetes with LADA (61). T cells from both type 1 diabetes and LADA commonly respond to four or more different molecular weight blot sections of islet proteins, whereas normal control subjects and antibody-negative type 2 diabetic patients generally respond to less than four blot sections (Fig. 3). But we have observed differences in the specific blot sections stimulating T cells from type 1 diabetes versus LADA. Some blot sections stimulate T cells from a high percentage of both type 1 diabetes and LADA patients. Other blot sections, especially in the lower molecular weight regions, more commonly stimulate T cells from type 1 diabetic than LADA patients (Fig. 4). These observations provide further evidence for important antigenic differences between LADA and type 1 diabetes.

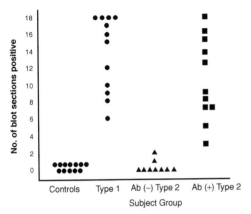

Figure 3 Peripheral blood mononuclear cell responses of 12 normal control subjects, 12 type 1 diabetic patients, 9 autoantibody-negative (Ab–) type 2 diabetic patients, and 11 autoantibody positive (Ab+) type 2 diabetic patients. The number of molecular weight regions positive for each individual is shown. The different symbols represent individual subjects. A positive response is taken as SI > 2.0. *Source*: Reproduced with permission from Ref. 60.

Use of cellular immunoblotting assay on a relatively large number of phenotypic type 2 diabetic patients has resulted in an interesting discovery. We have identified that some patients who are negative for autoantibodies (GADAs, IA-2 antibodies, insulin autoantibodies, and ICAs) have T-cell responses to islet antigens similar to the responses seen in type 1 diabetic patients (21). Like in the antibody-positive, phenotypic type 2 diabetic patients (LADA), these T-cell–positive but antibody-negative patients have a decreased stimulated C-peptide compared with antibody- and T-cell–negative phenotypic type 2 diabetic patients. We are currently investigating whether these antibody-negative, T-cell–positive patients seroconvert to antibody positivity over time or remain a distinct subset of autoimmune diabetes.

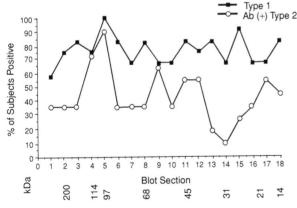

Figure 4 Peripheral blood mononuclear cell responses of type 1 diabetic patients compared with antibody type 2 diabetic patients (LADA). The percentage of subjects responding to each molecular weight region is shown. A positive responses is taken as SI > 2.0. Blot sections correspond to molecular mass regions > 200 kDa and < 14 kDa. *P < 0.05, significant differences. *Source*: Reproduced with permission from Ref. 60.

ROLE OF INSULIN RESISTANCE

Insulin resistance and decreased insulin secretion are the central pathophysiologic abnormalities in type 2 diabetes. Determinants of insulin resistance include several variables including age, BMI, ethnicity, physical activity, and medications. However, the role of insulin resistance and its contribution to the pathophysiology of LADA is controversial; the degree of insulin resistance in LADA has been reported to be less than in type 2 diabetes and comparable to type 1 diabetes (62,63). We have recently compared insulin resistance by using the homeostasis model (HOMA) in LADA, antibody-negative type 2 diabetes, and normal control subjects correcting for the effect of BMI. There was a positive correlation of BMI with insulin resistance in all three groups. Insulin resistance was remarkably similar in both LADA and antibody-negative type 2 diabetes patients when corrected for BMI (18).

GENETIC SUSCEPTIBILITY AND PROTECTION

Studies of both the animal models (the NOD mouse and the BB rat) and human type 1 diabetes confirm the presence of strong genetic control over both susceptibility to and protection from clinical disease in type 1 diabetes. The greatest risk and protection is conferred by the major histocompatibility complex region, HLA in humans; however, other genes are also involved in the process. Similarities and/or differences at the genetic level between type 1 diabetes and LADA would be of great interest (21).

HLA Associations

It is well established that HLA-DR3, -DR4, and -DQβ1*0201 and 0302 confer increased risk of type 1 diabetes. It is also known that other HLA alleles including DR2 and DQβ1*0301 and 0602 confer protection against type 1 diabetes. An increased frequency of HLA susceptibility alleles has been observed in LADA patients (20,64), but whether or not there are subtle differences between type 1 diabetes and LADA for specific alleles is controversial (20,64,65). The most consistent HLA-related finding is a relatively high frequency compared to type 1 diabetes of the protective allele DR2 and DQB1*0602 in subjects with LADA (66). One could, thus, possibly hypothesize that the type 1 diabetes disease process is more aggressive resulting in clinical presentation at a younger age in individuals with more susceptibility genes and less protective genes; and vice versa, the disease process is less aggressive resulting in clinical presentation at older ages in individuals with less susceptibility genes and/or more protective genes.

Another report suggested a relationship between HLA and insulin secretion in LADA patients. Stimulated C-peptide was lower in ICA[+] patients who were heterozygous for DR3 and DR4 compared to ICA[+] patients who were DR3/DR4[-] (67).

Non-HLA Associations

Allelic variations at several non-HLA loci with increased risk for and protection from classic type 1 diabetes have also been investigated in LADA patients. An increased frequency of the cytotoxic T-lymphocyte antigen-4 (CTLA-4) genotype A/G is seen in both type 1 diabetes and LADA, suggesting a similar role in both these types of diabetes (68). Similarly, allelic variation in the variable number of tandem repeats of the 5' region of the insulin gene has been reported in both type 1 diabetes and LADA, but the relative risk associated with the 1 S/S genotype was significantly stronger for LADA than for type 1 diabetes (69).

Microsatellite polymorphism in the major histocompatibility complex class I chain–related gene A (MICA) has been associated with different autoimmune diseases including type 1 diabetes. MICA5 is associated with type 1 diabetes under the age of 25 years, whereas MICA5.1 is associated with both LADA and type 1 diabetes over 25 years of age (65,70). Other associations reported include an allelic polymorphism within the promoter region of the tumor necrosis factor-α (TNF-α) gene, and a significantly lower frequency of the TNF2 allele in LADA compared with type 1 diabetes or nondiabetic control subjects (71).

CORRELATIONS OF CLINICAL PARAMETERS, AND GENETIC, METABOLIC, AND IMMUNOLOGIC VARIABLES

Clinical parameters, C-peptide levels, and islet cell–specific autoantibodies were evaluated in 54 LADA (onset of diabetes above 35 years of age, the detection of any circulating islet cell–specific autoantibody, and no indication for insulin therapy in the first 6 months after diagnosis), 57 classical adult-onset type 1 diabetic, and 190 type 2 diabetic patients (control group) (72). There were no differences in the various clinical parameters (lipid profile, frequency of hypertension, BMI, and waist-to-hip ratio) in the LADA group and the adult-onset type 1 patients. Although C-peptide levels did not differ at onset, they decreased less rapidly in the LADA group. There were no differences in the prevalence of predisposing HLA genotypes between these two groups; an increased DR3 DQβ1*0201 and DR4 DQβ1*0302 was found in LADA and adult-onset type 1 diabetes groups compared to controls. Data on the protective alleles DR2 DQβ1*0602 was, unfortunately, not presented in the study. Single autoantibody (ICA or GADA) positivity was more commonly seen in the LADA patients compared to adult-onset type 1 diabetes patients where a higher frequency of multiple autoantibodies was demonstrated. A similar difference in the autoantibody pattern was found comparing the newly diagnosed LADA with new childhood-onset type 1 diabetes. Further, the ICA positivity documented at onset disappeared in six patients having LADA with longer disease course. This observation may suggest that the tendency of ICA to disappear with increasing disease duration is similar in LADA and type 1 diabetes (73,74).

From the metabolic standpoint, it is assumed that loss of β-cell function is slower in autoimmune diabetes in adults than in childhood type 1 diabetes but faster than in classical antibody-negative adult-onset type 2 diabetes (31). However, some studies have shown comparable declines in β-cell function in autoimmune diabetes in adults and type 1 diabetes over the initial 2 to 3 years postdiagnosis (75–77). Interpretation of β-cell function data might be complicated by the observations that β-cell dysfunction tends to be more severe at diagnosis in younger children with type 1 diabetes, that intensive metabolic control slows the decline in β-cell dysfunction in type 1 diabetes, and older, more obese patients would be more insulin resistant and consequently would present with hyperglycemia with less β-cell dysfunction. The LADA and adult type 1 diabetes patients reported by Hosszufalusi et al. in the above study had similar phenotypes and hence probably similar insulin sensitivity to explain their similar C-peptide levels at diagnosis (72). But the adult type 1 diabetes showed a more rapid decline postdiagnosis compared to the LADA patients suggesting a more aggressive autoimmune attack against their β-cells (31).

THERAPEUTIC INTERVENTIONS

Whether or not the mechanisms of the immunological damage to and destruction of the pancreatic β-cells is same in all patients with autoimmune diabetes has important therapeutic implications. Immunomodulatory therapies, such as anti-CD3, have been identified to be efficacious in modulating the type 1 diabetes disease process (78). Because LADA is more common than classic childhood type 1 diabetes, it will be interesting to see whether these treatments are similarly effective in LADA.

Parenteral insulin therapy has been shown to protect against type 1 diabetes; this is observed in the NOD mouse, the BB rat, and in pilot studies in humans (79,80). Part of the mechanism underlying the protection in the BB rat appears to be due to a metabolic effect of insulin, and the protection provided by insulin in the BB rat is disease-specific (81). Insulin therapy begun early in life in the NOD mouse also protects against type 1 diabetes (82–84), and here the mechanism of protection is, at least in part, mediated by an immunologic effect of insulin. Early and aggressive insulin treatment of newly diagnosed type 1 diabetes patients, including short-term treatment with an artificial pancreas, has been shown to result in an increased frequency of remissions and higher C-peptide levels months to years later compared to conventional treatment (85). The Diabetes Control and Complications Trial (DCCT) provided the strongest data in man to suggest that parenteral insulin may slow or inhibit the type 1 diabetes disease process by a metabolic effect. A subset of patients with a higher initial C-peptide reserve, when randomized to intensive therapy, maintained significantly higher levels of C-peptide for a longer period of time compared to similar patients randomized to conventional therapy (86,87). The protective effect of intensive therapy on β-cell function is unlikely to be mediated by an immunologic effect of insulin since similar doses and types of subcutaneous insulin were received by the patients in both intensive and conventional treatment groups. It is much more likely that reduced glucotoxicity in the intensively treated subjects preserved β-cell function compared to patients in the conventional treatment group (87).

These above observations in type 1 diabetes provided the framework for two studies from Japan, in antibody-positive type 2 diabetes patients (86). The protective effect of insulin versus sulfonylurea on β-cell function in ICA$^+$ and in GADA-positive phenotypic type 2 diabetes subjects was assessed. Both studies showed better preservation of β cell function with insulin compared to sulfonylurea (88,89). Unfortunately, the Diabetes Prevention Trial—Type 1 (DPT-1) did not confirm the beneficial effect of parenteral insulin on the type 1 diabetes disease process (90). The divergent findings could be explained by any of several variables, including disease severity at the time of recruitment to the study (established diabetes versus high-risk subjects), age, disease subtype (LADA or classical type 1 diabetes), and ethnic background (Japanese or North American). Although surprising and disappointing, given the ability of parenteral insulin to prevent diabetes in the animal models and in small human pilot trials (91), this DPT-1 result emphasizes the necessity for basing treatment decisions in humans on properly designed and executed human trials. In our opinion, insufficient data currently exists to recommend insulin over other forms of therapy for Caucasian patients diagnosed with LADA.

The administration of GAD in a vaccine-like regimen has been reported to preserve C-peptide in a pilot study in LADA patients (92). Subsequently, the same dose of GAD administered twice, but 28 days apart, preserved C-peptide in classical childhood type 1 diabetes (93). Larger and more definitive studies to validate these early observations in both LADA and childhood type 1 diabetes are underway and/or planned.

Based upon the apparent antigenic differences between LADA and type 1 diabetes that have been observed, we have hypothesized that antigen spreading is more restrictive in autoimmune diabetes in adults than in childhood type 1 diabetes (31,60) and that some antigens may be more important in the type 1 diabetes versus LADA disease process and possibly vice versa. Specific antigens could be more important for the autoimmune attack against the β cells in childhood type 1 diabetes compared to autoimmune diabetes in adults.

If this hypothesis is true, it has important implications for future immunomodulatory therapy of autoimmune diabetes. The success of antigen-based therapies may depend upon whether tolerance to that antigen has been lost and whether it can be restored. Treatment with some antigens might be efficacious in both autoimmune diabetes in adults and childhood type 1 diabetes, such as the GAD treatment mentioned above, whereas other antigens might be selectively effective in childhood type 1 diabetes or LADA.

The importance of the patient population with phenotypic type 2 diabetes but with positive autoantibody markers of type 1 diabetes needs to be emphasized. Since the prevalence of type 2 diabetes is high and is increasing rapidly, even if only 10% are LADA patients, this is a population of patients two to three times larger than the classical childhood type 1 diabetes patient population. Effective immunomodulatory therapy that prevents diabetes or preserves residual β cell function in patients with autoimmune diabetes will be an important development.

These are exciting times for the fields of autoimmunity and type 1 diabetes. Translating into clinical medicine the latest findings from basic research at the cellular and molecular levels and from research in animal models is a major challenge (94,95). The National Institute of Health and the Juvenile Diabetes Research Foundation International are committed to a large clinical trials' program with the task of testing the efficacy of immunomodulatory therapy against the human type 1 diabetes disease process (94). This program, termed type 1 diabetes TrialNet, consists of clinical centers in the United States, Canada, Europe, and Australia, core laboratories, and a coordinating/data management center. This program oversees and conducts immunomodulatory intervention trials for type 1 diabetes. Several interventions in different populations are currently being evaluated. Future clinical trials under the auspices of TrialNet, the Immune Tolerance Network, and other such organizations will continue until safe and effective immunomodulatory therapy for human type 1 diabetes is found.

CONCLUDING REMARKS

Autoantibodies that are reactive to islet antigens are present at the time of diagnosis in almost all patients with type 1 diabetes. Additionally, ~ 10% of phenotypic type 2 diabetic patients also are positive for at least one of the islet autoantibodies. They also share many genetic similarities with type 1 diabetes. These similarities (genetic and immunological) between LADA and type 1 diabetes strongly suggest that LADA, like type 1 diabetes, is an autoimmune disease. But the antibody, T cell, and genetic differences between type 1 diabetes and LADA suggest the possibility that there are important differences in the underlying autoimmune disease processes of type 1 diabetes and LADA. In LADA diabetes occurs earlier in the β-cell–destructive process because of the greater insulin resistance; it is also likely that some of the observed differences are due to age-related effects on the immune system. Complexities arise also because of the variable definitions of LADA and type 1 diabetes, and consequently comparing the results of one study with another is problematic. The recent definition of LADA suggested by the Immunology of Diabetes Society (32) should help correct this problem. Intervention studies will provide the strongest data to determine whether or not type 1 diabetes and LADA are different. As immunomodulatory therapies that slow or halt the type 1 diabetes disease process are discovered, testing these therapies in LADA will be essential. If therapies are efficacious in both type 1 diabetes and LADA, the genetic and immunological differences described earlier will be superfluous. But if some therapies are effective only in type 1 diabetes, or in LADA patients, this would constitute the strongest evidence for important disease process differences between type 1 diabetes and LADA, and consequently accurately diagnosing type 1 diabetes versus LADA would become clinically important (21). If so, providers would need to screen all type 2 diabetes patients to identify those with antibodies to offer treatment to them.

REFERENCES

1. Alberti KG, Zimmet PZ. Definition, diagnosis and classification of diabetes mellitus and its complications. Part 1: Diagnosis and classification of diabetes mellitus: Provisional report of a WHO consultation. Diabet Med 1998;15:539–553.
2. Expert Committee on the Diagnosis and Classification of Diabetes Mellitus. Report of the Expert Committee on the Diagnosis and Classification of Diabetes Mellitus. Diabetes Care 1997;20:1183–1197.
3. Naik RG, Palmer JP. Late-onset type 1 diabetes. Current Opin Endocrinol Diabetes 1997;4: 308–315.
4. Bottazzo G-F, Florin-Christensen A, Doniach D. Islet-cell antibodies in diabetes mellitus with autoimmune polyendocrine deficiencies. Lancet 1974;ii:1279–1282.
5. MacCuish AC, Irvine WJ, Barnes EW, et al. Antibodies to pancreatic islet cells in insulin-dependent diabetics with coexistent autoimmune disease. Lancet 1974;ii:1529–1531.
6. Kuzuya T, Matsuda A. Classification of diabetes on the basis of etiologies versus degree of insulin deficiency. Diabetes Care 1997;20(2):219–220.
7. Service EJ, Rizza RA, Zimmerman BR, et al. The classification of diabetes by clinical and C-peptide criteria: A prospective population-based study. Diabetes Care 1997;20(2):198–201.
8. Van der Auwera B, Van Waeyenberge C, Schuit F, et al. DRB1*0403 protects against IDDM in Caucasians with the high-risk heterozygous DQA1*0301-DQB1*0302/DQA1*0501-DQB1*0201 genotype. Belgian Diabetes Registry. Diabetes 1995;44(5):527–530.
9. Neifing JL, Greenbaum CJ, Kahn SE, et al. Prospective evaluation of beta-cell function in insulin autoantibody-positive relatives of insulin-dependent diabetic patients. Metabolism 1993;42(4):482–486.
10. McCulloch DK, Palmer JP. The appropriate use of B-cell function testing in the preclinical period of type 1 diabetes. Diabet Med 1991;8(9):800–804.
11. Hathout EH, Thomas W, El-Shahawy M, et al. Diabetic autoimmune markers in children and adolescents with type 2 diabetes. Pediatrics 2001;107(6):E102.
12. Libman I, Pietropaolo M, Arslanian S, et al. Risk factors associated with type 2 diabetes in youngsters with type 1a (autoimmune) diabetes: Does it matter? Diabetes 2001;50(S2):A39.
13. Pihoker C, Brooks-Worrell BM, Greenbaum CJ, et al. Impact of islet reactive T cells and autoantibodies on clinical diagnosis of type 1, type 2, or atypical diabetes in children. Diabetes 2000;49(S1):A409.
14. Juneja R, Palmer JP. Type 1 1/2 diabetes: Myth or reality. Autoimmunity 1999;29:65–83.
15. Karjalainen J, Salmela P, Ilonen J, et al. A comparison of childhood and adult type I diabetes mellitus. N Engl J Med 1989;320(14):881–886.
16. Lorenzen T, Pociot F, Hougaard P, et al. Long-term risk of IDDM in first-degree relatives of patients with IDDM. Diabetologia 1994;37(3):321–327.
17. Irvine WJ, Gray RS, McCallum CJ, et al. Clinical and pathogenic significance of pancreatic-islet-cell antibodies in diabetics treated with oral hypoglycaemic agents. Lancet 1977;i:1025–1027.
18. Chiu HK, Tsai EC, Juneja R, et al. Equivalent insulin resistance in latent autoimmune diabetes in adults (LADA) and type 2 diabetic patients. Diabetes Res Clin Pract, 2007;77(2):237–244.
19. Libman IM, Becker DJ. Coexistence of type 1 and type 2 diabetes mellitus: "double" diabetes? Pediatr Diabetes 2003;4(1):110–113.
20. Naik RG, Palmer JP. Latent autoimmune diabetes in adults (LADA). Rev Endocr Metab Disord 2003;4:233–241.
21. Palmer JP, Hampe CS, Chiu H, et al. Is latent autoimmune diabetes in adults distinct from type 1 diabetes or just type 1 diabetes at an older age? Diabetes 2005;54:S62–S7.

22. Borg H, Gottsäter A, Landin-Olsson M, et al. High levels of antigen-specific islet antibodies predict future beta-cell failure in patients with onset of diabetes in adult age. J Clin Endocrinol Metab 2001;86:3032–3038.
23. Urakami T, Miyamoto Y, Matsunaga H, et al. Serial changes in the prevalence of islet cell antibodies and islet cell antibody titer in children with IDDM of abrupt or slow onset. Diabetes Care 1995;18:1095–1099.
24. Kobayashi T, Tamemoto K, Nakanishi K, et al. Immunogenetic and clinical characterization of slowly progressive IDDM. Diabetes Care 1993;16(5):780–788.
25. Juneja R, Hirsch IB, Naik RG, et al. Islet cell antibodies and glutamic acid decarboxylase antibodies but not the clinical phenotype help to identify type 1 1/2 diabetes in patients presenting with type 2 diabetes. Metabolism 2001;50:1008–1013.
26. Nakanishi K, Kobayashi T, Miyashita H, et al. Relationships among residual beta cells, exocrine pancreas, and islet cell antibodies in insulin-dependent diabetes mellitus. Metabolism 1993;42(2):196–203.
27. Yeung V, Chan JCN, Chow CC, et al. Antibodies to glutamic acid decarboxylase (anti-GAD) in Chinese IDDM patients. In: 15th International Diabetes Fedration Congress Proceedings, Kobe, Japan, 1994. p. 432.
28. Zimmet PZ. The pathogenesis and prevention of diabetes in adults: Genes, autoimmunity, and demography. Diabetes Care 1995;18:1050–1064.
29. Anonymous. Insulin-dependent? Lancet 1985;2:809–810.
30. Gleichmann H, Zorcher B, Greulich B, et al. Correlation of islet cell antibodies and HLA-DR phenotypes with diabetes mellitus in adults. Diabetologia 1984;27:90–92.
31. Palmer JP, Hirsch IB. What's in a name: Latent autoimmune diabetes in adults, type 1.5, adult-onset, and type 1 diabetes. Diabetes Care 2003;26:536–538.
32. Fourlanos S, Dotta F, Greenbaum CJ, et al. Latent autoimmune diabetes in adults (LADA) should be less latent Diabetologia 2005;48:2206–2212.
33. Kahn SE, Prigeon RL, McCulloch DK, et al. Quantification of the relationship between insulin sensitivity and ß-cell function in human subjects: Evidence for a hyperbolic function. Diabetes 1993;42:1663–1672.
34. Kahn SE. The importance of ß-cell failure in the development and progression of type 2 diabetes. J Clin Endocrinol Metab 2001;86:4047–4058.
35. Krischer JP, Cuthbertson DD, Yu L, et al. The Diabetes Prevention Trial-Type 1 Study Group: Screening strategies for the identification of multiple antibody-positive relatives of individuals with type 1 diabetes. J Clin Endocrinol Metab 2003;88:103–108.
36. Verge CF, Gianani R, Kawasaki E, et al. Number of autoantibodies (against insulin, GAD or ICA512/IA2) rather than particular autoantibody specificities determines risk of type I diabetes. J Autoimmun 1996;9(3):379–383.
37. Verge CF, Gianani R, Kawasaki E, et al. Prediction of type I diabetes in first-degree relatives using a combination of insulin, GAD, and ICA512bdc/IA-2 autoantibodies. Diabetes 1996;45(7):926–933.
38. Rowley MJ, Mackay IR, Chen QY, et al. Antibodies to glutamic acid decarboxylase discriminate major types of diabetes mellitus. Diabetes 1992;41:548–551.
39. Palmer JP. What is the best way to predict IDDM? Lancet 1994;343(8910):1377–1378.
40. Imagawa A, Hanafusa T, Miyagawa J, et al. A novel subtype of type 1 diabetes mellitus characterized by a rapid onset and an absence of diabetes-related antibodies. Osaka IDDM Study Group. N Engl J Med 2000;342(5):301–307.
41. Lernmark A. Rapid-onset type 1 diabetes with pancreatic exocrine dysfunction. N Engl J Med 2000;342(5):344–345.
42. Park Y, Lee HK, Koh CS, et al. The low prevalence of immunogenetic markers in Korean adult-onset IDDM patients. Diabetes Care 1996;19(3):241–245.
43. Fukui M, Nakano K, Shigeta H, et al. Antibodies to glutamic acid decarboxylase in Japanese diabetic patients with secondary failure of oral hypoglycaemic therapy. Diabet Med 1997;14(2):148–152.

44. Gottsater A, Landin Olsson M, Fernlund P, et al. Beta-cell function in relation to islet cell antibodies during the first 3 yr after clinical diagnosis of diabetes in type II diabetic patients. Diabetes Care 1993;16(6):902–910.

45. Hagopian WA, Karlsen AE, Gottsater A, et al. Quantitative assay using recombinant human islet glutamic acid decarboxylase (GAD65) shows that 64 K autoantibody positivity at onset predicts diabetes type. J Clin Invest 1993;91(1):368–374.

46. Kasuga A, Maruyama T, Ozawa Y, et al. Antibody to the Mr 65,000 isoform of glutamic acid decarboxylase are detected in non-insulin-dependent diabetes in Japanese. J Autoimmun 1996;9(1):105–111.

47. Willis JA, Scott RS, Brown LJ, et al. Islet cell antibodies and antibodies against glutamic acid decarboxylase in newly diagnosed adult-onset diabetes mellitus. Diabetes Res Clin Pract 1996;33(2):89–97.

48. Zimmet P. Antibodies to glutamic acid decarboxylase in the prediction of insulin dependency. Diabetes Res Clin Pract 1996;34 Suppl(1):S125–S31.

49. Turner R, Stratton I, Horton V, et al. UKPDS 25. Autoantibodies to islet-cell cytoplasma and glutamic acid decarboxylase for prediction of insulin requirement in type 2 diabetes. Lancet 1997;350:1288–1293.

50. Borg H, Marcus C, Sjoblad S, et al. Islet cell antibody frequency differs from that of glutamic acid decarboxylase antibodies/IA2 antibodies after diagnosis of diabetes. Acta Paediatr 2000;89: 46–51.

51. Borg H, Gottsäter A, Fernlund P, et al. A 12-year prospective study of the relationship between islet antibodies and ß-cell function at and after the diagnosis in patients with adult-onset diabetes. Diabetes 2002;51:1754–1762.

52. Seissler J, De Sonnaville JJJ, Morgenthaler NG, et al. Immunological heterogeneity in type 1 diabetes: Presence of distinct autoantibody patterns in patients with acute onset and slowly progressive disease. Diabetologia 1998;41:891–897.

53. Falorni A, Gambelunghe G, Forini F, et al. Autoantibody recognition of COOH-terminal epitopes of GAD65 marks the risk for insulin requirement in adult-onset diabetes mellitus. J Clin Endocrinol Metab 2000;85(1):309–316.

54. Hampe CS, Kockum I, Landin-Olsson M, et al. GAD65 antibody epitope patterns of patients with Type 1.5 differ from that of type 1 diabetes patients. Diabetes Care 2002;25: 1481–1482.

55. Padoa CJ, Banga JP, Madec A-M, et al. Recombinant Fab of human monoclonal antibodies specific to the middle epitope of GAD65 inhibit type 1 diabetes-specific GAD65Abs. Diabetes 2003;52:2689–2695.

56. Kobayashi T, Tanaka S, Okubo M, et al. Unique epitopes of glutamic acid decarboxylase autoantibodies in slowly proressive and acute-onset type 1 diabetes. J Clin Endocrinol Metab 2003;88:4768–4775.

57. Hillman M, Törn C, Thorgeirsson H, et al. IgG4-subclass of glutamic acid decarboxylase antibody is more frequent in latent autoimmune diabetes in adults than in type 1 diabetes. Diabetologia 2004;47:1984–1989.

58. Brooks-Worrell B, Dosch HM, Herold K, et al. Marked differences in T cell reactivity in recently diagnosed type 1 diabetes patients versus controls. In: 12th International Congress of Immunology and 4th Annual Conference of the Federation of Clinical Immunology Societies, Montreal, Canada, 2004.

59. Brooks-Worrell BM, Starkebaum GA, Greenbaum C, et al. Peripheral blood mononuclear cells of insulin-dependent diabetic patients respond to multiple islet cell proteins. J Immunol 1996;157:5668–5674.

60. Brooks-Worrell BM, Juneja R, Minokadeh A, et al. Cellular immune responses to human islet proteins in antibody-positive type 2 diabetic patients. Diabetes 1999;48(5):983–988.

61. Brooks-Worrell B, Gersuk VH, Greenbaum C, et al. Intermolecular antigen spreading occurs during the pre-clinical period of human type 1 diabetes. J Immunol 2001;166:5265–5270.

62. Behme MT, Dupré J, Harris SB, et al. Insulin resistance in latent autoimmune diabetes of adulthood. Ann N Y Acad Sci 2003;1005:374–377.

63. Zimnan B, Kahn SE, Haffner SM, et al. Phenotypic characteristics of GAD antibody-positive recently diagnosed patients with type 2 diabetes in North America and Europe. Diabetes 2004;53:3193–3200.

64. Chiu HK, Palmer JP. Autoimmune diabetes: More than just one flavor? J Endocrinol Invest 2004;27:480–484.

65. Sanjeevi CB, Gambelunghe G, Falorni A, et al. Genetics of latent autoimmune diabetes in adults. Ann N Y Acad Sci 2002;958:107–111.

66. Tuomi T, Carlsson A, Li H, et al. Clinical and genetic characteristics of type 2 diabetes with and without GAD antibodies. Diabetes 1999;48(1):150–157.

67. Groop L, Miettinen A, Groop PH, et al. Organ-specific autoimmunity and HLA-DR antigens as markers for beta-cell destruction in patients with type II diabetes. Diabetes 1988;37(1): 99–103.

68. Cosentino A, Gambelunghe G, Tortoioli C, et al. CTLA-4 gene polymorphism contributes to the genetic risk for latent autoimmune diabetes in adults. Ann N Y Acad Sci 2002;958:337–340.

69. Cerrone GE, Caputo M, Lopez AP, et al. Variable number of tandem repeats of the insulin gene determines susceptibility to latent autoimmune diabetes in adults. Mol Diagn 2004;8:43–49.

70. Törn C, Gupta M, Zake LN, et al. Heterozygosity for MICA5.0/MICA5.1 and HLA-DR3-DQ2/DR4-DQ8 are independent genetic risk factors for latent autoimmune diabetes in adults. Hum Immunol 2003;64:902–909.

71. Vatay Á, Rajczy K, Pozsonyi É, et al. Differences in the genetic background of latent autoimmune diabetes in adults (LADA) and type 1 diabetes mellitus. Immunol Lett 2002;84:109–115.

72. Hosszúfalusi N, Vatay A, Rajczy K, et al. Similar genetic features and different islet cell autoantibody pattern of Latent Autoimmune Diabetes in Adults (LADA) compared with adult-onset type 1 diabetes with rapid progression. Diabetes Care 2003;26:452–457.

73. Christie M, Delovitch TL. Persistence of antibodies to a 64,000-Mr islet cell protein after onset of type I diabetes. Diabetes 1990;39:653–659.

74. Marner B, Agner T, Binder C, et al. Increased reduction in fasting C-peptide is associated with islet cell antibodies in type 1 (insulin-dependent) diabetic patients. Diabetologia 1985;28: 875–880.

75. Carlsson A, Sundkvist G, Groop L, et al. Insulin and glucagon secretion in patients with slowly progressive autoimmune diabetes (LADA). J Clin Endocrinol Metab 2000;85:76–80.

76. Raz I, Elias D, Avron A, et al. B-cell function in new-onset type 1 diabetes and immunomodulation with a heat-shock protein peptide (DiaPep277): A randomized, double blind, phase II trial. Lancet 2001;358:1749–1753.

77. Tarn AC, Thomas JM, Dean BM, et al. Predicting insulin-dependent diabetes. Lancet 1988;i: 845–850.

78. Herold KC, Hagopian W, Auger JA, et al. Anti-CD3 monoclonal antibody in new-onset type 1 diabetes mellitus. N Engl J Med 2002;346:1692–1698.

79. Bertrand S, De Paepe M, Vigeant C, et al. Prevention of adoptive transfer in BB rats by prophylactic insulin treatment. Diabetes 1992;41:1273–1277.

80. Gotfredsen CF, Buschard K, Frandsen EK. Reduction of diabetes incidence of BB Wistar rats by early prophylactic insulin treatment of diabetes-prone animals. Diabetologia 1985;28: 933–935.

81. Gottlieb PA, Handler ES, Appel MC, et al. Insulin treatment prevents diabetes mellitus but not thyroiditis in RT6-depleted diabetes resistant BB/Wor rats. Diabetologia 1991;34(5):296–300.

82. Atkinson MA, Maclaren NK, Luchetta R. Insulitis and diabetes in NOD mice reduced by prophylactic insulin therapy. Diabetes 1990;39(8):933–937.

83. Muir A, Peck A, Clare Salzler M, et al. Insulin immunization of nonobese diabetic mice induces a protective insulitis characterized by diminished intraislet interferon-gamma transcription. J Clin Invest 1995;95(2):628–634.

84. Thivolet CH, Goillot E, Bedossa P, et al. Insulin prevents adoptive cell transfer of diabetes in the autoimmune non-obese diabetic mouse. Diabetologia 1991;34(5):314–319.

85. Shah SC, Malone JI, Simpson NE. A randomized trial of intensive insulin therapy in newly diagnosed insulin-dependent diabetes mellitus. N Engl J Med 1989;320(9):550–554.

86. Kobayashi T, Nakanishi K, Murase T, et al. Small doses of subcutaneous insulin as a strategy for preventing slowly progressive beta-cell failure in islet cell antibody-positive patients with clinical features of NIDDM. Diabetes 1996;45(5):622–626.
87. The Diabetes Control and Complications Trial Research Group. Effect of intensive therapy on residual beta-cell function in patients with type 1 diabetes in the diabetes control and complications trial. A randomized, controlled trial. Ann Intern Med. 1998;128:517–523.
88. Kobayashi T. Multicenter prevention trial of slowly progressive IDDM with small dose of insulin (the Tokyo Study). Diabetes Metab Res Rev 2001;17 (Suppl.):S29.
89. Kobayashi T, Maruyama T, Shimada A, et al. Insulin intervention to preserve beta cells in slowly progressive insulin-dependent (type 1) diabetes mellitus. Ann N Y Acad Sci 2002;958:117–130.
90. Diabetes Prevention Trial – Type 1 Diabetes Study Group. Effects of insulin in relatives of patients with type 1 diabetes mellitus. N Engl J Med 2002;346:1685–1691.
91. Keller RJ, Eisenbarth GS, Jackson RA. Insulin prophylaxis in individuals at high risk of type 1 diabetes. Lancet 1993;341:927–928.
92. Agardh CD, Cilio CM, Lethagen A, et al. Clinical evidence for the safety of GAD65 immunomodulation in adult-onset autoimmune diabetes. J Diabetes Complications 2005;19(4):238–246.
93. Ludvigsson J, Casas R, Vaarala O, et al. The Swedish GAD-vaccination Trial: Outcomes of a phase II safety and efficacy trial with DiamydTM for preservation of beta cell function in children with T1D. Oral Presentation (OP 41) at the 42nd Annual Meeting of EASD; Copenhagen, Malmoe, Denmark, Sweden, September 14–17, 2006.
94. Palmer JP. Immunomodulatory therapy of human type 1 diabetes: Lessons from the mouse. J Clin Invest 2001;108:31–33.
95. Shapiro AMJ, Lakey JRT, Ryan EA, et al. Islet transplantation in seven patients with type 1 diabetes mellitus using a glucocorticoid-free immunosuppressive regimen. N Engl J Med 2000;343:230–238.

3

Blood Glucose Monitoring: Glycated Hemoglobin, Fructosamine, Meters, and Sensors

T. S. Bailey
Advanced Metabolic Care & Research, Escondido, California, U.S.A.

The advances in diabetes care we see today are the product of years of technological advances in glucose measurement and insulin replacement coupled with a fundamental shift in the model of care—from provider-directed to self-management by the patient. The major obstacle to the normalization of glucose levels in type 1 diabetes continues to be the physiologic replacement of insulin. Chapter 5 in this book will discuss the latest strategies for insulin therapy.

This chapter will focus on technological breakthroughs in measuring biochemical markers of glucose control and their integration into the daily care of type 1 diabetes. These techniques for glycemic assessment have the potential to be exploited by persons with diabetes and those who care for them. However, all of this technology has yet to be harnessed to automatically calculate and deliver the correct insulin doses (i.e., "closed-loop" insulin therapy). Until such automation has been accomplished, there will be an increase in complexity and a commensurate increase in the need for education for all involved in diabetes care. For the near future, successful diabetes care will depend on educating and engaging our patients to employ the most appropriate available methods.

HISTORY AND BACKGROUND TECHNOLOGY

The measurement of glucose dates back to the nineteenth century (1). Urinary glucose was the first modality employed to monitor diabetes in patients. Technological advances by the Ames Division of Miles Laboratories in the 1950s made earlier cumbersome methods (such as Benedict's reaction test, which required heating urine) obsolete. The company initially developed a tablet-based method that produced a color change proportional to the glucose concentration. This color change was compared to a color chart and a semiquantitative estimation of glucose concentration was obtained. The technique was imperfect because the renal threshold for glucosuria is higher than desirable blood glucose levels and varies between individuals. Therefore, it detected only when glucose levels were already elevated.

This method was initially used in doctors' offices, but its application broadened to home use by patients as well.

A major advance in the 1960s was the development of "strips," where the enzymes glucose oxidase and peroxidase were embedded into a solid, flat material (CliniStix® and Tes-Tape®). A color change proportional to the glucose concentration was seen after dipping the strip or tape into the urine. Later, Dextrostix® strips were developed for glucose measurement in blood. The technique was cumbersome (apply a properly sized drop of blood, wait for a precise time, carefully wash, then blot) and the results were still interpreted visually.

Around 1970, a meter that could electronically "read" the Dextrostix by reflectance was first commercially introduced (2). This removed the subjective element where the user determined his or her result by comparing the strip color to a color on a chart. Instead, with a meter the result was indicated by a needle. Today's readers may be surprised that for most of the subsequent decades, this technology was promoted almost exclusively to health-care professionals.

In the 1980s, this technology first became widely available to patients. The units were designed to be portable and easier to use than previous models and competing companies advanced the technology. These advances included a digital readout (rather than having to read off the needle of a meter), an internal timer (rather than having to use the second hand of your watch), and easier blood sample removal methods (e.g., wipe rather than blot).

This technology was a key enabler of the landmark Diabetes Complications and Control Trial (DCCT) (3) published in 1993, which unequivocally demonstrated the benefits of intensive diabetes control compared with standard therapy on microvascular complications. The intensively managed subjects in the experimental group in this trial administered three or more insulin injections compared to one to two injections in the standard group. By trial protocol, the experimental subjects were required to test glucose levels a minimum of four times daily, while the control (standard care) subjects were encouraged not to check more than once daily. The DCCT trial not only confirmed the hypothesis that improved metabolic control is associated with lower microvascular complications, but also provided evidence that frequent monitoring and insulin dosing could accomplish this glycemic improvement safely.

The 1990s brought further refinements in glucose measurement. Reflectance meters were challenged by newer electrochemical methods. These techniques also used enzymatic reactions (predominantly glucose oxidase, but also glucose dehydrogenase or hexokinase). However, instead of measuring a color change, they measured an electrical change by an amperometric method. The amperometric method relies on the observation that electron transfer driven by the chemical reaction is proportional to the concentration of glucose present (4). This method allows smaller sample size and faster testing. Additionally, it eliminates the need for removing the sample from the strip (i.e., no blotting or wiping) and allows the blood to remain separate from the device (i.e., no cleaning required). In recent years, technology to provide faster, more accurate tests with smaller sample sizes has made numerous advances (5).

GLUCOSE MEASUREMENT ACCURACY

The performance standards for point-of-care testing of blood glucose have changed over time as the devices improved. Initially, the FDA goal was ±15% (1986), but in 1993 the recommendations were updated to ±5% (6). The international standard (ISO DIS 15197) states ±20%, but ±20 mg/dL for glucose levels less than 100 mg/dL (7). A commonly used analysis is the Clarke error grid (8). The Clarke error grid assigns a clinical significance to

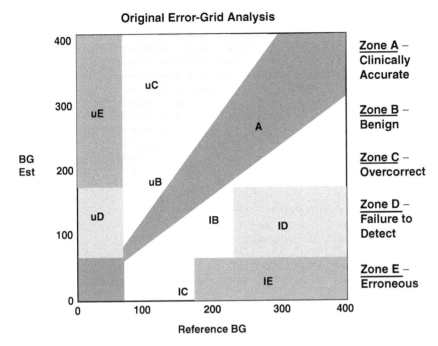

Figure 1 Clarke error-grid analysis.

each measurement error (e.g., data from a device showing an elevation when the reference device reads low would be assigned to region "C" because a patient might be led to "overcorrect" for a false elevation in glucose) (Fig. 1).

When evaluating a continuous glucose monitor, such error grids need to be modified because the direction of glucose movement must also be considered (8). Many factors can affect the accuracy of glucose testing, but newer technology is helping to eliminate these.

One factor leading to testing errors is the requirement for user calibration of the meter. This is usually accomplished by either entering a numerical lot code for test strips or placing a physical "key" into the meter. If the meter is not properly "coded," errors will occur, many having potential clinical significance. Some of the current meters have cleverly eliminated the need for this contrivance so the user is spared from the potential error of improper coding (9). Essentially, all glucose meters have a "control" solution available to verify the meters' accuracy. This solution has a known value and the testing supplies are packaged with the acceptable range of results for the meter. Users should periodically test their device and replace it if the results do not fall within the specified range.

Environmental factors such as temperature, altitude, and humidity may also affect the readings (10), as may hematocrit (11). Physical factors such as inadequate sample size or sugar on the skin surface may also interfere (12). There are a number of medications that may alter glucose levels (e.g., acetaminophen, ascorbic acid, mannitol), which may affect the glucose measurements (13). Recognition of these interfering substances is of critical importance in hospitalized patients with diabetes.

PLASMA VERSUS WHOLE BLOOD

Essentially, all samples for home glucose testing are whole blood. All meters were formerly calibrated to reflect this and as such provided (approximately 12%) lower values than plasma

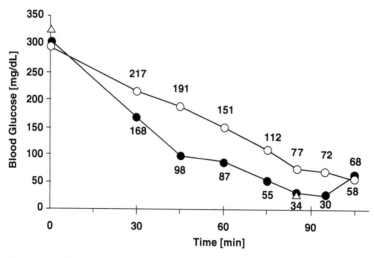

Figure 2 Alternate site testing—interstitial lag (15).

references (14). When manufacturers changed over to plasma calibration, patients noticed this and many initially preferred their older meters (because the values appeared lower). Today, meters are almost exclusively plasma-based. However, this continues to be relevant because many of the glycemic goals that were developed for patients were based on targets designed when older whole blood–calibrated meters were in clinical use.

ALTERNATE SITE TESTING

Alternate site (i.e., nonfinger) testing is now widely available. Low-volume sampling with a variety of improvements in collection technique (e.g., capillary action wicking and ability to add additional sample over time) and decrease in specimen size requirement has enabled this. This greatly increases the surface area of the body available to patients who test frequently. For those, such as musicians, who use their fingers at work, this is a significant advantage. However, since the measurements are made in a compartment more distal to blood (i.e., interstitial fluid), there is an inherent delay. Figure 2 shows an example of this (15).

This delay is of particular importance when glucose levels are rapidly decreasing (which could lead to a false overestimation) or increasing (which could lead to a false underestimation of actual glucose levels). Patients are instructed to perform standard capillary testing when this is suspected. A situation similar to this occurs with continuous glucose monitoring (CGM).

HbA1c TEST

Since the publication of the DCCT (3) in 1993, HbA1c test has been elevated from a laboratory test to an actual patient outcome. This is justified by the strong association of HbA1c elevation with microvascular complications. Diabetes complications occur too slowly in most patients with diabetes to be studied as an endpoint in clinical trials of new therapies. HbA1c, on the other hand, reflects ambient glucose levels in the past 1 to

3 months. It is currently the most acceptable surrogate for predicting whether a therapy being tested is likely to result in a reduction of the chronic complication of diabetes.

Following the publication of the DCCT, there was a movement to standardize the various glycosylated hemoglobin tests that were being performed. The majority of testing is now traceable to DCCT, thanks to the National Glycohemoglobin Standarization Program (NGSP). However, the International Federation of Clinical Chemistry has long been working on an improved assay which provides values that are up to 2% lower than the NGSP values clinicians are accustomed to working with (16).

The results of changing HbA1c reporting methodology on HbA1c outcomes were found in a study in Sweden. Because of a change in testing methodology patients' glycemic control appeared to improve after conversion to a test that reported higher values. Following a subsequent change that reported lower values, patients' glucose regulation deteriorated. This happened as a result of the psychological effects of apparent worsening and improvement that was due solely to the reporting methodology (17). There is concern that any change in reference range to values that are lower than those in current use will lead similarly to worsening glycemic control.

Other proposed changes are to report HbA1c in terms of predicted mean glucose levels or as DCCT risk equivalents. The optimal method to report HbA1c should allow health-care providers to have a common goal level to work toward that is supported by the large epidemiologic studies of diabetes complications.

OTHER BLOOD MARKERS

Proteins other than hemoglobin are glycosylated and have been investigated for possible utility in the management of diabetes. The best known non–HbA1c-glycated protein is commonly called fructosamine. Fructosamine levels change with glucose levels more quickly than do HbA1c. Although this has been available for many years from commercial laboratories, it is not recommended for routine use in diabetes (18). A home-testing version of this test was commercialized, but is no longer available. Weekly testing of this by patients with type 2 diabetes was shown to have a beneficial effect (19).

1,5-Anhydroglucitol (AG) is a monosaccharide derived from eating a normal diet. 1,5-Anhydroglucitol (commercially available as Glycomark™) levels are fairly constant with normal glucoses. However, with hyperglycemia, glucosuria occurs and 1,5-anhydroglucitol levels fall in proportion to the degree and duration of glucosuria. These changes occur more rapidly compared to HbA1c and therefore may be useful to rapidly detect changes in glucose control (20). In relatively well-controlled patients with diabetes, they may also be a good index of postprandial hyperglycemia (21).

CGM

All those who treat patients with diabetes have on occasion been presented with the records of a patient who, checking only once daily, "connects the dots." This patient usually proudly displays what appears to be a very stable, flat line glucose profile and may assume that this indicates good diabetes control. That same person, checking glucoses more frequently, invariably realizes that there is a great deal more variability that he had originally suspected. Continuous glucose monitors increase the frequency of presentation of glucose values to hundreds per day with consequent exposure of even greater, previously undetected variability.

The practice of glucose monitoring in patients with diabetes is now undergoing a significant update. The increased sampling frequency allows "connecting the dots" so users can now see the glucose trajectory following a meal or insulin and the changes in slope of the curve (i.e., the change in velocity of glucose changes). This new information will allow users to figure out what needs to change to improve control. The technology presently has two distinct form factors: one where the biosensor is temporarily implanted into the interstitial space (22–24) and another where the sensor is extracorporeal and interstitial fluid is transported via microdialysis to make contact with the sensor (25,26). Fully implantable systems which continue to function for months to years are being developed (27). The specific details of each of these systems are beyond the scope of this book and are likely to change over the next few years. This chapter will concentrate on the more general principles of continuous monitoring.

The logistics of using a temporarily implanted interstitial continuous glucose monitor is as follows:

1. A "sensor" is inserted through the skin into the subcutaneous space. The sensor is inserted with little or no discomfort with an insertion device and measures glucose levels for 3 to 7 days.
2. A "transmitter" is inserted into or attached to the sensor to send information wirelessly to a "receiver."
3. After a warm-up period of 2 to 10 hours (this varies by brand) during which the sensor equilibrates to its surroundings, the monitor is calibrated with a standard glucose meter.
4. The "receiver" receives the glucose information from the transmitter, processes it, and displays the results on a screen in a variety of formats.
5. Periodically (most commonly twice daily), the monitor requests a recalibration to compensate for possible "drift" of the sensor.
6. At the end of the sensor's life, the device requests a change in sensor. The transmitter and receiver are reused.
7. The information is stored in the "receiver" and can be uploaded to a computer for later review by the user or a caregiver.

Figure 3 illustrates how one such CGM device (Dexcom STS) operates.

The underlying operating principles of the devices that are currently available and in development in the United States are similar in that they rely on the enzyme glucose oxidase to sense ambient glucose levels. However, they differ in ways that may influence their performance. Following are the key areas in which they may be compared:

1. Catheter size and method of insertion.
2. Initial time to come into calibration (i.e., how long it takes to report the first reading after sensor insertion).
3. Method of calibration. (It is important to realize that any error in the glucose meter used to calibrate the continuous monitoring device will affect subsequent readings by the device.)
4. Sensor drift (i.e., how frequently it will require recalibration).
5. Functional life (i.e., how often the sensor needs to be changed).
6. Regulatory clearance for meter replacement versus adjunctive use with a glucose meter.
7. Lag time during rapid glucose changes. (This is mostly a characteristic of interstitial versus blood monitoring. However, microdialysis devices may have an additional delay due to the time required to reach the extracorporeal sensor.)

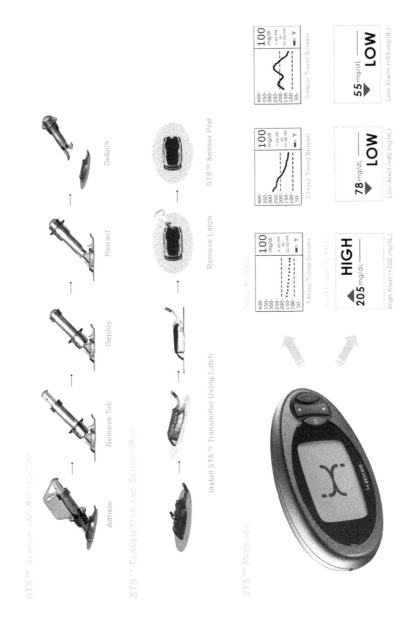

Figure 3 Dexcom STS use diagram.

8. Vulnerability to interfering substances. (The most commonly encountered is acetaminophen.)
9. Sensitivity and specificity of low- and high-glucose alerts.
10. Usefulness of on-screen data display.
11. Availability of software to upload the data for more detailed analysis.

In the author's experience, proper instruction on use of the data screens and how to set the low- and high-glucose alerts improves the utility of the CGM. All monitors display the most recent glucose reading on the initial screen. However, they differ in how the trends are presented.

One approach is to display an upward-pointing arrow if glucose is rising and a downward-pointing arrow if glucose is declining. If the rise or fall is more rapid, two arrows may be shown. While this is useful and easy-to-interpret, it may be misleading. For example, in a person with a glucose level of 70 and a decline in glucose of 59 mg/dL/min, some monitors would display no arrows (i.e., potentially misleading the use to conclude that glucose levels are stable, as the rate of change is < 1 mg/dL/min). However, this patient may be at-risk for hypoglycemia that is not disclosed by such arrows alone.

Another approach is a line graph showing the glucose points plotted over the prior 1 to 24 hours. The 1-hour screen shows short-term trends clearly. However, reviewing overnight glucoses is better accomplished by a longer (e.g., 9-hour) screen view. Data periods exceeding 1 day are difficult to view on the small displays of these devices.

The trend graph provided by a continuous glucose monitor gives much more information than what would be available from a standard glucose meter. When a standard meter shows the blood sugar level to be "normal," a continuous monitor can reveal whether this "normal" reading is rapidly increasing or decreasing. For example, if the glucose is "90" but the trend over the past 30 minutes has been a rapid decrease from "250," the patient could realize that a snack is required immediately to stop the rapid drop. It is important to confirm all such findings with a standard meter reading, but the trend appears to be generally reliable.

The educational curriculum for these patients will be different and more sophisticated than standard glucose monitoring. For many patients, it may be as intuitive as "stay between the lines." However, scenarios such as "glucose normal but rising slowly by 0.75 mg/dL/min," "glucose high but falling rapidly by 2 mg/dL/min," and "glucose mildly low but rising by 0.5 mg/dL/min" represent situations likely to be encountered by our patients and will form an important part of the training provided with these products. Future investigations will validate the optimal patient approach to CGM data. Presently, the common situations where continuous monitors appear to be helpful include unexpected hypoglycemia and unanticipated glucose rises.

Unexpected hypoglycemia leads to the fear of hypoglycemia by both patient and provider. This can present a significant barrier to the intensification of diabetes regulation. Patients using continuous monitors can have early warning of this by setting alarms and viewing their graphs. A consistent finding in studies evaluating continuous glucose monitors has shown that there been a decrease in both hyperglycemia and hypoglycemia. An example of this is illustrated in Figure 4. This shows an increase in glucose values in the normal range (23). There are data to suggest that in patients with lower HbA1c values the primary effect of continuous monitoring is to decrease the frequency of hypoglycemia (28).

Setting the low alarm in patients who have hypoglycemia unawareness (see Chap. 11) may be one of the most important uses of this technology. During the day, a slow drop in blood glucose, which could have led to mental impairment, might be detected and treated. Similarly, during the night, the alarm could wake a person prior to a hypoglycemic event.

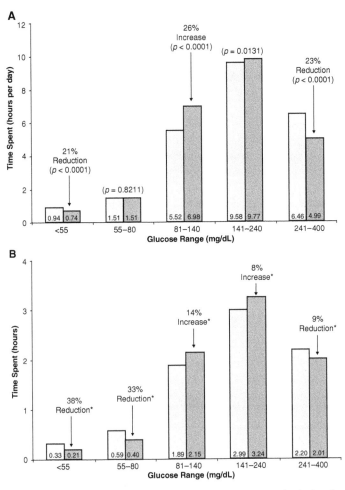

Figure 4 Chart from Garg (23) showing less hypoglycemia during day (A) and night (B).

Patients with hypoglycemia unawareness may need to set the low alert to 100 mg/dL (or higher) to successfully prevent hypoglycemia. Patients may initially be frustrated with frequent alarms. However, the increased safety should outweigh any inconvenience.

A further refinement that has been used in some devices is a "predictive alarm." This uses the rate of glucose change and projects it linearly forward to alert the user a set interval prior to when the algorithm predicts when glucose levels will go beyond chosen low and high limits. Properly setting this type of alarm could reduce the risk of hypoglycemia not signaled by arrows alone referred to above.

Unanticipated hyperglycemia is still handled by many patients using an approach known as "sliding scale." This refers to patients using infrequently sampled glucose levels (which do not convey any information as to whether glucose is rising or falling) to determine insulin doses (i.e., the higher the glucose, the higher the insulin dose). Experts now agree that such a simplistic approach (i.e., without regard to residual insulin activity or direction and rate of glucose change) is ill-advised (29).

However, a patient using a continuous monitor can perform a more sophisticated variant of this (e.g., a "touch-up" bolus) safely. Patients may overtreat highs by "stacking" (multiple insulin doses over a short time interval), which could lead to hypoglycemia.

However, with patient education regarding the delayed onset and prolonged duration of insulin activity, this does not appear to be a problem in author's experience. A recent multicenter randomized, controlled clinical trial demonstrated that by using continuous monitoring technology for 12 weeks without extensive training there was a decrease in HbA1c in subjects with relatively high baseline HbA1c levels (30). An additional benefit of continuous monitoring is seeing the result of a miscalculation within minutes, potentially prior to symptoms.

Using the continuous monitor as a guide to eating might seem obvious. However, during our experience conducting clinical trials of continuous monitoring technology, we found a near-universal surprise as to the magnitude of the glucose excursions following meals. This led patients to deliver insulin boluses earlier and to choose fewer or different meal carbohydrates.

Exercise is another situation where a continuous monitor can be of assistance. Current monitors continue to function during exercise and may be of great help in assisting patients with diabetes to keep glucose levels stable during vigorous activity. However, current systems may not be stable during certain contact sports and cannot function fully submerged.

Drifting will occur with each sensor but some sensors may have less drift than others. The effect of calibrating more frequently might intuitively appear to be beneficial, but this has not been established for all systems. Many sensors are potentially vulnerable to interference by acetaminophen so patients need to be warned about this common component to many over-the-counter remedies.

It is important to remember that CGM is a new technology. While there is evidence that it may replace standard testing for self-management (31), the current systems are indicated for adjunctive use only. Therefore, a finger-stick glucose should always be taken prior to treating a high value with insulin. This is particularly important during rapid fluctuations, as this may be a time where there may be a significant lag period between interstitial and blood glucose levels.

DATA MANAGEMENT

The recent advances in diabetes technology and therapeutics have greatly increased the complexity of diabetes management for both patients and their care providers. While our patients with type 1 diabetes can appreciate the benefits of CGM, advanced insulin pump therapy, and newer noninsulin medications (such as pramlintide), what they really want is an easier way to manage the disease. However, until further progress is made in islet cell replacement (i.e., an "artificial" or transplanted pancreas), it is likely that diabetes data management will grow in importance.

Prior to release of the results of the DCCT trial in 1993, health-care professionals with an interest in diabetes were accustomed to practicing by "faith" in good control. Their extensive personal experience led them to believe that patients keeping closer tabs on their diabetes had fewer complications. The logbook has been an important component of diabetes treatment since the sugar levels were tracked for the first time in the first young boy treated with insulin in 1922 at the University of Toronto. Dr. Elliot Joslin of the Joslin Diabetes Center in Boston promoted recording important events in a person's life into a diary so that both the patient and his/her health-care team could refer to it for treatment decisions.

Figure 5 illustrates a typical logbook. As you can see, this may be difficult to read. Apart from legibility or effort, most human brains are unable to quickly extract complex patterns from mountains of data or inadequate data brought into a clinic. Research comparing

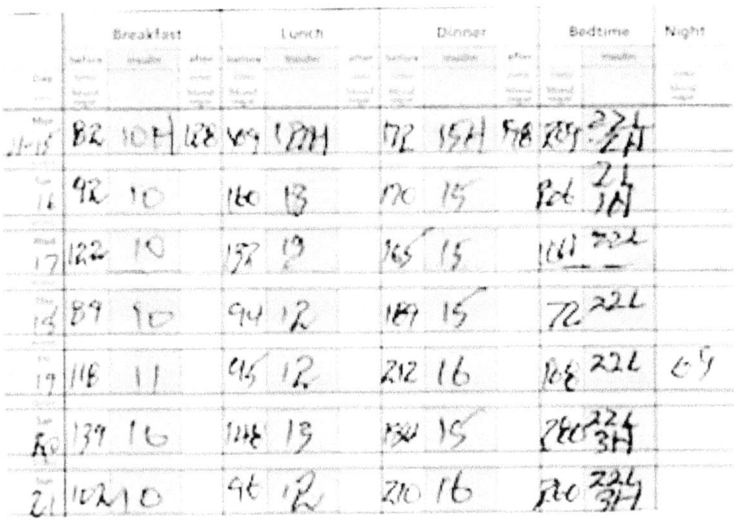

Figure 5 Typical logbook.

written logs to the data (contained in the memory of meters) has also shown that many of these values are altered or fabricated (32).

The logbook methodology is as follows:

1. Patients keep a record of everything that affects their blood sugar since the last visit (insulin doses, foods consumed, activity, stress, etc.).
2. The diabetes care provider (during a visit frequently lasting a total of less than 15 minutes) reviews all of this data and gives advice and prescribes changes in therapy for the patient to follow until the next visit.
3. The next visit is scheduled and steps 1 and 2 repeated at intervals depending on the status of the patient.
4. Blood sugar levels improve significantly after each visit.

The DCCT used such logbooks and incorporated the requirement that subjects in the experimental ("intensive") group monitor their blood glucose a minimum of four times (preprandially and at bedtime). Adjusting insulin doses based on these readings was initially left up to the individual investigator. However, a consensus on insulin adjustment strategy was promoted by Skyler (33) and had a wide influence. This form of data management was validated by the DCCT investigators who maintained better control in the intensive treatment group for the duration of the trial. This strategy of adjustment of insulin doses based on a retrospective review of patterns seen in patients' logbooks is now commonplace in diabetes clinics (34).

With this approach, patients are offered advice based on observed patterns of failure. For example, a patient on insulin who has consistently elevated glucose levels at bedtime with acceptable predinner values might be instructed to increase the dose of rapid-acting insulin or reduce carbohydrate intake at dinner. This may be a reasonable solution for people with diabetes with a consistent lifestyle. However, to those with complex lifestyles it offers little flexibility.

Retrospective review of glucose data identifies consistent miscalculations and insulin-dosing errors but fails to provide timely advice to patients as a day unfolds. A prospective approach incorporating techniques of carbohydrate counting, insulin dose "wizards" (currently available with insulin pumps), and CGM is preferable in motivated patients. However,

Sample Smart Chart

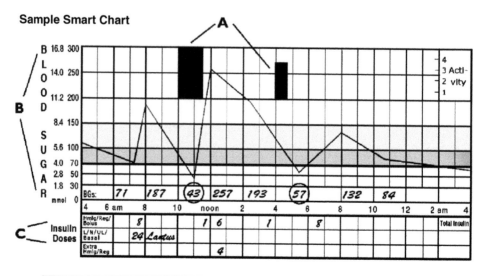

A - Activity and exercise   B - Blood glucose readings   C - Insulin doses
D - Foods and carbs   E - Comments

Figure 6   Smart Chart image. (Courtesy of Diabetesnet.com)

the need for detailed and accurate records in such patients actually increases because the patterns are more complex.

In this author's experience, a provider's failure to review patient-generated records frequently leads to patients foregoing record-keeping entirely. A lack of records to review leaves providers with little upon which to render advice. Additionally, patients and providers may become frustrated with information overload in the context of clinic visits that are too short to make sense of their records. The two approaches currently available to assist with more effective data management are manual charting systems (Fig. 6) and automated device uploading and charting. The remainder of this chapter will discuss how computer technology can contribute to enhanced data management.

The first diabetes management software was created by Rodbard and colleagues in the early 1980s (35) as glucose meters came into common use. Software from device manufacturers and other independent developers subsequently appeared. Initially only glucose levels were tracked. Presently medications, activity, and meals can also be entered. Both PC-based and Internet software have been extensively reviewed (36, 37).

These software programs have the following common characteristics:

1. They upload glucose values from the glucose meter, insulin pump, or other device.
2. They create charts and graphs to enable detection of patterns.
3. They provide an accurate record of diabetes treatment activity that is stored in the device.

Those who find keeping track of their money a hassle often benefit from a computer program that assists them with their personal finances. Similar to the way a computer organizes financial data, it can also organize blood glucose and other diabetes data. The ability to upload data to a computer is nearly universal with today's meters, pumps, and continuous monitors. However, tapping into the information in a device requires a method of transmitting it to the software that will store and analyze it.

All of the following methods have been utilized: (*i*) Connecting the device directly to the computer with a cable (generally plugs in to a serial or USB port), (*ii*) infrared wireless transfer, and (*iii*) radiofrequency (RF) wireless transfer (e.g., proprietary protocol or Bluetooth®). Some systems use one of the above methods to connect to a centralized database without the use of a computer. The transmission may take place via the Internet, cellular phone, or standard telephone lines (i.e., POTS).

Each device has a proprietary cable (or wireless transfer capability). This means that a different cable is usually required for each brand or model you wish to upload. The interface for each device is usually obtained from the manufacturer and usually comes with software. With Macintosh computers there are fewer choices, as most software is designed to work under Windows. The use of a centralized database system (e.g., MediCompass®; www.imetrikus.com) allows patients to upload glucose data from their home and healthcare professionals to view the data from their office. It also allows merging glucose values from different meters (e.g., the meters the patient uses at home, at work, and at the gym) and from different meter brands. Such integrated systems can also eliminate the switchbox and cables that are required in offices that work with multiple devices (Figs. 7 and 8).

Although integrating data from multiple glucose meters is now well established, there are far fewer choices to integrate the glucose data with data uploaded from insulin pumps and continuous glucose monitors. With the increasing sophistication of insulin

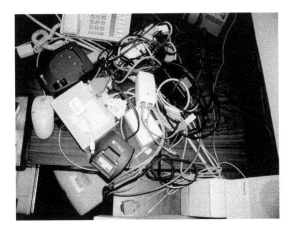

Figure 7 Switchbox mess.

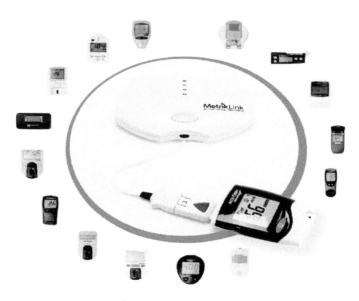

Figure 8   MetrikLink.®

pumps, the need for uploading the devices grows, since the information can no longer be so readily accessed by punching the devices' buttons. Insulin pumps with "smart" features or "wizards" have encouraged patients to enter carbohydrate intake, providing yet another important data point to examine. One barrier to uploading devices other than meters in a busy clinic setting is time. Each such device can take up to 5 minutes to upload. As patients can have multiple devices, the process can be time-consuming. This is a further reason to encourage uploading of devices by patients at home prior to each visit. It is important to remember that improved ability to upload data from devices is not the end but a new beginning of the quest for optimal glycemic control.

There are many graphs that are useful to better understand blood sugar readings. The standard (also referred to as "modal") day graph arranges blood sugar readings from the meter so it looks like a whole week or even months of values happen in 1 day. This chart is important because it shows at what time of the day blood sugar levels are in or out of control. This helps pinpoint where the problem is and clearly illustrates the times of day where there is no information and more testing should be done. This chart also has a goal area (the shaded area) so it's easy to tell at a glance if a blood sugar value is too high, too low, or within the goal range. Figure 9 shows an illustration of this graph. Breakfast and lunch glucoses are in-range, pre-dinner glucoses are rarely checked, and evening glucoses are frequently elevated.

Pie graphs with before-meal or after-meal blood sugar levels the percentages of time blood sugar levels are high, low, or within the blood sugar goal range. These charges are great motivational tools because they immediately show how well a patient is doing and help keep him on track. They also can show how meals are affecting blood sugar. Figure 10 shows an example of a pie graph.

Figure 11 illustrates a glucose line graph. All glucose levels are graphed in chronological order in a glucose line chart. It lets you see long-term trends in blood sugar and whether the values are in or out of goal range. If there is high variability in glucose levels it may look like a seismograph. This patient appears to be improving over time.

Combining the glucose line graph with insulin data can be useful to recognize the interaction of these components. Figure 12 shows these factors graphed together.

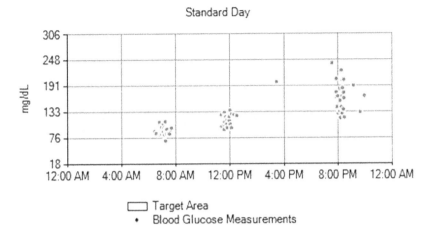

Figure 9   Standard day graph.

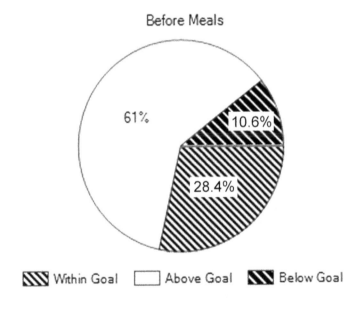

Figure 10   Pie graph.

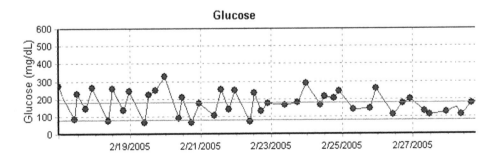

Figure 11   Line graph.

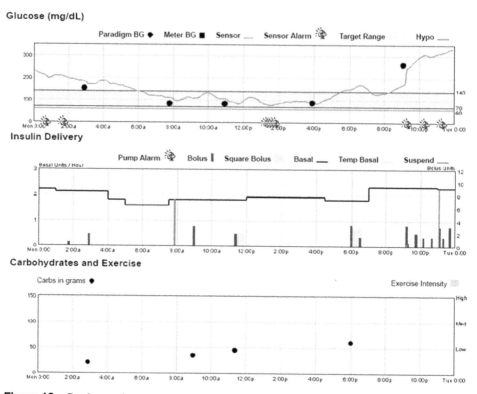

Figure 12 Combo graph.

Descriptive statistics can be helpful to describe glucose datasets and complement graphical charts. Mean glucose correlates well with HbA1c and looking at mean glucose by time of day can be helpful (Fig. 13).

There is no consensus yet on the best metric to describe glucose variability. This is likely to be of increasing importance as there are data suggesting that glucose variability may be associated with oxidative stress (38), which may in turn lead to developing diabetes complications. A simple approach to describing the variability is to use standard deviation (SD). This has the advantage of being already available in most diabetes software. SD reflects the spread around the average with a single number. You can calculate this based on values from entire days or just specific times of day (e.g., before breakfast readings). Dr. Irl Hirsch of the University of Washington created a useful and easy benchmark—the SD multiplied by 2 should not exceed the mean. For super control, the SD multiplied by 3 should be less than the mean (39). If your SD is high, this means that better coordination of meals, activity, and treatment might be needed.

There are other more sophisticated alternatives to SD. These include mean amplitude of glycemic excursion (MAGE) (40), M value (41), J index (42), and mean of daily difference (MODD) (43). Although these are more difficult to manually calculate, more common use of computerized analysis will allow them to be used more easily.

The primary benefit of CGM is likely to be real-time use of the data. Uploading and examining short-term stored data alone with the prior technology of Medtronic CGMS has not been shown to be of consistent benefit (44). However, examination of this retrospective data may be useful in selected patients. Patients with nighttime hypoglycemia and morning high blood sugars pose a diagnostic and therapeutic challenge. The testing of overnight glucose levels is not popular among patients. Determining whether this is due to the dawn

Summary - Blood Glucose

	Total	Avg Tests/ Day	Mean	Std Dev	Min	Max	Targets					
							# Below	# In Target	# Above	% Below	% In Target	% Above
All Unmarked	227	3.7	155	65	23	589	20	87	120	8.8	38.3	52.9
Pre Breakfast	55	9	116	24	65	112	7	39	9	12.7	70.9	16.4
Post Breakfast	0	0	0	0	0	0	0	0	0	0	0	0
Pre Lunch	55	9	130	25	76	175	3	31	21	5.5	56.4	38.2
Post Lunch	0	0	0	0	0	0	0	0	0	0	0	0
Pre Dinner	55	9	127	39	98	243	0	7	48	0	12.7	87.3
Post Dinner	0	0	0	0	0	0	0	0	0	0	0	0
Bedtime	58	9	139	98	77	133	8	10	40	13.8	17.2	69.0
Night	4	1	118	55	65	178	2	0	2	50.0	0	50.0
Marked	0	0	0	0	0	0	0	0	0	0	0	0

Figure 13 Statistics chart.

phenomenon, Somogyi effect, or incorrect insulin dosing can easily be accomplished by a continuous monitor. In patients who use an insulin pump this is a great way to test and optimize the overnight basal insulin infusion rates.

The appropriate use of glucose data, both intermittent and continuous, is essential to the optimal intensive management of diabetes. It has shown the potential to reduce HbA1c, hyperglycemic excursions, and dangerous hypoglycemia. Proper training of the patient in glucose monitoring and more consistent and meaningful review of the wealth of retrospective data by the diabetes care provider are of critical importance. Integrating the latest technology into the care of patients with type 1 diabetes will facilitate the prevention of the long-term complications associated with hyperglycemia and help to reduce the short-term risks of hypoglycemia.

REFERENCES

1. Davison JM, Cheyne GA. History of the measurement of glucose in urine: A cautionary tale. Med Hist 1974;18(2):194–197.
2. Available at www.mendosa.com/history.htm. Accessed on July 30, 2006.
3. The DCCT Research Group. The effect of intensive treatment of diabetes on the development and progression of long-term complications in insulin-dependent diabetes mellitus. N Engl J Med 1993;329:977–986.
4. Heller A. Amperometric biosensors. Curr Opin Biotechnol 1996;7:50–54.
5. Newman JD, Turner APF. Home blood glucose biosensors: A commercial perspective. Biosens Bioelectron 2005;20:2435–2453.
6. Available at www.fda.gov/diabetes/glucose.html# 13. Accessed on October 4, 2006.
7. International Organization for Standardization, Geneva 2000. ISO/DIS 15197 Draft International Standard: Determination of Performance Criteria for In Vitro Blood Glucose Monitoring Systems for Management of Human Diabetes Mellitus.
8. Clarke WL. The Original Clarke Error Grid Analysis (EGA). Diabetes Technol Ther 2005;7(5): 776–779.

9. Baum JM, Monhaut NM, Parker DR, et al. Improving the quality of self-monitoring blood glucose measurement: A study in reducing calibration errors. Diabetes Technol Ther 2006;8(3): 347–357.

10. Fink KS, Christensen DB, Ellsworth A. Effect of high altitude on blood glucose meter performance. Diabetes Technol Ther 2002;4(5):627–635.

11. Tang Z, Lee JH, Louie RF, et al. Effects of different hematocrit levels on glucose measurements with handheld meters for point-of-care testing. Arch Pathol Lab Med 2000;124: 1135–1140.

12. Available at www.fda.gov/cdrh/cdrhhhc/bgm.html. Accessed on October 4, 2006.

13. Tang Z, Du X, Louie RF, et al. Effects of drugs on glucose measurements with handheld glucose meters and a portable glucose analyzer. Am J Clin Pathol 2000;113:75–86.

14. Available at www.fda.gov/diabetes/glucose.html. Accessed on December 30, 2006.

15. Jungheim K, Koschinsky T. Risky delay of hypoglycemia detection by glucose monitoring at the arm. Diabetes Care 2001;24:1303–1304.

16. Sacks D (for the ADA/EASD/IDF working group of the HbA1c assay). Global harmonization of Hemoglobin A1c. Clin Chem 2005;51:681–683.

17. Hanas R. Psychological impact of changing the scale of reported HbA1c results affects metabolic control. Diabetes Care 2002;25:2110–2111.

18. Goldstein DE, Little RR, Lorenz RA, et al. Tests of glycemia in diabetes. Diabetes Care 2004;27:1761–1773.

19. Edelman SV, Bell JM, Serrano RB, et al. Home testing of fructosamine improves glycemic control in patients with diabetes. Endocr Pract 2001;7:454 –458.

20. McGill JB, Cole TG, Nowarzke W, et al. Circulating 1,5-anhydroglucitol levels in adult patients with diabetes reflect longitudinal changes of glycemia. Diabetes Care 2004;27:1859–1865.

21. Dungan KM, Buse JB, Largay J, et al. 1,5-Anhydroglucitol (1,5-AG) and postprandial hyperglycemia as measured by Continuous Glucose Monitoring System (CGMS) in inadequately controlled patients with diabetes. Diabetes Care 2006;29:1214–1219.

22. Feldman B, Brazg R, Schwartz S, et al. A continuous glucose sensor based on wired enzyme[TM] technology—results from a 3-day trial in patients with type 1 diabetes. Diabetes Technol Ther 2003;5:769–779.

23. Garg S, Zisser H, Schwartz S, et al. Improvement in glycemic excursions with a transcutaneous real-time continuous glucose sensor. Diabetes Care 2006;29:44–50.

24. Gross TM, Bode BW, Einhorn D et al. Performance evaluation of the MiniMed continuous glucose monitoring system during patient home use. Diabetes Technol Ther 2000;2:49–56.

25. Maran A, Poscia A. Continuous subcutaneous glucose monitoring: The GlucoDay system. Diabetes Nutr Metab 2002;15:429–433.

26. Heinemann L, Continuous glucose monitoring by means of the microdialysis technique: Underlying fundamental aspects continuous subcutaneous glucose monitoring. Diabetes Technol Ther 2003;5:545–561.

27. Garg SK, Schwartz S, Edelman SV. Improved glucose excursions using an implantable real-time continuous glucose sensor in adults with type 1 diabetes. Diabetes Care 2004;27:734–738.

28. Garg S, Jovanovic L. Relationship of fasting and hourly blood glucose levels to HbA1c values: Safety, accuracy, and improvements in glucose profiles obtained using a 7-day continuous glucose sensor. Diabetes Care 2006;29:2644–2649.

29. Hirsch IB, Farkas-Hirsch R. Sliding scale or sliding scare: It's all sliding nonsense. Diabetes Spectr 2001;14:79–81.

30. Deiss D, Bolinder J, Riveline JP, et al. Improved glycemic control in poorly controlled patients with type 1 diabetes using real-time continuous glucose monitoring. Diabetes Care 2006;29: 2730–2732.

31. Zisser H, Bailey TS, Jovanovic L. Diabetes self-management guided by continuous glucose monitoring: Results of a pilot study. American Diabetes Association Annual Meeting, Washington, DC, June 2006, OR-69.

32. Mazze, RS, Shamoon H, Pasmantier R, et al. Reliability of blood glucose monitoring by patients with diabetes mellitus. Am J Med 1984;77:211–217.

33. Skyler JS, Skyler DL, Seigler DE. Algorithms for adjustment of insulin dosage by patients who monitor blood glucose. Diabetes Care 1981;4:311–318.
34. Pearson J, Bergenstal R. Pattern management: An essential component of effective insulin management. Diabetes Spectr 2001;14:75–78.
35. Pernick NL, Rodbard D. Personal computer programs to assist with self-monitoring of blood glucose and self-adjustment of insulin dosage. Diabetes Care 1986;9:61–69.
36. Park JY, Daly JM. Evaluation of diabetes management software. Diabetes Educ 2003;29: 255–267.
37. Available at www.mendosa.com/software.htm. Accessed on December 30, 2006.
38. Monnier L, Mas E, Ginet C, et al. Activation of oxidative stress by acute glucose fluctuations compared with sustained chronic hyperglycemia in patients with type 2 diabetes. JAMA 2006;295:1681–1687.
39. Hirsch IB. Blood glucose monitoring technology: Translating data into practice. Endocr Pract 2004;10:67–76.
40. Service FJ, Molnar GD, Rosevear JW, et al. Mean amplitude of glycemic excursions, a measure of diabetic instability. Diabetes 1970;19:644–655.
41. Schlichtkrull J, Munck O, Jersild M. The M-value, an index of blood-sugar control in diabetics. Acta Med Scand 1965;177:95–102.
42. Wojcicki J. J-index. A new proposition of the assessment of current glucose control in diabetic patients. Horm Metab Res 1995;27:41–42.
43. Molnar GD, Taylor WF, Ho MM. Day-to-day variation of continuously monitored glycaemia: A further measure of diabetic instability. Diabetologia 1972;8:342–348.
44. Yates K, Milton AH, Dear K, et al. Continuous glucose monitoring–guided insulin adjustment in children and adolescents on near-physiological insulin regimens- a randomized controlled trial. Diabetes Care 2006;29:1512–1517.

4
Diabetes Education, Nutrition, Exercise, and Special Situations

Jo Ann Ahern
Animas Corporation, West Chester, Pennsylvania, U.S.A.

EDUCATION

Diabetes education is required for all who are diagnosed with diabetes regardless of kind of diabetes or the age of the patient. Diabetes education does not ensure that patients will follow instructions and do everything that they are asked to do. Education is necessary but patients should be able to make the decision as to what they are willing to do to maintain or improve their health. Educators need to remember that just because someone decides that they will not follow directions for care, education was wasted. Everyone deserves to make an informed decision. Diabetes self-management training (DSMT) should be reimbursed as part of the care of the patient with diabetes since it is an enormous part of the treatment plan.

The scope of practice for diabetes educators defines the specialty and provides a framework for appropriate and effective practice of the specialty. This statement on the scope of practice for diabetes educators is not a static set of rules and definitions; rather, it is a fluid framework that adjusts to reflect the multidisciplinary nature of diabetes care, the evolving body of knowledge and evidence for effective interventions, and the ever-changing (and increasingly challenging) health-care environment.

DIABETES EDUCATOR'S SCOPE OF PRACTICE

All health-care providers need sufficient diabetes knowledge to provide safe, competent care to persons with or at risk for diabetes. As management of diabetes becomes increasingly complex, it is imperative that diabetes health-care professionals are well educated and appropriately credentialed. Expertise in diabetes care develops through experience, continuing education, individual study, and mentorship.

Diabetes educators use established principles of teaching and learning theory and lifestyle counseling to help clients confidently and effectively manage the disease. Instruction is individualized for persons of all ages, incorporating cultural preferences, health beliefs, and preferred learning styles of the client.

Behavior change directed at successful diabetes self-management was formally adopted as the desired outcome of DSMT in 2002 (24). Seven specific self-care behaviors, known collectively as *The AADE 7 Self-Care Behaviors*^{TM}, along with five core outcome measures, have been defined to guide the process of DSMT (25, 26).

The primary goal of diabetes education is to provide knowledge and skill training that helps individuals identify barriers and facilitates problem-solving and coping skills to achieve effective self-care behavior and behavior change. It is the position of the American Association of Diabetes Educators (AADE) that all educators should measure the AADE 7 Self-Care Behaviors, both for individuals and in the aggregate, at least twice: pre- and postintervention. The AADE 7 Self-Care Behaviors are listed below:

1. Healthy eating
2. Being active
3. Monitoring
4. Taking medications
5. Problem solving
6. Healthy coping
7. Reducing risks

Additional follow-up measurements are ideal and should be applied as appropriate to the practice setting. By adopting the AADE 7 Self-Care Behaviors, educators are able to determine their effectiveness with individuals and populations, compare their performance with established benchmarks, and measure and quantify the unique contribution that DSMT plays in the overall context of diabetes care.

AADE OUTCOMES MEASUREMENT STANDARDS

In the September/October issue of *The Diabetes Educator* (vol. 29, issue 5) AADE published its position statement (1) on standards for outcomes measurement of diabetes self-management education.

Seven diabetes self-care behavior measures determine the effectiveness of diabetes self-management education at individual, participant, and population levels. Diabetes self-care behaviors should be evaluated at baseline and then at regular intervals after the education program. The continuum of outcomes, including learning, behavioral, clinical, and health status, should be assessed to demonstrate the interrelationship between DSME and behavior change in the care of individuals with diabetes.

Individual patient outcomes are used to guide the intervention and improve care for that patient. Aggregate population outcomes are used to guide programmatic services and for continuous quality improvement activities for the DSME and the population it serves.

PRACTICE OPTIONS

Three practice options, which may overlap, are available to health-care professionals who choose to specialize in diabetes care:

1. Diabetes educator
2. Certified diabetes educator (CDE)
3. Board certified in advanced diabetes management (BC-ADM)

These classifications are differentiated by educational preparation, formal credentialing, professional practice regulations, and the clinical practice environment. It is the position of the AADE that all diabetes educators work toward formal certification. The diabetes educator and CDE are chiefly concerned with and actively engaged in the process of DSMT. The BC-ADM incorporates skills and strategies of DSMT into the more comprehensive clinical management of people with diabetes. Differences in the preparation, scope, and practice of diabetes educators (certified or not) and the BC-ADM may make dual credentialing desirable for some. For example, a diabetes educator or CDE may also have the BC-ADM credential, provided he or she meets the academic and practice requirements for BC-ADM certification. Conversely, the BC-ADM may not necessarily be a diabetes educator as defined here. A more comprehensive description of each classification is given below (2).

Diabetes educators are health-care professionals who have achieved a core body of knowledge and skills in the biological and social sciences, communication, counseling, and education and who have experience in the care of people with diabetes. Mastery of the knowledge and skills required to become a diabetes educator are obtained through formal and continuing education, individual study, and mentorship. The role of the diabetes educator can be assumed by professionals from a variety of health disciplines, including, but not limited to, registered nurses, registered dietitians, pharmacists, physicians, mental health professionals, podiatrists, optometrists, and exercise physiologists. The diabetes educator is an integral partner in the diabetes care team.

The diabetes educator understands the impact of acute or chronic problems on a person's health behaviors and lifestyle, and on the teaching/learning process. Such appreciation is essential for the development of a comprehensive plan for continuing education and cost-effective, self-care management.

Members of the various health disciplines who practice diabetes education bring their particular focus to the educational process. This widens or narrows the scope of practice for individual educators as is appropriate within the boundaries of each health profession, which may be regulated by national or state agencies or accrediting bodies. Regardless of discipline, the diabetes educator must be prepared to provide clients with the knowledge and skills to effectively manage his or her diabetes. Diabetes educators must possess a body of knowledge that spans across disciplines in order to provide comprehensive DSMT. For example, dietitians who are diabetes educators provide instruction for insulin injection, insulin dosing, and medication side effects as well as providing nutrition counseling. Exercise physiologists in the diabetes educator role may help clients develop a meal plan, and pharmacists may provide counseling and instruction about foot care.

Diabetes educators may assume responsibilities beyond providing DSMT to individuals. Program management; case management; clinical management; health-care consultancy with other providers, organizations, and industry; public and professional education; public health and wellness promotion; and research in diabetes management and education are all important roles assumed by diabetes educators.

CDEs, in addition to fulfilling the requirements of a diabetes educator, meet the academic, professional, and experiential requirements set forth by the National Certification Board for Diabetes Educators (NCBDE) (27). The NCBDE defines the criteria for certification as a diabetes educator. As part of the application process, a diabetes educator must document that he or she meets all the criteria for certification. An accepted applicant must demonstrate competency in the required body of knowledge and skills by means of a written examination. Certification is valid for a period of 5 years, and is maintained either through repeat examination or through documented participation in relevant continuing education activities every 5 years.

BC-ADM is a credential available since 2001. The BC-ADM credential is the first advanced-practice certification offered to members of more than one discipline. Nurse Practitioners, Clinical Nurse Specialists, dietitians, and registered pharmacists may apply. Recognizing that nonnursing health-care professionals participate in diabetes care, the task force acknowledged the need for an advanced diabetes manager credential that includes nutrition and pharmacy as well as nursing.

Four discipline-specific examinations are offered for the BC-ADM credential, reflecting the practice of comprehensive clinical management of individuals with diabetes. Candidates must document at least 500 hours of recent advanced-practice diabetes care. They must demonstrate skill in performing complete and/or focused assessments, recognizing and prioritizing complex data, and providing therapeutic problem-solving, counseling, and regimen adjustments for people with diabetes.

The educational preparation required to take the exams is as follows: a master's degree in nursing is required for clinical nurse specialists and nurse practitioners, dietitians must have a relevant clinical master's degree, and registered pharmacists must have a doctorate of pharmacy degree. Upon verification of eligibility, candidates sit for a discipline-specific written examination administered by the American Nurses Credentialing Center (ANCC). Certification is valid for 5 years. Recertification is by reexamination or through qualified continuing education activities as defined by the ANCC. Additional information about certification and recertification can be obtained directly from the ANCC (28).

The BC-ADM practice is characterized by autonomous assessment, problem identification, planning, implementation, and evaluation of diabetes care, within the guidelines for BC-ADM practice set by the individual discipline. The process of using assessment data to independently derive a diagnosis or problem list is a key distinguishing aspect of BC-ADM practice. A diabetes care professional with a BC-ADM credential may or may not be a CDE. As diabetes education is an integral part of diabetes care and management, the professional with the BC-ADM credential necessarily incorporates aspects of DSMT into his or her practice, either directly or through referral to another qualified diabetes educator.

NUTRITION

The American Dietetic Association recommends a diet that emphasizes fruits, vegetables, whole grains, and fat free milk. This diet includes lean meats, poultry, fish, beans, eggs, and nuts. It is low in saturated fats, trans fats, cholesterol, salt, and added sugars. There is no perfect diet for everyone and diet should be individualized for each person based on age, activity, and preferences. My Pyramid can be found on the American Dietetic Association's website and the patient can input his or her own information and receive recommendations for dietary consumption.

Carbohydrate counting is generally accepted as the "state of the art" in diabetes management. Every patient with diabetes should be taught carbohydrate counting from the onset/diagnosis of diabetes. Carbohydrate counting is easy and practical and anyone can understand the concept. All food items have carbohydrates listed on the package somewhere. Patients need to be taught to look at the *total carbohydrates* since this is the most critical to blood glucose levels. Patients of any age are quite good at counting carbohydrates; even the elderly are able to master this task. If patients understand how many carbohydrates to consume, they are able to manage blood glucose levels and control weight. Women should not consume more than 45 to 60 g of carbohydrate per meal and 15 to 30 g for snacks. This should be individualized based on physical activity. If an elderly woman moves very little, she may need fewer than 45 g of carbohydrate per meal. If a woman is athletic, she may need more than 60 g of carbohydrate per meal, but this is a good starting point. Men need 60 to 75 g of carbohydrate per meal and 30 to 45 g for snacks. This also needs to be adjusted based on the activity level and age of the man.

Carbohydrate, protein, and fat all raise blood glucose levels. Carbohydrate raises glucose levels more quickly than protein or fat and usually has a peak effect of 90 to 120 minutes after the meal is consumed. Protein raises glucose levels closer to 4 hours after the meal and fat closer to 8 hours after the meal. This is critical to know in order to take the appropriate amount of insulin to cover the meal. Most insulin users have an insulin:carbohydrate ratio. This means that they take a certain amount of insulin to cover a certain amount of carbohydrate. They must be taught, however, the effect of high protein meals and high fat meals. The average starting point for an adult is one unit of insulin for 15 g of carbohydrate. This needs to be adjusted based on postprandial glucose levels. If glucose levels 1 to 2 hours after the meal are greater than 180 mg/dL (3), the insulin:carbohydrate ratio is not adequate. This, of course, is assuming that the preprandial glucose level is 70 to 120 mg/dL and the person bolused at least 15 minutes before the meal. Small changes can be made if the person is treated with an insulin pump as the pump can be programmed with small changes of the insulin:carbohydrate ratio. If a person were taking 1 unit/15 g of carbohydrate and was > 180 mg/dL 1.5 to 2 hours after the meal, the insulin:carbohydrate ratio could be changed to 1:12. This would also need to be tested until appropriate postprandial glucose levels are reached. If a person is consuming a large amount of fat at the meal, the bolus may need to be increased and extended. When a person with diabetes consumes a meal such as pizza, he or she will need to add extra carbohydrates to their estimate and set a combination bolus with a percent given immediately and a percent extended over several hours. My suggestion to patients eating a meal such as pizza is to add 20 to 30 g of carbohydrate to their estimate and take 70% before the meal and 30% over the next 5 to 6 hours. This helps to cover the initial rise of glucose from the carbohydrates and the later increase in absorption of the fat content. People usually continue to make adjustments to this until they achieve success, that is, glucose levels less than 180 mg/dL after the meal and 70 to 120 mg/dL before the next meal. A correction factor also needs to be calculated into the bolus dose of insulin. The pump will also do this once the correction factor/sensitivity factor is calculated for the patient. The patient would enter the glucose, if it is not already there, and the pump will calculate the amount of insulin it takes to reach the target glucose (my suggestion is 100 mg/dL for the target) so that the glucose comes closer to the desired range. If a patient is on injections, it is more difficult to determine all these calculations and draw them up in a syringe as you cannot calculate to an exact amount this way. Most people have to do this on multiple daily injections, but the outcome is not as good as it is with a pump simply because the dose is an estimate and not exact and syringes can only measure down to 0.5 unit where pumps can measure all the way to the 0.05 unit of insulin. It is simply not possible to duplicate this with injections.

When all is said and done, we simply eat too much in this country and this needs to be addressed in our nutrition counseling. In a survey of > 2000 adults with diabetes, the most frequently cited barrier to achieving self-management goals was adherence to diet and exercise (4). We eat too much fat and not enough vegetables and fruits, and do not exercise enough (5). Everyone is looking for the easy way out, a pill, that will fix it all for them. We know that medical nutrition therapy does make a difference (6). Diabetes medical nutrition therapy trials and outcome studies have demonstrated reductions in HbA1c of approximately 1% in type 1 diabetes (3). When a health-care provider advises a patient on weight loss (not just telling them they need to lose weight), patients are nearly three times as likely to act on the recommendation (7). Patients are more satisfied with their interactions with health-care providers when they receive information, support, and resources, especially when our messages are positive, nonjudgmental, and understanding of the difficulties of changing behavior (8). Patients should be referred to a dietitian who is knowledgeable and skilled in developing an individualized diabetes meal plan.

EXERCISE

Exercise is an essential part of any plan of care (9). It should be emphasized to all patients with diabetes that this is as important as the other aspects of care. It is something that is generally overlooked and not discussed in a busy office visit, but patients need to understand the importance of this aspect of diabetes management. Patients often have a misconstrued idea of what exercise is. They can incorporate exercise into their daily life. It does not mean they need to join a gym or jog every day, though this would be good. They can take the stairs instead of the elevator, park far away from the store or workplace so that they have to walk further, wear a pedometer to work and get up and walk periodically, walk for 10 minutes after lunch, go visit a coworker on a different floor or up the hall, stand up at every commercial on TV and do some jumping jacks. These are all small ways to incorporate exercise into daily routines.

Exercise training raises high density lipoprotein cholesterol, lowers blood pressure, and leads to a 20 to 40% increase in insulin sensitivity by enhancing insulin action in skeletal muscles (10). Therefore, all diabetic patients should be encouraged to engage in 30 minutes of modest aerobic exercise (such as brisk walking, aerobics, swimming, or bicycling) three to four times per week. The intensity should be gauged to produce an increase in pulse rate to 60 to 70% of maximum, which can be calculated as 220 minus age. This level of exercise is referred to as "conversational exercise" because it is not intense enough to prevent the patient from conversing with a partner during the workout.

Exercise usually lowers blood glucose levels. If someone is a real competitive athlete, glucose levels will go up during competition due to adrenaline being released during this activity. Many times, the same person will have a low glucose level at a practice but a high one at a game even in the same sport. It takes a lot of insulin dose adjustments before normal glucose levels are achieved with exercise. There are many ways to deal with this. First, do the exercise without changing anything to see what happens. Many people prefer to take their pumps off for exercise. This can usually be worked out if the sport is not too long, like baseball or cross country running. If the patient is on injections, it is more difficult to address, but a plan needs to be developed. This patient may need to lower the bolus prior to the previous meal or snack or he/she may need to decrease the long acting insulin during the sport season. This makes it difficult to figure out what to do if there is no exercise that day as long-acting insulins (Lantus, Levimir) last for several days so changing based on the same day simply does not work for the patient. He or she would probably need to increase the fast-acting insulin on off days to counteract high glucose levels.

For athletes competing in sports, it is advisable to remove the pump during the sport (if using a pump), but reattach it as soon as the sport is over and replace at least 1 hour of basal insulin as a bolus. This will keep the glucose from rising within the first hour after the sport is finished. The Diabetes Research in Children Network (DirecNet) studied this and found that if the pump was kept on at the usual basal rate, hypoglycemia occurred, but if it was removed, hyperglycemia occurred very soon after the exercise was completed (11). Therefore, to prevent the hypoglycemia during exercise, pump should be removed or basal decreased significantly, but insulin needs to be replaced soon after exercise to prevent hyperglycemia. Exercise also cause delayed hypoglycemia in most patients with diabetes. In order to prevent this, patients are instructed to decrease basal rate at bedtime to 70 to

80% of their usual dose for 4 to 5 hours. This prevents nocturnal hypoglycemia in these patients. It was shown by Bussau, et al., that a sprint at the end of practice or a game reduces hypoglycemia due to increase in catecholamines (12). Since many athletes do this as part of their sport, it is no wonder that they come off the field with extremely high glucose levels that need to be corrected. Sprinting does raise glucose and many sports require sprinting.

Health-care providers must recommend exercise to their patients. The success rate is not very good for patients continuing an exercise plan, but if it is not discussed, the success rate is even poorer (13). Exercise is extremely difficult to maintain as is diet but if patients are not encouraged, they surely will not see any necessity for it. It should be addressed at every visit as a part of the visit. Sometimes hearing things over and over does eventually make a difference to a patient. Even if the motivation wears off, the patient will usually follow a plan for a while and if they are seen every 3 months, they may have more time that they exercise than they do not exercising. In a study at the Joslin Diabetes Center located at the University Health Care Center in Syracuse, NY, patients were asked to develop their own meal and exercise plan. At 2 and 6 months respectively, 89% and 92% of the participants felt that they were following the meal plan either some or most of the time. One hundred percent of respondents were able to determine their own exercise plan, with 98% indicating they could adhere to the plan, and 85.7% felt that the new plan would be easier than previous ones. At 2 and 6 months respectively, 70% and 73% felt that they were following their exercise plan either some or most of the time. Individualized meal and exercise plans can be successfully created by the patients themselves (14). In an integrative literature review, Dr. Nancy Allen, examined the literature on diabetes research using social cognitive theory (15) to determine its predictive ability in explaining exercise behavior and to identify key interventions that enhance exercise initiation and maintenance. The results showed that a statistically significant relationship between self-efficacy and exercise behavior was found in correlational studies. Results from the predictive study support the predictability of self-efficacy for exercise behavior. Self-efficacy (16) was predictive of exercise initiation and maintenance over time. The evidence for successful interventions to increase self-efficacy and exercise behavior over time was inconclusive (17).

In conclusion everyone is in agreement that exercise is an important and even essential part of any diabetes management plan. It is also one of the most difficult parts of the regimen for patients to adhere to.

TRAVEL

Traveling with diabetes is always an adventure. Many people have a job that requires travel and many others travel for pleasure. If a patient is traveling on an airplane, he or she needs to do the following according to the American Diabetes Association and the Transportation Security Administration (TSA):

Notify the screener that you have diabetes and are carrying your supplies with you. Please note that while TSA is not currently requiring a prescription label, it recommends having the label available to identify the medication in order to expedite the security check-point screening process. The following diabetes-related supplies and equipment are allowed through the checkpoint once they have been screened:

- Insulin and insulin loaded dispensing products (vials or box of individual vials, jet injectors, pens, infusers, and preloaded syringes) that are clearly identified with a prescription label containing a name that matches the passenger's name on his or her ticket.

- Other liquid prescription medicines such as Smylin, Byetta, or a Glucagon Emergency Kit that are clearly identified with a prescription label containing a name that matches the passenger's name on his or her ticket.
- Note that essential nonprescription liquid medicines (such as regular insulin, where in some states a prescription to dispense is not required) should be clearly labeled.
- Multiple containers of liquids and gels (including cake mate) to treat hypoglycemia. If containers are more than 3 oz, then passengers need to declare these items to security checkpoint personnel.
- Unlimited number of unused syringes when accompanied by insulin or other injectable medication.
- Blood glucose meters, blood glucose meter test strips, continuous blood glucose monitors, lancets, alcohol swabs, meter-testing solutions, and monitor supplies.
- Insulin pump and insulin pump supplies (cleaning agents, batteries, plastic tubing, infusion kit, catheter, and needle).
- Urine ketone test strips.
- Unlimited number of used syringes when transported in Sharps disposal container or other similar hard-surface container.

In addition to the information providers above, it is recommended that passengers review TSA's 9/26/06 Q&A (PDF) (http://www.diabetes.org/uedocuments/PersonswithDisabilitiesQuestionsandAnswers.pdf) regarding changes to liquids ban at airport security checkpoints.

Pump Wearers

Although insulin pump manufacturers indicate that pumps can safely go through airport security systems, pump wearers may request a visual inspection rather than walking through the metal detector or being hand-wanded. Note that this may subject you to closer scrutiny or a "pat-down."

- Advise the screener that the insulin pump cannot be removed because it is connected to a catheter inserted under your skin.
- Insulin pumps and supplies must be accompanied by insulin with a label clearly identifying the medication.

If You Experience Hypoglycemia During the Security Procedure

Immediately inform screeners if you are experiencing low blood sugar and are in need of medical assistance.

If You Request a Visual Inspection of Your Supplies

You have the option of requesting a visual inspection of your insulin and diabetes associated supplies. Keep in mind that

- you must request a visual inspection before the screening process begins otherwise your medications and supplies will undergo X-ray inspection.
- you should separate your medication and associated supplies from your other property in a pouch or bag.
- medications should be labeled so they are identifiable.

- in order to prevent contamination or damage to medication and associated supplies and/or fragile medical materials, you will be asked at the security checkpoint to display, handle, and repack your own medication and associated supplies during the visual inspection process.
- any medication and/or associated supplies that cannot be cleared visually must be submitted for X-ray screening. If you refuse, you will not be permitted to carry your medications and related supplies into the sterile area.

Contact TSA

If you have an immediate need while being screened, you should ask for a screener supervisor. You may also contact the TSA contact center to report unfair treatment or to obtain additional information by calling toll-free 866-289-9673 during the following hours of operation (all times are Eastern Standard Time):

- Monday through Friday 8 a.m.–10 p.m.
- Saturday, Sunday, and Holidays 10 a.m.–6 p.m.

Complaints about discriminatory treatment (http://airconsumer.ost.dot.gov/DiscrimComplaintsContacs.htm) by federal security screeners should be directed to TSA. TSA accepts complaints by mail to Transportation Security Administration, TSA Headquarters, 12th Floor, Room 1203 N, TSA-1, 400 Seventh St., SW, Washington, DC 20590.

In addition to filing a complaint with a federal agency, passengers alleging discriminatory treatment by air carrier personnel (pilots, flight attendants, gate agents, or check-in counter personnel) may download and print a complaint form and follow instructions provided by Department of Transportation's (DOT's) Web site (http://airconsumer.ost.dot.gov/problems.htm). They should also notify their airline carrier. Other consumer complaints may be directed to the Department of Transportation's Office of Consumer Protection Division, 400 Seventh St., S.W., Washington, DC, 20590, U.S.A. More information on where passengers may file complaints for travel service problems, contact DOT by calling 1-800-255-1111.

The association recommends packing at least twice the number of supplies needed during travel, and bringing a quick-acting source of glucose to treat low blood glucose, as well as an easy to carry snack such as a nutrition bar. Carry or wear medical identification and carry contact information for your physician while traveling. It may also be helpful to have contact information for a health-care professional available at your destination, and be prepared to adjust medication when traveling in different time zones.

- You should separate your medication and associated supplies from your other property in a pouch or bag.
- Medications should be labeled so they are identifiable.
- In order to prevent contamination or damage to medication and associated supplies and/or fragile medical materials, you will be asked at the security checkpoint to display, handle, and repack your own medication and associated supplies during the visual inspection process.
- Any medication and/or associated supplies that cannot be cleared visually must be submitted for X-ray screening. If you refuse, you will not be permitted to carry your medications and related supplies into the sterile area.

Contact TSA

If you have an immediate need while being screened, you should ask for a screener supervisor.

In addition, blood glucose levels tend to increase while traveling in any mode, therefore, increase the basal rate by approximately 30% while traveling. If on injections, increase the bolus doses and may need more doses during travel. When traveling across time zones and wearing a pump, the time needs to be changed on arrival. This is essential to maintain basal rates at the right times of day. If on injections with Lantus or Levimir, these need to be adjusted by approximately 2 hr/day. If on NPH, it may need to be given as much as 3 hours earlier or later depending on the time zone.

If traveling to high altitudes, 3000 to 5000 m (10,000 to 16,000 ft), barometric pressure decreases linearly with increasing altitude (18). Inspired Po_2 at the summit of Mount Everest (8848 m) is < 30% of that at sea level (19). Acclimatization refers to the physiological changes that occur consequent to prolonged exposure to the hypoxia and low barometric pressure of altitude, and it includes hyperventilation, with the resultant respiratory alkalosis being reduced over time by compensatory renal bicarbonate excretion. Although erythrocyte levels also increase, this occurs much more slowly, over the course of several weeks (18). It is also important to note that acclimatization does not imply normalization because, despite continued hyperventilation, alveolar Po_2 levels remain well below that at sea level even in fully acclimatized individuals.

Those who seem to do well and are successful on these climbs are those who are in excellent control (HbA1c < 7%) and have no complications (20–22). Acute mountain sickness can occur causing dizziness and nausea. This can effect glucose control. Symptoms of acute mountain sickness may mask symptoms of hypoglycemia in some people with diabetes (20). Diabetes control deteriorated in climbers consistently due to elevation and decreases in temperature. Climbing requires much preparation and consideration of the consequences.

Traveling should be fun and it should be an adventure, but to keep it that way, much planning needs to take place. Patients should discuss travel plans with their health-care provider well before taking the trip. This greatly reduces the risk of problems related to travel in those with diabetes (23). Make sure that all the guidelines that the ADA puts forth are followed. Always take twice as many supplies as necessary.

WEATHER

Most people with diabetes do not understand the effect of weather on blood glucose control. When the weather is cold, glucose level may rise due to constriction of blood vessels. This constriction decreases the absorption of insulin from the subcutaneous tissue. Sometimes glucose level may drop during cold weather due to the amount of shivering that someone does. Shivering decreases glucose levels due to increased metabolic rate. Hot weather tends to lower glucose levels due to the dilation of the blood vessels. This helps the insulin to be absorbed faster than usual. Glucose levels frequently drop in the spring when temperatures begin to rise. This is something to be aware of so that it can be avoided or, at least, greatly limited.

HYPERGLYCEMIA

If a patient is treated with an insulin pump and glucose levels are elevated to > 250 mg/dL in the fasting state, the patient must be instructed to change the site immediately since he or she does not know how long insulin has not been infused for. If the patient is staying at home, he or she can correct the glucose and wait 1 to 2 hours for it to decrease to the normal range. If this does not happen, site needs to be changed immediately. The danger of not doing this is ketoacidosis and it can be avoided with careful attention to glucose levels > 250 mg/dL. At other times of the day, the correction should be made and glucose retested in 1 to 2 hours to make sure that glucose is coming down into the normal range. If moderate or large ketones are present or nausea, the correction should be doubled, as patients are very insulin resistant in this stage of ketosis. I strongly suggest that the patient then double the basal rate for 2 to 3 hours to bring the glucose back into the normal range quickly. If hyperglycemia occurs in those on injections, they simply need to correct with fast-acting insulin based on their correction factor.

SICK DAYS

When a patient with diabetes is ill, glucose levels tend to rise due to increased levels of cortisol. If glucose levels are elevated and a patient is on a pump, basal insulin should be increased by means of a temporary rate with an increase of 30 to 50%. If not on a pump, more frequent doses of fast-acting insulin need to be given every 3 to 4 hours. Some patients become hypoglycemic when ill. In this case, the temporary rate should be decreased by 30 to 50% until glucose levels begin to rise. If glucose levels remain low and insulin is discontinued for more than 1 hour, ketones can occur. If glucose continues to drop despite decreasing or stopping insulin, and patient is nauseous and/or vomiting, a small dose of glucagon (20 to 30 units) can be given to raise glucose level for a few hours. This may keep someone out of the hospital and at home where they are much more comfortable.

MENSTRUATION

In most women, glucose levels tend to rise the week before onset of menses. A different basal rate can be set into the pump to accommodate this rise in glucose. The basal profile can be changed back once menses begins. This makes life a little easier when the different basal profiles are already in the pump so that the woman does not need to do it on a monthly basis. If on injections, fast-acting insulin probably needs to be increased to cover meals and higher glucose values before onset of menses. The basal insulin is difficult to adjust because it takes a couple of days to equilibrate and this could cause hypoglycemia when menses occurs.

SMOKING

Everyone is aware of the long-term effects of smoking and these are all increased in those with diabetes. The acute effects of smoking are frequently overlooked. When someone with diabetes smokes a cigarette, blood vessels constrict and insulin is poorly absorbed. Most people who smoke grab a cigarette right after consuming a meal. This is extremely problematic since the insulin is not getting absorbed well, but the food is. This leads to high postprandial glucose levels. When smoking ceases, the blood vessels dilate causing the patient to absorb insulin quickly. This happens after the food has been digested causing subsequent low blood glucose levels. Patients who smoke with diabetes, therefore, have very erratic glucose levels with many hypo and hyperglycemic episodes.

MARIJUANA USE

Use of marijuana is similar to smoking cigarettes except it has the added effect of increasing appetite so people eat more food and either forget to cover it with insulin or just do not care. It is also difficult to detect hypoglycemia when high on marijuana.

COCAINE USE

When using cocaine, most people lose their interest in eating at all. They also forget to take insulin and begin to care only about the next fix. This is tragic for anyone, but for someone with diabetes it is particularly worrisome. If insulin is taken but the person does not eat, hypoglycemia occurs. If insulin is ignored, ketoacidosis occurs. Both are worrisome and scary.

ALCOHOL USE

Use of alcohol is tricky as well. This is the most commonly used drug. The problems with alcohol and diabetes are as follows:

1. Drinking alcohol masks the symptoms of hypoglycemia.
2. While detoxing alcohol the liver will not perform its usual job of glycogenolysis. If glucose falls dangerously low, the liver will not counter-regulate as it is too busy detoxing the alcohol and this is its first priority. It is important to remember that this is the one time that counter-regulation will not occur. Basal rates should be decreased by approximately 20% when going to sleep after a night of drinking. In this way, hypoglycemia is avoided. If a patient is on injections, a snack would need to be consumed before going to sleep. More than two alcoholic beverages should not be consumed by anyone but especially those with diabetes as it can be much more dangerous for him or her.

REFERENCES

1. http://www.aadenet.org/pdf/PS-Outcomes.pdf.
2. http://www.aadenet.org/AboutUs/.
3. American Diabetes Association. Nutrition Recommendations and Interventions for Diabetes-2006 (position statement). Diabetes Care 2006;29:2140–2157.
4. Glasgow RE, Hampson SE, Strycher LA, et al. Personal-model beliefs and social environmental barriers related to diabetes self-management. Diabetes Care 1997;20:556–561.
5. Nelson KM, Reiber G, Boyko EJ. Diet and exercise among adults with type 2 diabetes: Findings from the Third National Health and Nutrition Examination Survey (NHANES III). Diabetes Care 2002;25:1722–1728.
6. Pastors JG, Warshaw H, Daly A, et al. The evidence for the effectiveness of medical nutrition therapy in diabetes managment. Diabetes Care 2002;25:608–613.
7. Galuska DA, Will JC, Serdula MK, et al. Are health care professionals advising obese patients to lose weight? JAMA 1999;282:1576–1578.
8. Wadden TA, Anderson DA, Foster GD, et al. Obese women's perceptions of their physicians' weight management attitudes and practices. Arch Fam Med 2000;9:854–860.

9. Steppel JH, Horton ES. Exercise in the management of type 1 diabetes mellitus. Rev Endocr Metab Disord 2003;4:355–360.

10. Mayer-Davis EJ, D'Agostino R, Karter AJ, et al. Intensity and amount of physical activity in relation to insulin sensitivity. JAMA 1998;279:669–674.

11. Diabetes Research in Children Network (DirecNet) Study Group, Tsalikian E, Kollman C, Tamborlane WV, et al. Prevention of hypoglycemia during exercise in children with type 1 diabetes by suspending basal insulin. Diabetes Care 2006;29:2200–2204.

12. Bussau VA, Ferreira LD, Jones TW, et al. The 10-s maximal spring; a novel approach to counter an exercise mediated fall in glycemia in individuals with type 1 diabetes. Diabetes Care 2006;29: 601–606.

13. Mirrato EH, Hill JO, Wyatt HR, et al. Are health care professionals advising patients with diabetes are at risk for developing diabetes to exercise more? Diabetes Care 2006;29:543–548.

14. Kearns JW, Kemmis K, Ploutz-Snyder R, et al. IT'S MINE: Initiating treatment success—my individualized nutrition and exercise plan. Diabetes Educ 2005;31:199, 210–203, 204–205.

15. Bandura A. Social Foundations of Thought and Action: A Social Cognitive Theory. Englewood Cliffs, NJ: Prentice-Hall, 1986.

16. Bandura A. Self-efficacy: The Exercise of Control. New York: WH Freeman, 1997.

17. Allen NA. Social cognitive theory in diabetes exercise research: An integrative literature review. Diabetes Educ 2004;30:805–819.

18. Brubaker P. Adventure travel and type 1 diabetes: The complicating effects of high altitude. Diabetes Care 2005;28:2563–2572.

19. West JB. The physiologic basis of high-altitude diseases. Ann Intern Med 2004;141:789–800.

20. Moore K, Vizzard N, Coleman C, et al. Extreme altitude mountaineering and type 1 diabetes: The Diabetes Federation of Ireland Kilimanjaro Expedition. Diabet Med 2001;18:749–755.

21. Pavan P, Sarto P, Merlo L, et al. Extreme altitude mountaineering and type 1 diabetes: The Cho Oyu alpinisti in Alta Quota expedition. Diabetes Care 2003;26:3196–3197.

22. Pavan P, Sarto P, Merlo L, et al. Metabolic and cardiovascular parameters in type 1 diabetes at extreme altitude. Med Sci Sports Exerc 2004;36:1283–1289.

23. Burnett JC. Long and short haul travel by air: Issues for people with diabetes on insulin. J Travel Med 2006;13:255–260.

24. Mulcahy K, Maryniuk M, Peeples M, et al. Diabetes self-management education core outcomes measures. Diabetes Educ 2003;29(5):768–770, 773–784.

25. Peeples M, Mulcahy K, Tomky D, et al. National Diabetes Education Outcomes System (NDEOS). The conceptual framework of the National Diabetes Education Outcomes System (NDEOS). Diabetes Educ 2001;27(4):547–562.

26. Mensing C, Boucher J, Cypress M, et al. National standards for diabetes self-management education. Diabetes Care 2005;28(Suppl 1):S72–S79.

27. National Certification Board for Diabetes Educators. Information about certification as a Certified Diabetes Educator. NCBDE, 330 East Algonquin Road, Suite 4, Arlington Heights, Illinois 60005. Available at http://www.ncbde.org.6/www.ncbde.org.6.

28. American Nurses Credentialing Center. Information on Board Certification in Advanced Diabetes Management, BC-ADM, credential. ANCC, 8515 Georgia Ave, Suite 400, Silver Spring, MD 20910-3492 (800-284-2378). Available at www.nursingworld.org/ancc/certification/cert/certs.html. Accessed on January 27, 2005.

5
Insulin Therapy in Adults with Type 1 Diabetes Mellitus

M. F. Magee
MedStar Diabetes & Research Institutes at Washington Hospital Center and Georgetown University School of Medicine, Washington, DC, U.S.A.

J. J. Reyes-Castano and C. M. Nassar
MedStar Diabetes & Research Institutes at Washington Hospital Center, Washington, DC, U.S.A.

INTRODUCTION

Insulin is the cornerstone of pharmacotherapy for the estimated 0.73 to 1.46 million persons with type 1 diabetes mellitus (DM1) in the United States. While the peak incidence of DM1 is around the time of puberty, about 25% of cases will present after 35 years of age (1). As progressively more aggressive targeted glycemic, blood pressure, and LDL cholesterol treatment strategies impact both microvascular and macrovascular diabetes complications and comorbidities, there is an ever increasing need for effective insulin therapy strategies for treatment of the individual with DM1. In conjunction with lifestyle and self-care management, meticulous attention, by both the patient and the health-care provider, to the insulin regimen prescribed through the use of either multiple daily insulin (MDI) dosing or a continuous subcutaneous insulin infusion (CSII) pump will enable attainment of HbA1c and blood glucose (BG) targets.

That an HbA1c of ≤ 7% can be achieved in the person with DM1 has been clearly demonstrated in the Diabetes Control and Complications Trial (DCCT). Furthermore, this study demonstrated that improved glycemic control with intensive insulin therapy in patients with DM1 leads to graded reduction in retinopathy, nephropathy, and neuropathy (2), as discussed in chapter(s) on complications (see Chaps. 8, 9, 10). The Epidemiology of Diabetes Interventions and Complications (EDIC) follow-up study of DCCT subjects has more recently demonstrated that intensive insulin therapy also reduces cardiovascular morbidity and mortality (3).

As early as 1993, the DCCT research group recommended that intensive diabetes treatment be instituted in most individuals with DM1, unless contraindications to doing so existed. Furthermore, the DCCT demonstrated that intensive therapy is most effective in preventing complications when introduced during the first 5 years of diabetes. In 303 subjects with early DM1 and residual beta-cell function who were randomly assigned to intensive or conventional therapy, those receiving intensive therapy were slower to lose residual beta-cell function than the conventional therapy group (risk reduction 57%) (4). In addition, intensive therapy in those with residual beta-cell function resulted in a lower HbA1c, a 50% reduction in risk for retinopathy progression, and a lower risk for severe hypoglycemia compared to those who received intensive therapy but did not have residual beta-cell function. It seems abundantly clear that intensive therapy should be implemented as early as possible, and be maintained for as long as possible in DM1.

The health-care provider must tailor an individualized insulin regimen for each person with DM1 to enable targeted BG control. In order to be successful in this regard, it is essential to have an understanding of the normal physiologic pattern of insulin secretion, the currently available insulin preparations and safe and effective methods for both initiating and adjusting the insulin therapy regimen. This chapter will provide a discussion of each of these key elements of insulin therapy for adults with DM1.

PHYSIOLOGIC INSULIN SECRETION

While the person with DM1 has an absolute deficiency in ability to secrete insulin from the pancreatic beta cell, it is helpful to understand physiologic insulin secretion as we prescribe an insulin regimen to optimally meet the daily needs of the DM1 patient (5,6).

Basal Insulin

The normal concentration of insulin measured by radioimmunoassay in the peripheral venous plasma of fasting humans who do not have diabetes is 0 to 70 μU/mL (0–502 pmol/L) (5). Basal insulin secretory profiles reveal a pulsatile pattern of hormone release, with small secretory bursts occurring about every 9 to 14 minutes (7), superimposed upon greater amplitude oscillations of about 80 to 150 minutes. The amount of insulin secreted in the basal state averages 1 U/hr.

The Prandial Insulin Response

Meals, particularly those incorporating carbohydrates and/or other nutritional stimuli of insulin secretion may induce up to a 4- to 10-fold increase in insulin secretion when compared to the basal state, which usually lasts for 2 to 3 hours before returning to the baseline. Rise in BG concentration following intravenous administration of glucose cause a burst in secretion that peaks within 3 to 5 minutes and subsides within 10 minutes and is known as "first phase" insulin release (FPIR) (8,9). If the BG concentration remains high, then the rise in insulin secretion is sustained in a second-phase of insulin release. The average amount of insulin secreted per day in a normal human is about 40 U (287 nmol) (5).

Loss of pulsatile insulin secretion is one of the earliest signs of beta-cell dysfunction in patients destined to have DM1 (10). By the time of diagnosis, beta-cell insulin secretion is negligible to absent. Therefore, one should assume that the individual with DM1 has absolute insulin deficiency and will *always* require exogenous insulin therapy to prevent ketogenesis and uncontrolled hyperglycemia due to gluconeogenesis.

When prescribing insulin for the person with DM1, one will attempt to mimic these physiologic basal–bolus patterns of insulin secretion. In order to safely and effectively do so, the prescriber must have a sound knowledge of currently available insulins.

TYPES OF INSULINS

With advances in recombinant DNA technology, it is now possible to produce large quantities of insulin with an amino acid structure identical to that of human insulin using strains of genetically altered *Escherichia coli* bacteria or yeast. All forms of insulin have identical physiologic effects. Insulins differ in their rapidity of time to onset of action, the time from subcutaneous injection to peak of action, and their duration of action (Table 1).

When insulin is injected, six monomers are associated in a hexameric form. The time it takes for the hexamer to dissociate into monomers, which can be absorbed across the capillary basement membrane is a strong determinant of the time of onset of action, peak levels in the circulation, and duration of action. For example, regular insulin must first dissociate into dimers, then into monomers, a process that takes 30 to 60 minutes following administration of a subcutaneous shot. This phenomenon accounts for the need to dose regular insulin 30 to 45 minutes prior to a meal if it is to attenuate the postprandial glycemic excursion. On the other hand, rapid-acting insulin analogs dissociate more quickly into monomeric form following injection. This results in their shorter time to onset of action and ability to dose with the meal, or even at the end of a meal (11,12).

COMPONENTS OF THE PHYSIOLOGIC INSULIN REGIMEN

Insulins are divided for practical purposes into two broad categories, basal and bolus, based on their pharmacokinetics. Physiologic insulin replacement attempts to mimic normal insulin secretion patterns, and is used to meet an individual's total daily insulin requirement that consists of the sum of basal, prandial, and correction dose insulin requirements (13–15).

Basal insulin refers to exogenous insulin per unit of time necessary to prevent unchecked gluconeogenesis and ketogenesis. It provides a constant background level of insulin that controls BG overnight while the patient sleeps and between meals when they are not eating and the meal bolus insulin action has waned. When dosed appropriately, basal insulin should not cause hypoglycemia if/when the patient does not eat or ingests less food than was anticipated during a meal. In treating DM1, basal insulin needs will most commonly be met by: injection of once daily insulin glargine; once or twice daily insulin detemir; or by rapid-acting or regular insulin delivered subcutaneously via an insulin pump.

The term bolus insulin incorporates both prandial and correction doses of insulin. Bolus insulin is *preferentially* provided as one of the rapid-acting insulin analogs, e.g., aspart, glulisine and lispro, or may be provided as short-acting regular insulin. Prandial or meal insulin refers to insulin which covers the postmeal glycemic excursion. Efforts are made to match meal insulin doses to anticipated carbohydrate intake, which will be achieved either by a consistent carbohydrate meal plan or by "carbohydrate counting." The latter refers to counting the number of grams of carbohydrate to be taken in a meal and calculating an appropriate dose of insulin to take with the food. An individualized carbohydrate to insulin ratio is based upon an estimate of known insulin sensitivity. (Further details are discussed below in the section on pattern management.)

Correction- or supplemental-dose insulin is used to treat hyperglycemia that occurs before or between meals despite administration of routine daily doses of basal and prandial insulin, and is taken *in addition to* these standing doses. When the patient with diabetes is ill or stressed, total daily insulin requirements commonly increase. This increase in insulin requirement is a result of release of insulin counter-regulatory hormones, predominantly cortisol and catecholamines, and to a lesser extent glucagon and growth hormone, which

Table 1 Salient Features of Insulin Preparations (18,34,122)

Category	Generic	Brand name	Time to onset	Time to peak	Duration of action	Special considerations
Basal insulins						
Long acting (preferred)	Glargine	Lantus®	2–4 hr	No pronounced peak	20–24 hr	Usually once daily dosing. If antihyperglycemic action wanes in hours prior to administration of once daily shot, dose twice daily
	Detemir	Levemir®	2 hr	No pronounced peak	6–24 hr	If low total daily insulin requirement (< 0.1 unit/kg/day) or antihyperglycemic action wanes in hours prior to administration of once daily shot, dose twice daily
Intermediate acting	NPH	Humulin® N; Novolin® N	2–4 hr	4–10 hr	12–18 hr	Peaks and troughs often limit ability to titrate for intensive management; not generally recommended for MDI therapy
Bolus insulins						
Rapid acting (preferred)	Lispro Aspart Glulisine	Humalog® Novolog® Apidra™	5–15 min	30–90 min	4–6 hr	Preferred prandial/meal insulins; give with, at end of or up to 20 min following meal (lispro & glulisine)
	Inhaled insulin	Exubera®	7 min	1 hr	4–8 hr	Taken with each meal. 1 mg blister ~ 3 units of regular insulin; 3 mg blister ~ 8 units of regular insulin
Short acting	Regular	Humulin® R; Novolin® R	30–60 min	2–4 hr	6–8 hr	If used, must be taken 30–45 min before meal in order to control postprandial glycemic excursion

The time course of action of any insulin may vary considerably in different individuals or at different times in the same individual. It will also depend also on the dose given, site of injection, blood supply, temperature, and level of physical activity.

are released in the physiologic endogenous stress response. If correction-dose insulin is needed at bedtime, it should be administered at a reduced dose compared to other times of day to reduce risk of nocturnal hypoglycemia.

Patients with DM1 have absolute insulin deficiency and therefore require basal insulin replacement *at all times* to prevent diabetic ketoacidosis (DKA), even when they are unable to eat. Withholding basal insulin from the patient with DM1 results in a rapid rise in BG, by as much as 29 to 60 mg/dL/hr, with accompanying onset of ketonemia in approximately 2 to 3 hours, leading inevitably to DKA (16).

Basal Insulins: Long-Acting and Intermediate-Acting Insulins

Even during an overnight fast, the normal pancreas continues to secrete insulin. Basal insulin suppresses hepatic glucose production and ketogenesis and maintains near normoglycemia in the fasting state. When administered subcutaneously, basal insulins have a delay of 2 to 6 hours from time of injection into the subcutaneous depot that determines their individual time to onset and duration of action. In the setting of DM1, subcutaneous basal insulin is most commonly used in combination with bolus prandial insulin doses administered prior to each meal in the MDI regimen. Basal insulins for subcutaneous injection may be broadly categorized into long-acting and intermediate-acting insulins. The salient features of each of the currently available basal insulins (Table 1) will now be overviewed.

Long-Acting Insulins

Insulin Glargine (Lantus®). Glargine is a recombinant human insulin analog. It differs from human insulin in that asparagine at position A21 is replaced by glycine, and two arginines are added to the C-terminus of the beta chain. Because of these changes, insulin glargine is soluble in an acidic environment and forms a stable hexamer precipitate in the neutral pH environment upon injection into subcutaneous tissue. The hexamer precipitate allows for a delay in the onset of action and a constant release of insulin over a 24-hour period with no pronounced peak (17). It thus serves to provide basal insulin action over the course of a day. The mechanism of action of glargine is similar to that of human insulin, and on a molar basis its glucose-lowering effects are similar to those of human insulin. Because glargine is provided in an acid solution, it cannot be mixed with other forms of insulin as it would alter their absorption profiles. Its acidity also accounts for discomfort with injection in a small proportion (2.7%) of users (18). In clinical trials in patients with DM1, glargine when compared to twice daily NPH insulin has been associated with a reduced risk of hypoglycemia (particularly nocturnal hypoglycemia). Hypoglycemia is less likely to occur with once daily glargine dosing when it is taken in the morning (19). In about 10% to 20% of patients with DM1, glargine must be taken twice daily to provide 24-hour coverage of basal insulin needs. In a smaller proportion of patients, there may be a modest peak approximately 2 hours after injection. In a comparison study between insulin glargine and detemir in adults with type 2 diabetes mellitus (DM2), insulin glargine showed a better adjusted HbA1c than that seen with insulin detemir (6.92% vs. 7.13%, respectively, $p = 0.035$) (20).

Insulin Detemir (Levemir®). Also, a recombinant human insulin analog, detemir, which has a 14-carbon fatty acid (myristic acid) covalently bound to lysine at position B29 and threonine at position B30, is omitted. Fatty acid acylation enhances detemir's affinity to albumin. Albumin binding allows for a protracted duration of effect predominantly via delayed absorption from the subcutaneous adipose tissue depot at the injection site (21,22). Detemir's duration of action is longer than that of neutral protamine Hagedorn (NPH) insulin (Table 1). In one study, a detemir dose of 0.29 U/kg provided the same effect as 0.3 U/kg NPH, but with a longer duration of action (16.9 hours vs. 12.7 hours, respectively) (23). The duration of action for insulin detemir increases dose dependently from 5.7 hours at a low dose (0.1 U/kg) to 23.2 hours at a high dose (1.6 U/kg) (23). Detemir's duration of action in some cases is less than 24 hours. This is particularly so when the total daily insulin requirement is low (< 0.1 U/kg/day) as may be the case in DM1. Therefore in persons with DM1, particularly those who are lean, detemir may need to be dosed twice daily to effectively meet basal insulin requirements.

Detemir has been shown to effect glycemic control in several controlled noninferiority clinical trials in DM1 patients on a basal-bolus regimen when used either twice or once daily (24–27). Detemir is associated with less risk of hypoglycemia, particularly nocturnal hypoglycemia when compared to NPH insulin (24–28).

Data have demonstrated consistently across clinical trials to date in DM1 that patients treated with detemir have less weight gain than those using NPH (24–27). Data regarding weight comparison for detemir versus glargine have not yet been published for DM1. For DM2, it has recently been reported in a large observational (PREDICTIVE) study's German subgroup analysis that modest clinical weight reduction (0.8 ± 0.2 kg, $p < 0.0001$) was observed when patients were transitioned from a glargine ± oral agent regimen to detemir (29). In addition, less weight gain was observed when detemir was compared to glargine for 26 weeks in a recent report from the 2006 International Diabetes Foundation meeting in adults with DM2 (+1.3 kg vs. 2.6 kg, respectively) (20). The mechanism underlying detemir's modestly favorable weight effects have not been elucidated to date. It has been suggested that enhanced activity in the brain may suppress appetite and/or that it may exhibit greater effects in the liver than in the periphery, thus restoring a more physiological mode of insulin action (30,31).

Intermediate-Acting Insulin

NPH insulin (Humulin® N; Novolin® N). NPH or isophane insulin is a crystalline suspension of insulin with protamine and zinc. Combination with protamine and low concentrations of zinc enhance the aggregation of insulin into dimers and hexamers after subcutaneous injection. A depot is formed after injection and the insulin is released slowly, providing an intermediate-acting insulin with a slower onset of action and a longer duration of activity (12–16 hours) than that of regular insulin. The duration of action of NPH insulin is variable; rarely some patients may require only one NPH injection daily; while others require three or more injections daily. NPH insulin is equipotent to the other basal insulins. NPH has variable absorption and peaks both of which can predispose to hypoglycemia, particularly when a meal is delayed or food intake is curtailed. For these reasons, NPH insulin is not commonly used in an MDI regimen for DM1 (32).

Bolus Insulins: Rapid-Acting Insulin Analogs and Regular and Inhaled Insulins

Rapid-Acting Insulin Analogs

Rapid-acting insulins are generally *preferred* as the bolus insulin of choice in intensive glycemic control regimens. Their rapid time to onset of action allows injection immediately before meals, whereas regular insulin must be given 30–45 minutes before meals to optimally match the glycemic excursions after a meal. The rapid-acting analogs glulisine and lispro are also indicated for injection at the end of or up to 15 minutes following a meal, which confers the potential for increased flexibility in meal scheduling and allows the person with DM1 to take the meal-time insulin following eating (11,12). This latter feature is particularly useful when the caloric intake for a given meal is not certain, e.g., when eating out or when ill, as the analog may be dosed after the meal to match actual carbohydrate intake.

Conversely, the one clinical setting in which rapid-acting analogs may not be preferred is when they are to be given to meet all of the patient's insulin requirements for a period of time, e.g., during acute illness, or when nothing is to be taken by mouth after midnight for a procedure the next day or when there will be a prolonged NPO period following surgery after an insulin drip is discontinued. The rapid-acting analogs have a relatively shorter duration of action (up to 4 hours) when compared to regular insulin. It is therefore preferable to continue basal insulin or use an insulin drip under such circumstances when at all possible. If this cannot be done, then rapid-acting insulin analogs must be dosed every 4 hours to prevent DKA, or the patient can take regular insulin every 6 hours until the usual basal insulin regimen can be resumed. This consideration is more likely to be an issue of concern in the hospital rather than in the outpatient setting. (Further discussed under sick day adjustments below.)

A meta-analysis of 42 randomized controlled trials (involving 5925 patients with DM1) that compared rapid-acting insulin analogs to regular insulin showed only a minor benefit of the rapid-acting insulin analogs in terms of HbA1c reduction (33). A moderate increase in the dose of basal insulin may be required when a patient is switched from regular insulin to a rapid-acting insulin for premealtime dosing, in order to meet insulin requirements between meals when the action of the rapid-acting analog has waned that were previously being met by the tail of action of regular insulin.

Regular insulin and the rapid-acting analogs are equipotent. In clinical trials comparing regular insulin to the rapid-acting insulin analogs, improvements in overall glycemic control have been similar; however, the rapid-acting insulin analogs may be superior to regular insulin in improving overall glycemic control when they are used via CSII (34).

The rapid-acting insulins are also particularly useful in addressing unexpectedly high BG levels (e.g., between meals or in the setting of stress) because they will lower glucose levels more rapidly and without the prolonged effect of regular (35–37).

The teratogenicity and long-term safety profile of rapid-acting insulins in pregnancy are unknown, except for insulin aspart, which has been recently granted a category B pregnancy rating for DM1 by the Food and Drug Administration (FDA) (38).

Insulin Lispro (Humalog®). It is also of recombinant DNA origin. It is Lys (B28), Pro (B29) insulin. The effect of this amino acid rearrangement is to reduce the capacity of the insulin to self-aggregate in subcutaneous tissues, resulting in behavior similar to that of monomeric insulin. This allows more rapid absorption from the subcutaneous depot following injection. Given intravenously, the pharmacokinetic profiles of lispro and human regular insulin are similar. Lispro was the first available rapid-acting insulin analog that closely matches circulating insulin levels to the time course of the increase in plasma glucose seen after ingestion of a carbohydrate-rich meal. Frequency of hypoglycemia is lower with premeal lispro than with regular insulin (6.4 episodes/30 days vs. 7.2 episodes/30 days, respectively) (39). The rapid onset of action of insulin lispro is not blunted by mixing with NPH insulin just before injection (40). A meta-analysis of patients with DM1 found that the incidence of severe hypoglycemia was 30% lower in patients treated with insulin lispro ($n = 2327$) when compared to regular insulin ($n = 2339$). Insulin lispro can also be administered via external CSII pumps. Pharmacodynamically, insulin lispro has an onset of glucose-lowering activity in 5 to 15 minutes and reaches mean peak plasma concentrations at 60 minutes when given SC. It has a duration of action of about 2 to 4 hours. After SC administration, the half-life of insulin lispro is about 1 hour. Intermittent SC injections of insulin lispro may be given within 15 minutes prior to or immediately after a meal because of its fast onset of action (41).

Insulin Aspart (Novolog®). It differs from human insulin by substitution of aspartic acid for proline at position B28. This substitution also leads to a more rapid onset and duration of action analogous to those seen with insulin lispro when compared to regular insulin. Insulin aspart is administered by SC injection and is also approved for delivery via external CSII pump. Insulin aspart has an onset of action of about 15 minutes. It is therefore given immediately before meals (start meal within 5–10 minutes after injection). Insulin aspart has a peak glucose lowering effect at 60 minutes and exhibits a duration of action of roughly 2 to 4 hours. The half-life of insulin aspart following SC injection is about 80 minutes (34).

On January 29, 2007 the FDA approved a pregnancy category B rating for insulin aspart [rDNA origin] injection, indicating that adequate clinical studies of its use in pregnant women have not revealed increased risks to the fetus. The approval was based on data from a study conducted at 63 sites in 18 countries ($n = 322$), showing that changes in glycated hemoglobin and rates of maternal hypoglycemia were comparable with insulin aspart and human regular insulin. Although the study was not large enough to evaluate the risk for congenital malformations, the use of insulin aspart compared with human regular insulin yielded fewer preterm deliveries ($P < .053$), consistently low rates of major hypoglycemia, a decreased risk for neonatal hypoglycemia (glucose < 2.6 mmol/L) requiring treatment, and reduced risks to the fetus. Outcomes with insulin aspart are comparable to those of human regular insulin.

Insulin Glulisine (Apidra™). It is produced by recombinant DNA technology utilizing a nonpathogenic laboratory strain of *E. coli* (K12). Insulin glulisine differs from human insulin in that asparagine at position B3 is replaced by lysine and the lysine at position B29 is replaced by glutamic acid. Insulin glulisine may be mixed with NPH insulin (Apidra should be drawn into the syringe first). Insulin glulisine is administered by subcutaneous injection and can be used for administration via external CSII pumps. Insulin glulisine has an onset of action of approximately 5 to 15 minutes, and also has a peak glucose lowering effect at 1 hour. The apparent half-life of insulin glulisine after subcutaneous administration is 42 minutes, compared to 86 minutes for regular human insulin. Intermittent SC injections of insulin glulisine may be given within 15 minutes before to 20 minutes after starting a meal (34).

Short-Acting Insulin [Regular Insulin (Humulin® R; Novolin® R)]

Regular Insulin. It consists of zinc insulin crystals in monomeric form in a clear solution. After subcutaneous injection it tends to self-associate, first into dimers and then into hexamers that must then dissociate prior to absorption as only the monomers and dimers can be absorbed to any appreciable degree (42). This results in a 30- to 60-minute delay in the time to its onset following subcutaneous injection, which practically speaking limits its flexibility in terms of convenience of time of administration relative to meals for the patient. Furthermore, since the peak glycemic response to a mixed meal is between 2 to 4 hours after ingestion, regular insulin may peak too late to allow targeted control of postprandial hyperglycemia (43). Finally, there is also a potential for hypoglycemia to develop as a late sequelae some hours after a meal, due to regular's longer duration of action, which often further limits ability to titrate it to tight postmeal BG goals. Regular insulin can be administered via the intravenous, intramuscular, or SC routes, and it is used in CSII pumps.

The onset of action of regular insulin (100 U/mL) after SC administration begins approximately 30 minutes after injection with maximal effects occurring 2 to 4 hours later. The apparent plasma half-life following SC administration is approximately 1.5 hours with a duration of action of 6 to 8 hours. SC regular insulin must be given 30 to 45 minutes before a meal to allow matching of the insulin action to the postprandial BG rise (34,44,45).

Regular insulin is approved for intravenous (IV) administration. When given IV, its onset of action is within 15 minutes with maximal effects occurring 15 to 30 minutes after injection. The plasma half-life of IV regular insulin is approximately 5 to 6 minutes and its duration of action is 30 to 60 minutes. This short half-life and duration of action has important practical implications. When a patient with DM1 is being treated with an IV insulin infusion, e.g., for DKA, it is imperative to give the first shot of SC insulin at the time of drip discontinuation with sufficient lag time prior to stopping the IV to allow time to onset of the insulin that was given SC. This step must be taken, as there is rapid dissipation of the IV insulin's action when the drip is stopped, in order to prevent gluconeogenesis and ketogenesis.

Finally, regular insulin has been developed for administration via inhalation (see below) and is in product development for possible delivery as an oral spray for absorption via the buccal mucosa.

Inhaled Insulin (Exubera®). Inhaled insulin has been approved for use in the management of DM1 in adults (46). It causes a rapid rise in serum insulin concentration (similar to that which occurs after subcutaneous aspart or glulisine are injected, and faster than that seen with subcutaneous regular insulin) (46–52). It has a slightly longer duration of action than the rapid analogs.

The FDA has to date approved one inhaled insulin product and delivery device, Exubera. In this system, insulin powder is packaged in a foil blister, which is inserted into the device. A 1-mg capsule of Exubera provides the equivalent of about 2.7–3 U of insulin; the 3-mg capsule provides about 8 U. When the device is activated, the blister is pierced and the insulin powder is dispersed into a cloud in a chamber, which the patient then inhales through a mouthpiece. The bioavailability of this inhaled insulin preparation is approximately 10% to 20% that of a subcutaneously injected insulin dose. Decreased bioavailability is due to a combination of factors: loss of the insulin powder (~30%) through retention in the blister and the inhalation device, deposition in the oropharynx (~20%), and the tracheobronchial tree (~10%). Forty percent of an inhalation is delivered to the alveolar spaces from where it passes across the alveolar capillary membrane to the circulation. Exhalation of particles, breakdown by enzymes, and elimination by macrophages also have some impact on bioavailability. Bioavailability may vary among insulin delivery systems, amongst patients, and even within the same patient (53–56).

In a 6-month randomized trial of DM1 patients (mean age 29 ± 14) in which premeal inhaled ($n = 163$) was compared with SC regular insulin ($n = 165$), mean glycosylated hemoglobin was reduced to a similar degree in the inhaled and SC insulin groups [−0.3% and −0.1%, respectively; adjusted difference −0.16% (CI −0.34 to 0.01)], with a similar percentage (23.3% in the inhaled insulin group vs. 22% in the SC group) of subjects achieving A1c < 7. Although 2-hour postprandial glucose reductions were comparable between the groups, fasting plasma glucose levels declined more in the inhaled than in the subcutaneous insulin group [the mean adjusted change in FPG was −35 mg/dL in the inhaled group, whereas in the subcutaneous group, there was a slight increase in FPG (4 mg/dL); adjusted treatment group difference -39.53 mg/dL (CI -57.50 to -21.56)]. Inhaled insulin was associated with a lower overall hypoglycemia rate [9.3% (inhaled) vs. 9.9% (subcutaneous) (risk ratio [RR] 0.94 [CI 0.91–0.97])] but higher severe hypoglycemia rate [6.5% vs. 3.3% (RR 2.00 [CI 1.28–3.12])] when compared to regular insulin before meals (57).

A systematic review of six randomly controlled trials comparing inhaled insulin with rapidly acting injections (three in DM1 and three in DM2) concluded that glycemic control was equivalent, but that patient satisfaction and quality of life was greater with inhaled insulin (58). These studies were limited in length (12 and 24 weeks), therefore long-term safety and/or pulmonary effects could not be established.

Clinical trials of to date, have been designed as noninferiority studies, therefore ability of inhaled insulin to enable attainment of glycemic goals (A1C < 6.5–7.0%) known to be effective in preventing long-term complications has not yet been fully assessed.

From the nonpulmonary perspective, both intradose variability in insulin absorption and the difficulty in making precise dose adjustments [Exubera allows variation by 1 mg (three regular insulin equivalent units) at a time] may preclude the use of inhaled insulin for DM1 patients managed with intensive insulin regimens. Two other inhaled insulin delivery devices that are in development and clinical trials testing at present will each use a novel delivery system that may allow increased flexibility in dosing moving forward. The DM1 patient who uses inhaled insulin also needs to take SC basal insulin.

Safety issues related to Exubera may be classified as nonpulmonary and pulmonary. Nonpulmonary risks include hypoglycemia, which is similar to that seen with use of other insulins. Several studies have found an increase in insulin antibodies with inhaled insulin (59,60), compared with those receiving subcutaneous insulin (51,61–64). Patients with DM1 had higher levels of antibodies than those with DM2. The presence of insulin antibodies had no correlation with HbA1c level, change in insulin dose, or incidence of hypoglycemia (65). The clinical significance of the presence of these insulin-binding antibodies is not yet established (66).

With regards to pulmonary effects, inhaled insulin has been under intense and ongoing scrutiny in terms of potential impact on pulmonary function as it has moved through the development, clinical trials, and approval processes. The most common pulmonary symptom associated with inhaled insulin is a nonproductive cough, that is reported more frequently in patients taking inhaled insulin than in those in the comparison group receiving subcutaneous insulin or oral agents [risk ratio, 3.52 (CI, 2.23–5.56); 16.9% vs. 5.0%, respectively]. There were no differences between patients with DM1 or DM2. Cough occurred within seconds to minutes after administration of inhaled insulin; it was mild and was not associated with changes in pulmonary function. Cough was noted early in the treatment course (within the first month) and diminished in frequency and severity over time (67). Cough may be seen in up to 21% of persons using Exubera inhaled insulin, compared to 4% to 8% for patients not using it (68).

Diabetes mellitus is known to affect the lung. The underlying mechanism(s) that cause change are unclear (69). Mediators of inflammation, such as IL-1, IL-6, and TNF are associated with insulin resistance (70). Reduction in inflammatory markers with tight glucose control has been reported (71) implicating diabetes itself as a cause of systemic inflammation. It is possible that this inflammatory process is involved in the pathophysiology of diabetes related lung disease. It has also been postulated that lack of insulin in lung tissue causes increased oxidative stress and the production of free radicals (72). Pulmonary function test (PFT) changes are seen in diabetes patients. When compared with nondiabetic adults, individuals with diabetes mellitus have some reduction in pulmonary function, namely lower average values for FVC and FEV_1. Glycemic control is not felt to be as important to this deterioration as is the duration of the diabetes (73). Sandler and associates demonstrated that the lower mean DLCO/alveolar ventilation in diabetes patients was associated with a lower pulmonary capillary blood volume, hypothesized to be due to pulmonary microangiopathy, premature lung aging, or glycosylation-induced alterations in hemoglobin-carbon monoxide reaction rates (74).

In clinical trials, DM1 patients receiving inhaled insulin had a decline in FEV_1 from baseline when compared to those in a comparison group treated with SC regular insulin [weighted mean difference, -0.031 L (CI -0.043 L to -0.020 L)]. The modest decline in FEV_1 seen with inhaled insulin was statistically significant. The decrease in FEV_1 was slowly progressive over the first 6 months but stabilized in studies of up to 2 years' duration. Among patients with DM1, inhaled insulin was associated with a greater decrease in DLCO from baseline than was SC insulin [weighted mean difference, -0.902 mL/min/mmHg (CI, -1.546 to -0.258 mL/min/mmHg)]). The decline in diffusing capacity of the lung for carbon monoxide (DLCO) was evident in studies of 24 weeks duration or less, although there was no difference in the 2-year study. In a 12-week crossover trial, DLCO returned to baseline after patients were switched back to SC insulin. Among patients with DM2, there was no difference in DLCO from baseline between the inhaled insulin group and the comparison group in studies up to 2 years in duration (67). The modest decrease in DLCO does not have any recognized clinical correlates.

Before starting inhaled insulin, a baseline spirometry should be obtained. Following initiation of inhaled insulin therapy, repeat spirometry is recommended at 6 months and then yearly as long as there is no deterioration in pulmonary function.

Inhaled insulin is contraindicated in patients with any degree of pulmonary compromise. Pathology of the lung as well as other exogenous factors play a crucial role in the absorption, delivery, and systemic exposure of inhaled insulin. Several pulmonary conditions impact systemic exposure to inhaled insulin. In chronic smokers, the alveolar-capillary membrane is more permeable, increasing absorption of insulin by two- to fivefold; chronic obstructive pulmonary disease increases exposure by about 50%. Asthma decreases it by 20% to 30%. Acute smoking attenuates absorption, perhaps due to reversible constriction of the airways (75). Active smokers should not be started on inhaled insulin, and previous smokers must demonstrate at least 6 months of abstinence. It is also known that passive smoking decreases exposure to inhaled insulin by 20% to 30%.

DETERMINANTS OF INSULIN EFFICACY

Factors Determining Absorption of Subcutaneously Administered Insulin in the Ambulatory Patient

Understanding variables that influence rates of absorption of insulin from the subcutaneous injection depot enables one to develop a clear understanding of how they will act to impact BG and of the importance of consistent timing of doses with regards to time of day and to meals. The degree of absorption of any insulin dose, both among patients and in the same patient, can vary from day to day by as much as 25% to 50%, leading to unexplained fluctuations in glycemic control (76,77). This effect is greatest with long-acting insulins and least with regular, lispro, aspart, and glulisine insulin. There is some suggestion that day-to-day variability of absorption is less with insulin determir compared to glargine, but the clinical significance of this observation has not been established (78).

Factors that influence insulin absorption include: the time course of dissociation of injected insulin in the SC depot, size of the SC depot, site of the injection, SC blood flow, impact of exercise on uptake from the injection site, presence of hypertrophy or atrophy in the SC injection site, and the presence of anti-insulin antibodies.

Time Course of Dissociation

As has already been mentioned, the time it takes for the insulin to dissociate into monomers, which can be absorbed directly across the capillary basement membrane is a strong determinant of its time to onset of action, to peak levels in the circulation, and its duration of action. For example, regular insulin must first dissociate into dimers, then into monomers, a process that takes 30 to 60 minutes following administration of a SC shot and is maximal 2 to 4 hours following delivery of the dose. On the other hand, rapid-acting insulin analogs dissociate more quickly into monomeric form following injection, which results in their shorter time to onset of action and an ability to dose these analogs with a meal (11,12).

Insulin Type

The type of insulin administered determines the time of onset, peak activity, and duration of action of subcutaneous administration, as discussed in detail earlier in this chapter and as summarized in Table 1.

Size of the Subcutaneous Insulin Depot

Variability in absorption is increased and net absorption is reduced with increasing size of the subcutaneous depot (76). While it is not common for the adult with DM1 to be on high doses of insulin, in the patient who is taking large number of units of insulin in a given dose, e.g., over 50 to 100 U in a single injection, it is preferred to split the shot into two equally divided doses to decrease the size of the depot, thereby promoting efficacy and reducing absorption variability.

Injection Technique

Both the angle of needle entry and the depth of penetration affect the rate of insulin absorption. Very shallow insertion can cause a painful intradermal injection that will not be well absorbed. In comparison, a perpendicular injection in a lean area may result in an intramuscular injection, from which absorption is more rapid (79,80).

The recommended insulin injection technique is to use an area of the body in which about 2.5 cm (1 in.) of subcutaneous fat can be pinched between two fingers. The syringe, with a 0.5-inch microfine (27 G) or ultrafine (29 G or 31 G) needle, is inserted perpendicular to the pinched-skin up to the hilt and the insulin is then injected. The needle should be held in place for several seconds before being withdrawn to avoid insulin leakage after withdrawal of the needle.

Site of Injection

Potential sites for injection are the upper arms, abdominal wall, thighs, and buttocks. Insulin is absorbed most rapidly from the abdominal wall, slowest from the leg and buttock, and at an intermediate rate from the arm. At any of these sites, the rapidity of insulin absorption varies inversely with subcutaneous fat thickness (77,81).

Rate of Subcutaneous Blood Flow

The degree of absorption is also impacted by the rate of subcutaneous blood flow. Insulin absorption is reduced by smoking (82) and increased by any increase in skin temperature induced by such things as exercise, saunas or hot baths, and local massage (83–86). These variations are more marked with regular and rapid-acting insulins than with long-acting insulins (85).

POTENTIAL COMPLICATIONS OF INSULIN THERAPY

Potential complications directly related to insulin itself which both the health-care provider and the patient should be aware of are hypoglycemia, weight gain, exacerbation of retinopathy, insulin allergy, and lipodystrophy, each of which will now be discussed.

Hypoglycemia

The normal physiologic response to hypoglycemia includes early suppression of insulin secretion, release of glucagon and catecholamines, and later release of cortisol and growth hormone. It is important to understand that persons with DM1 have alterations in the physiologic suppression of insulin and release of glucagon expected in response to low BG, which impairs ability to return BG levels to normal. These pathophysiologic alterations are present in as few as 5 years after DM1 develops. In addition, hypoglycemia itself impairs the autonomic nervous system activation that is expected when hypoglycemia occurs, further impairing the patient's response. For a full discussion of the pathophysiology of insulin counterregulatory responses in DM1, see Chapter 1.

Hypoglycemia is the most serious complication of intensive insulin replacement regimens and often will be the factor that limits ability to achieve intensive targeted glucose control. In the DCCT, patients in the intensive treatment group had a threefold greater risk (62%) of severe hypoglycemia when compared to those in the conventional treatment group (19%) ($p < 0.001$) (2). It is therefore important to make efforts to prevent hypoglycemia from occurring in adults with DM1.

Practically speaking, mild hypoglycemic reactions that the patient senses and can treat are not uncommonly associated with intensive insulin therapy. Severe hypoglycemia with neuroglycopenia can however lead to confusion, aggressive behavior, loss of consciousness, seizures, coma, and death. Severe reactions may also result in motor vehicle accidents and serious falls with traumatic injuries. Certain patients, particularly those adults with long-standing DM1 and autonomic neuropathy, may not subjectively sense any symptoms of hypoglycemia even in the presence of dangerously low-glucose concentrations. The presence of recurrent severe hypoglycemia is an indication to liberalize BG targets, i.e., raise both the lower and upper limits of the target BG range in order to prevent such occurrences. Risk of insulin-induced hypoglycemia can be reduced if the patient is carefully educated about recognition of his/her individual warning signs of hypoglycemia and/or of their blunting or absence as applicable, and know how to treat hypoglycemic reactions appropriately. If hypoglycemic unawareness is present, a family member and/or work colleague or friend(s) should be instructed in recognition of the signs and symptoms of hypoglycemia and in use of a glucagon emergency kit. In patients with advanced end-stage microvascular or macrovascular diabetes complications in whom the benefit of intensive glucose control is less clear, one may also consider liberalization of BG targets in order to avoid increased risk of hypoglycemia that is inherent in intensive insulin treatment regimens. Despite the higher risk of severe hypoglycemia with intensive insulin therapy, in the DCCT serial neuropsychological testing showed no long-term changes in cognitive function (2).

In DM1 patients treated with Exubera, the frequency of all hypoglycemic episodes was similar to those treated with SC regular insulin over 12 and 24 weeks of therapy (5.58% vs. 5.4%, respectively) (61,62). However, the rate of severe hypoglycemia [defined as that requiring assistance by another, involving a neurological symptom (memory loss, confusion, irrational behavior, unusual difficulty walking, seizure, loss of consciousness) and associated with an SMBG < 50 mg/dL or in the absence of SMBG, that which was reversible with oral carbohydrate, SC glucagon or IV glucose] was twice as frequent with insulin Exubera [6.5 vs. 3.3; RR 2.00 (CI 1.28 to 3.12)], compared with SC regular (87).

Treatment for mild hypoglycemia consists of 15 to 30 g of a rapidly absorbed source of carbohydrate such as 4 ounces of juice or regular soft drink, 4 ounces of skim milk, a small tube of gel cake frosting, or commercially available glucose tablets or gels. A finger-stick (FS) BG check and the ingestion of carbohydrate is repeated every 15 to 20 minutes until the BG level has returned to normal. Rapid-acting carbohydrate should be followed by a snack or by a meal that was missed or is due in order to prevent hypoglycemic recurrence.

In addition to the availability of glucose tablets, hard candy, or other sources of a readily absorbable form of carbohydrate, it is recommended that all patients with DM1 should have emergency glucagon kits available at home and at work, assuming that there are people who can be trained in their use. In the event of an unconscious hypoglycemic reaction, 0.5 to 1 mg of glucagon given intramuscularly rapidly raises the plasma glucose concentration to an acceptable range and avoids the difficulties and dangers associated with attempting to get a comatose, stuporous, or disoriented individual to ingest glucose by mouth. Again, once the patient has sufficiently recovered from the episode, a snack or meal should be eaten.

Weight Gain

Improvement in glucose control with a reduction in glycosuria is often associated with weight gain as loss of calories in the urine is reduced. Increased food intake to treat or prevent recurrent hypoglycemia can also contribute to weight gain. Insulin itself may stimulate appetite. Recent data from clinical trials for insulin detemir consistently show slightly less weight gain when compared to NPH (24,25,28,88) (as discussed in the insulin section earlier in this chapter). Mechanism(s) underlying a potential for less weight gain with insulin detemir are unknown. Data from mouse models suggest that dysregulation of insulin action at the level of the insulin receptor and downstream signaling targets in the central nervous system (CNS) are associated with obesity and diabetes. In the brain, intact insulin signaling via the IRS-PI 3-kinase pathway is essential for nutrient homeostasis and appetite regulation as pharmacological inhibition of insulin signaling, especially in the hypothalamus, leads to obesity-induced diabetes. Keeping in mind that clinical trials have shown that insulin detemir therapy is characterized by weight stability or even modest weight loss, it has been hypothesized that in addition to activating the insulin-signaling cascade in peripheral tissues detemir may also activate cerebral insulin signaling. It is known that albumin directly penetrates into the cerebrospinal fluid across choroids plexus epithelial cells. In this model, it is postulated that detemir's cerebral action may be enhanced due to its attached fatty acid chain (30). The long-term clinical significance of this modest but reproducible weight advantage that has been seen in clinical trials with detemir remains to be determined.

Exacerbation of Retinopathy

Intensive therapy slows the rate of development and progression of mild to moderate retinopathy. In addition, in the DCCT it was found that retinopathy occasionally worsens in the first year after initiation of intensive therapy, which manifests as an increase in the number of soft exudates (due to retinal infarcts in the superficial layers) (2,89). This is felt to represent the closure of small retinal blood vessels that were narrowed but previously patent. Correction of hyperglycemia lowers plasma volume, which places marginal vessels at-risk. Increased availability of insulin-like growth factor-1 (IGF-1) may also contribute (90).

Despite the early exacerbation of retinopathy seen in the DCCT, there was clear evidence of benefit from intensive therapy when patients with mild to moderate nonproliferative retinopathy were followed for 9 years. Specifically, the incidence of worsening retinopathy in intensively treated patients was higher than in those receiving conventional therapy at 1 year (7.4% vs. 3%) but much lower at 9 years (25% vs. 53%) (2).

Insulin Allergy

Allergy to recombinant human (rDNA) and biosynthetic insulin preparations is a rare complication of insulin therapy. Insulin antibodies of high titers were observed in many patients treated with early insulin preparations containing proinsulin, C-peptide, and other peptide contaminants. Immunoglobulin G-insulin antibodies in very high titers can lead to immune-mediated insulin resistance, which is now extremely rare (91).

Currently, the prevalence of allergic reactions during insulin treatment is around 2%, but less than one-third of reported events are considered related to insulin itself (92).

Transition from animal insulins to rDNA insulins has markedly decreased the incidence of allergic reactions. Allergenicity of the insulin molecule itself is felt to be attributed to the chemical structure of the terminal part of the beta chain. Other causes of insulin therapy associated allergic responses are other components of insulin preparations, including protamine, additives such as cresol or zinc, and latex (91).

Insulin antibodies of the immunoglobulin G and immunoglobulin E type are reported in low titers in patients treated exclusively with human insulin. Frequency and levels of immunoglobulin G-insulin antibodies are identical in patients treated either with biosynthetic or semisynthetic human insulin preparations. Allergic symptoms to human insulin are now found in less than 1% of de novo–treated patients. Overall immunological complications of insulin therapy have decreased significantly during the last two decades and are now predominantly observed in patients with interrupted insulin therapy.

The most common manifestation of allergic reactions to insulin consists of local wheal-and-flare reactions at the site of injection. Occasionally, more generalized allergic reactions occur, and even more rarely anaphylactic reactions. Mild local allergic reactions to insulin can be treated by first trying a switch to an alternative insulin preparation, or with antihistamines or by the addition of low doses of dexamethasone to the insulin vial. More severe reactions require desensitization. In the future, anti-immunoglobulin E treatment with omalizumab may offer another alternative to these patients (92).

Lipodystrophy: Lipoatrophy and Lipohypertrophy

Repeated insulin injections at a site sometimes lead to dystrophic change. Atrophy of subcutaneous fatty tissue known as lipoatrophy. Lipoatrophy is an immune complication of insulin therapy, which is not often seen seen since the development of the current human insulin preparations and insulin analogs. It was reported previously in 10% to 55% of patients treated with nonpurified bovine/porcine insulin preparations, but has almost disappeared since the advent of human insulins (91). In fact, injection of these newer preparations directly into the atrophic area often resulted in restoration of normal contours.

Even with the purified human insulins, hypertrophy of subcutaneous fatty tissue may be a problem if one injects repeatedly at the same site. This complication of insulin therapy may be largely avoided by broad rotation of SC shot or CSII pump insertions sites. Lipohypertrophy that is problematic may be treated by liposuction.

PHYSIOLOGIC REPLACEMENT THERAPY INSULIN REGIMENS

Conventional Insulin Therapy

Conventional insulin therapy is used to describe simpler, usually fixed dose insulin regimens, such as single daily injections, or two injections per day of regular and NPH insulin, either mixed together in the same syringe or provided as a premix of insulins, which are given in prespecified doses before breakfast and dinner. Such regimens are based on the concept that each of the insulin components in the two doses is covering insulin needs for one-quarter of the day and results in a single peak of insulin absorption. Such mixed-split regimens are not physiologic. In addition, conventional insulin therapy is unlikely to enable achievement of target HbAlc levels in patients with DM1 and are no longer recommended unless the adult with DM1 cannot or will not comply with an intensive insulin regimen.

Intensive Insulin Therapy

In patients with DM1 and deficiency of endogenous insulin production, the exogenous insulin regimen will be designed to simulate as closely as possible the multiphasic profile of insulin secretory responses to meals and snacks present in normal subjects in order to enable targeted glycemic control. The term intensive insulin therapy is used to describe more complex insulin administration regimens in which basal insulin therapy is combined with bolus doses of insulin given three or more times daily timed to correspond with ingestion of meals and/or snacks. When the intensive insulin therapy is delivered by SC injection, the regimen is known as a multiple daily injection (MDI) regimen. Intensive insulin therapy is also delivered by continuous subcutaneous insulin infusion (CSII) using an external insulin pump. Currently in the United States, approximately 25% to 30% of persons with DM1 are treated with insulin pumps.

In MDI, basal insulin is delivered as once or twice daily long-acting or twice daily intermediate-acting insulin and in CSII basal insulin is delivered in continuous fashion. In both MDI and CSII, bolus/meal insulin is delivered as discrete doses in conjunction with food intake, by shot in the MDI regimen and by activation of a bolus for delivery by the insulin pump in CSII.

In one trial comparing CSII using insulin aspart versus MDI with insulin aspart and glargine, CSII therapy resulted in lower glycemic exposure [40% lower for CSII than MDI as measured by area under the curve (AUC) glucose $\geq$ 80 mg/dL and AUC glucose $\geq$ 140 mg/dL] without increased risk of hypoglycemia [CSII: 92% (73% for nocturnal hypoglycemia), MDI: 94% (72% for nocturnal hypoglycemia)], as compared with MDI (93).

Considerations in the Decision to Intensify Insulin Therapy

As mentioned earlier in this chapter, studies suggest that intensive therapy should be started as early as possible following the diagnosis of DM1 and that it has clear benefits for patients with DM1 when implemented at any time in the course of the disease. It is important to consider the practical aspects of such a regimen in the discussion with the adult patient with DM1 who is to intensify insulin therapy. Following are the issues for consideration:

- A commitment by the patient to follow the regimen is required. It will be necessary to manage and coordinate diet, activity, insulin administration, and BG monitoring. Algorithms for insulin administration in MDI management of DM1 involve frequent monitoring of the BG concentration, generally at a frequency of four or more times per day.
- The incidence of hypoglycemia may be increased up to threefold in patients with DM1 managed with intensive insulin regimens (94).
- Weight gain is more likely with intensive insulin therapy regimens, which can limit patient compliance, particularly in women. Addition of pramlintide (Symlin®) to the therapeutic regimen can help mitigate postprandial hyperglycemia and may allow weight loss rather than gain as hyperglycemia is controlled in some patients. Its ability to increase satiety, slow gastric emptying, and suppress glucagon secretion can impact postprandial hyperglycemia when used in combination with insulin therapy. (Pramlintide is discussed fully in Chap. 6.)
- The cost of intensive insulin therapy is about three times that of conventional treatment, based upon an analysis of the DCCT (95). On the other hand, intensive therapy is associated with a lower incidence of costly chronic complications. Formal economic analyses have demonstrated that intensive therapy is cost-effective for the treatment of diabetes (96).

MDI Insulin Regimen

Long-Acting Basal Insulin Once (or Twice) Daily with Rapid-Acting Bolus Insulin Before Each Meal

This MDI basal-bolus insulin regimen simulates the pattern of insulin production, which occurs physiologically in the person without diabetes. Basal insulin action will most commonly be provided by insulin glargine or detemir. Insulin glargine will generally be given once daily for control of fasting and premeal glucose levels. This dose is given at the same time daily and may be delivered either at bedtime, or with breakfast or dinner. It is a practical consideration to allow the patient to select which of these times of day he/she would be most likely to consistently take the basal insulin glargine dose to assure adherence to the regimen. In a small percentage of patients, the duration of action of glargine is not a full 24 hours, which then necessitates twice daily shots to provide continuous basal insulin action. Insulin detemir is given once or twice daily. Typically for the lean patient with DM1 whose total daily insulin requirement is modest (and particularly if under 0.1 U/kg/day), twice daily dosing of insulin detemir is used. As discussed in the insulin section above, clinical trials dosing of detemir in DM1, which demonstrated safety and efficacy were carried out using both once and twice daily dosing of detemir. When dosed twice daily, insulin detemir is typically given with breakfast and at bedtime or at dinner time, depending upon which of the latter times would evenly distribute the timing of the twice daily doses. When used once daily, insulin detemir is typically dosed in the same fashion as described for insulin glargine, although it should be noted that currently in the United States, it is formally indicated only for PM dosing when prescribed once daily.

In the patient who is taking either insulin glargine or detemir as a once daily dose, a pattern whereby a rise in BG levels in the hours prior to the time for administration of the basal insulin dose for the day, that is not attributable to the intake of food or reduction in the prior meal's insulin dose, suggests that the basal insulin action is waning and that twice daily dosing is indicated.

Bolus doses of rapid-acting insulin analog are preferred in the MDI regimen due to their rapid time to onset of action, which allows dosing with the meal, rather than regular insulin, which must be given with a 30 to 45 minute lag time if dosed premeal. The rapid-acting analogs will provide insulin coverage to control postmeal glycemic excursions. They may also be given if a carbohydrate containing snack is to be taken. As mentioned earlier and as discussed below under insulin adjustment recommendations for variations in meal portion size and carbohydrate content in detail, the meal bolus of insulin is generally matched to the carbohydrate content of the meal, either through implementation of a consistent carbohydrate diet or by using carbohydrate counting to match insulin dose to the meal's carbohydrate content. (Also see Chap. 4 for further discussion of this topic.)

Alternative MDI Regimens

Alternative MDI regimens using NPH insulin have been described; however, they are generally *not used widely* for treating persons with DM1 since the advent of the long-acting basal insulins, which when dosed once or twice daily have essentially no peak effect, thereby conferring lesser risk of hypoglycemia than an NPH-containing insulin regimen. In such regimens, three shots of NPH given at breakfast, dinner, and bedtime are used to meet the basal insulin requirement combined with two shots of rapid-acting bolus insulin delivered with breakfast and with dinner. The third dose of NPH insulin at bedtime in this MDI regimen takes into account the observation that in individuals with DM1, the duration of action of the intermediate-acting insulin given before dinner is insufficient to control BG in the early morning hours. Attempts to increase the dose of intermediate-acting insulin at dinner would expose the patient to a greater risk of hypoglycemia in the middle of the night, hence the incorporation of a modest dose of NPH at bedtime provides sufficient insulin action to control glycemia in the morning while minimizing risk of nocturnal hypoglycemia.

Practical Guidelines for Calculation of Insulin Doses for the MDI Regimen

When undertaking calculation of insulin doses for initiation of therapy for any insulin regimen, one must be cognizant of the variability in total daily insulin requirements among individuals and within a given individual, and of the variation in a given insulin's lag time to onset of action, time to peak, and duration of action. It is also necessary to be aware in the event of making a switch from one type of regimen to another of the level of BG control prior to the time of change. In all of the practical guidelines presented in this chapter for insulin dosing, dosing suggestions are based on evidence presented in the literature and a conservative consensus of opinion designed to assure safety and avoid hypoglycemia at the time of introduction of the new insulin regimen. Close monitoring of FS BG values and insulin doses at the time of such transitions *must* be undertaken in order to monitor safety and effectiveness of the insulin regimen and to facilitate adjustments as needed to enable attainment of glycemic control targets.

Initiating Insulin Therapy in DM1

Most newly diagnosed patients with DM1 can be started on a total daily dose (TDD) of 0.2 to 0.4 U of insulin/kg/day, although many may ultimately require 0.5 to 1.0 U/kg/day (97). In the event of newly diagnosed DM1 with presentation in DKA, the total daily insulin requirement will be determined at the time of discontinuation of intravenous insulin infusion treatment. Approximately half (40–50%) of the calculated total daily insulin dose is given as basal either as once per day long-acting basal insulin (glargine or detemir) or as twice daily detemir insulin. The once daily long-acting basal insulin, as previously mentioned is generally given either at bedtime or in the morning; however, it may also be given at dinner time if this will be most convenient for the patient. The remainder of the TDD is then given as rapid-acting (preferred) or regular insulin, divided into before-meal bolus doses. The dose of bolus insulin to be taken before each meal is then allocated as 10% to 15% of the total daily insulin requirement with each meal and a smaller percentage, e.g., 3% to 5% with a snack. If there is a clear difference in the carbohydrate content or insulin requirement for given meals, then the distribution of prandial insulin may be tailored to accommodate the difference(s), e.g., if postbreakfast hyperglycemia is a challenge and lunch typically a smaller meal, one may choose to apportion 20% to 25% of the daily prandial insulin for breakfast, 10% to 15% for lunch, 15% to 20% for dinner, and 3% to 5% for the bedtime snack. Premeal dosages of bolus insulin can also be calculated based on the dietary intake (i.e., 1–2 units of insulin per 10–15 g of carbohydrate). These doses will subsequently be adjusted per usual meal size and content, as well as per how activity and exercise patterns impact individual BGs, as described in the insulin adjustment section below.

Converting from a Conventional Insulin Therapy Regimen to an MDI Regimen

It is generally advisable to reduce the total daily basal insulin dose (units) when long-acting basal insulin is to be started at the time of conversion from twice daily NPH by 20% from the previous total daily basal NPH doses. This is particularly important if any episodes of hypoglycemia have been occurring and/or there has been a tendency for BGs to be at the lower limit of the patient's target range on the prior intermediate insulin regimen in order to prevent hypoglycemia. If switching from twice daily doses of NPH insulin to once daily insulin glargine when the BGs have not been well-controlled, one may prescribe a glargine dose that is equivalent to the total number of units of NPH insulin that were being given daily.

If the patient switches from short-acting insulin (regular) to rapid-acting insulin (lispro, aspart, or glulisine), the dose of the rapid-acting insulin may need to be reduced and the dose of basal insulin may need to be increased, to compensate for the pharmacokinetic differences among these types of insulins, and in particular for the longer tail of regular insulin action that may provide some insulin effect between meals that the rapid-acting analog will not.

CSII by External Insulin Pump

An alternative method of delivering an intensive insulin therapy basal–bolus regimen is by CSII via an external pump. The insulin is delivered through a fine catheter from the pump to a subcutaneous insertion site. The pump delivers insulin as a preprogrammed, variable rate basal infusion as well as patient-directed boluses given before meals or snacks or in response to elevations in BG concentration outside the prespecified target range.

The basal insulin infusion rate for the adult patient with DM1 commonly falls between 0.2 to 1 U/hr, although it can be higher. The basal rate can be programmed either to continue at a constant rate over the 24-hour period or more commonly to increase and decrease at predetermined times of the day to prevent anticipated excursions in the BG concentration, for example, morning rises in glucose associated with the dawn phenomenon. Typically the patient with DM1 will require anywhere from 3 to 4 or more alternative basal rates to enable tight glycemic control. Pumps provide the ability to use multiple alternative basal profiles to deal with recurrent patterns that require adjustment of insulin doses (e.g., menstruation, weekend lifestyle, and a variety of levels of exercise/activity). In addition they offer profiles, such as dual wave bolus or extended bolus to accommodate anticipated variations in eating patterns, e.g., for eating a large or extended multicourse meal.

Only rapid-acting or regular insulin is used in the insulin pump. Adjustments to the basal insulin infusion rate or changes in the size and timing of the insulin boluses generally allow more timely responses in BG concentration than are seen when adjustments are made to doses of intermediate-acting or long-acting insulin. All of these features confer a potentially greater flexibility for the patient in terms of lifestyle and insulin dosing. It has been suggested that use of lispro insulin may lead to a lower risk of hypoglycemia than the other rapid insulin analogs and/or regular insulin in pumps (98,99).

Considerations in the Decision to Start CSII Pump Therapy

There are some practical considerations that the patient and provider must consider together when weighing a decision to use an insulin pump:

- Patients treated with insulin pump therapy must *always* monitor glucose frequently (four or more times daily) and must *always* be alert to the possibility of failure of the infusion system, otherwise unexplained hyperglycemia develops.
- The pump insertion set must be changed every 24 to 72 hours to assure uninterrupted insulin delivery and to prevent insertion site infections as described below.
- There is a risk of infection at the subcutaneous insertion site. Infections may occur on average once annually per patient even when best of practices for insertion and site care are used. Such infections are usually minor and can be treated by changing the site of infusion and using a topical antibiotic; a short course of oral antibiotics may also sometimes be required. If an insertion site abscess develops, surgical drainage in conjunction with antibiotic treatment will be necessary.
- Because rapid-acting insulin is most commonly used, pump failure as a result of mechanical malfunction or catheter-related problems can quickly result in severe hyperglycemia with ketoacidosis that will develop in a matter of hours, as mentioned earlier, in the patient with DM1 (100,102).
- The initial cost of an insulin pump itself is high ($4500–6000 in 2007). One must then also purchase pump supplies on an ongoing basis. The relatively recently released patch, OmniPod pump system requires a lesser initial payment for the PDA device that controls Pod functions and programs insulin dosing (~ $600). Single 72-hour use Pod units are then purchased in prospective fashion on a monthly basis for about $35 each, spreading out cost. Most health-insurance payors will cover 80% to 100% of the cost of a CSII pump system and supplies.
- Some patients consider pump to be uncomfortable, embarrassing, or otherwise awkward.

Calculation of Initial Insulin Doses for CSII Pump Therapy

Basal will typically be delivered to meet between 40% and 50% of the patient's total daily insulin requirement. The balance of the daily requirement is given as premeal bolus doses, which will control postprandial glucose excursions. In a patient with reasonably controlled previous MDI injection regimen (e.g., A1c < 7.0%), the initial total daily dose of insulin (TDDI) administered by pump may be 10% to 20% less than the TDD of the previous regimen, as absorption of insulin from the subcutaneous delivery site is more efficient. Conversely, patients with a prior trend to hyperglycemia may start with the same TDD as they had been using with their SC injection regimen. In general, as in the MDI regimens described earlier, approximately one-half of the total daily insulin dose is administered as basal insulin apportioned equally at the time of start up into an hourly delivery rate by dividing the desired total daily basal insulin dose by 24 hours to determine the number of units of insulin to be delivered per hour. For most patients, basal rates are in the range of 0.01 to 0.015 U/kg/hr (i.e., for a 60-kg woman approximately 0.6 to 0.9 U/hr), but they can range from under 0.5 to more than 2.0 U/hour. Premeal boluses for pump initiation may be estimated as follows: 20% for breakfast, 10% for lunch, 15% for dinner, and 5% for bedtime snack, or may be determined by carbohydrate counting and an individualized insulin-to-carbohydrate ratio (103).

The total daily basal rate can alternatively be calculated by multiplying the patient's weight (in kg) by 0.3. Assuming that this basal rate represents 50% of the total daily insulin requirements for the person with DM1, an equivalent number of units of insulin used for basal delivery can be distributed between meal insulin boluses as described for MDI above or again will alternatively be calculated using carbohydrate counting ratios.

Controlled clinical trials have indicated that on an average, intensive insulin regimens that use multiple insulin injections lead to levels of glucose control similar to those achieved with the insulin pump. On the other hand, there are some patients who never achieve adequate control with multiple daily injections but experience dramatic improvements with pump therapy. According to the Clinical Practice Recommendations of the American Diabetes Association (104), the insulin pump should be used only by candidates strongly motivated to improve glucose control and willing to work with their health-care provider in assuming substantial responsibility for their day-to-day diabetes self-management.

Implantable Insulin Infusion Pumps

A surgically implanted programmable pump is available in the European Union (EU) and is under investigation in the United States. Studies in patients with both DM1 and DM2 have found that this pump system results in glycemic control equivalent to that of MDI injections (105,106).

The implantable pump has the advantage, compared with intensive regimens using injections or external pumps, of a lower incidence of severe hypoglycemia (4 episodes/100 patient-years vs. 33 episodes/100 patient-years with multiple daily injections in patients with DM1) (105) and less day-to-day fluctuation in BG concentrations, less weight gain, and better quality of life. These advantages may occur, in part, because implantable pumps deliver into the peritoneal cavity or intravascularly, where absorption into the hepatic portal circulation provides more physiologic insulin delivery to the liver. Systemic insulin levels are lower than those that result when subcutaneous (SC) insulin shots are used.

Implantable pumps are prone to catheter blockage that may be due to either their slow rate of insulin delivery (107) or increased macrophage activation in some patients (108,109). In addition, anti-insulin antibodies occur more commonly with continuous intraperitoneal insulin infusion (CPII) than with CSII (110).

INSULIN DOSING ADJUSTMENTS AND PATTERN MANAGEMENT

With experience and close observation of BG results and insulin doses, the health-care provider and the patient can identify patterns that will suggest a need for adjustment in insulin doses to enable attainment of BG targets and A1c goals in the adult DM1 patient who is on an intensive insulin therapy regimen, whether it be with MDI or CSII. Pattern management refers to the practice of reviewing a patient's BG logs, identifying patterns, and/or trends where BG is outside or might be expected to deviate from designated target ranges, and taking corrective action to reach or maintain these ranges.

Numerous clinical circumstances can lead to changes in insulin requirements. These circumstances commonly involve: variations in food intake (portion size and carbohydrate content) and/or timing, exercise frequency, timing and level of intensity, days the patient is ill or stressed, changes in concomitant medications, (e.g., addition or withdrawal of glucocorticoids to/from the treatment regimen), and stage of the menstrual cycle. Even in the patient who adheres to the comprehensive diabetes management regimen, there will be times when BG levels will shift, resulting in high and/or low BG patterns. Finally, pregnancy will necessitate tight glycemic control and frequent adjustments in insulin doses to keep glucoses in target range. Management of pregnancy in the adult with DM1 is discussed in detail in Chapter 12 and will therefore not be discussed here.

In all of these circumstances it will be appropriate for the health-care provider and the patient to evaluate the reasons that have led to suboptimal control in order to make adjustments in the subcutaneous insulin or lifestyle regimen to enable attainment and maintenance of target BG levels. It is also extremely useful, when possible, to make anticipatory insulin adjustments when a recurring circumstance, e.g., exercise will occur in order to avoid loss of control moving forward.

Successful pattern management requires a close collaboration between the patient and the diabetes-care provider team. The DCCT and recent clinical trials in DM2 have demonstrated that, with appropriate education and the provision of insulin treatment algorithms, adult patients are able to self-titrate their insulin doses to achieve treatment targets identified by the patient and their care team (111,112).

The goals of pattern management are several fold. It will identify BG trends that are outside target ranges by time of day; all variables that may have contributed to hyperglycemia or hypoglycemia; and provide strategies for safe and effective adjustments in insulin dose(s) that will return BG to, or maintain BG within desired ranges. For practical purposes, insulin adjustment guidelines may be broken into core and advanced adjustments. Basic insulin adjustment guidelines will target correction of low- and high-BG levels, including those which occur on "sick" days, and incorporate core lifestyle considerations in order to (i) optimize the match between prandial insulin and carbohydrate intake to enable postprandial glycemic control and (ii) necessary changes in insulin doses for routine exercise. Advanced insulin adjustment guidelines will address such circumstances as travel, perimenstrual patterns, glucocorticoid therapy, and dialysis days.

Establishing Individual BG Goals and Times of Day for BG Monitoring

When embarking on the process of pattern management, one must first establish glycemia-related targets (Table 2) and times of day that FS BG measurements will be performed for the individual patient. It is key to establish with the patient that the recommended goals are acceptable. Selecting mutually agreeable BG goals will help to assure adherence to the prescribed regimen.

Individual targets must always be set for fasting and postprandial glucose and for HbA1c. It may be necessary to lay out stepwise goals for reaching targets over time, particularly if current levels of control are far removed from recommended values, or the patient has concerns regarding the recommended targets. Fear of hypoglycemia as a result of increase in insulin doses and "not feeling right/well" if BG values are lowered to beyond a perceived threshold level are examples of reasons patients may cite as concerns regarding

Table 2 Recommended Glycemia-Related Targets (123,124)

Glycemic target	ADA	AACE
Fasting glucose	90–130	< 110
Postprandial glucose	< 180 mg/dL	< 140
A1C	< 7%; as close to 6% as possible	< 6.5%
Glycemic variability	Mean BG should be ≤ 2 SDs from the mean BG	

intensification of the insulin regimen that may necessitate stepping of goals and further education to enable them to become comfortable with increasing insulin doses.

One additional concept that is increasingly recognized as a glycemia-related target is glycemic variability. This measure quantifies variation in BG range over the time period of analysis. The concept of glycemic variability acknowledges the fact that HbA1c is an average of BGs in the 2 to 3 months preceding its measurement and that a normal value does not necessarily mean that all BGs have been within the prespecified target range. For example, if a patient has had numerous episodes of both hypoglycemia and hyperglycemia, the HbA1c may appear to be at target because it represents an average of all BG values whether they be high, low, or within the target range. Glucose fluctuation, particularly during postprandial periods and during other times when BG values swing, has been shown to exhibit a triggering effect on oxidative stress when compared to chronic sustained hyperglycemia. Free radical production in turn is implicated in the pathways that lead to hyperglycemic-induced vascular damage (113). Mean amplitude of glucose excursion (MAGE) correlates with free radical production and magnitude of glucose fluctuations (114).

Standard deviation from the average BG may be used in clinical practice as a marker for MAGE. An initial goal for glycemic variability is suggested by Hirsch as twice the standard deviation (SD) should be less than the average BG level (SD × 2 < average BG). Even more desirable would be an average glucose level exceeding three times the SD (SD × 3 < average BG) (115). The SD is calculated and reported by many of the currently available BG monitor software programs.

All glycemia-related goals are also subject to modification in the presence of extenuating clinical circumstances such as blunted glycemic awareness, particularly if there is a history of hypoglycemia-related unconscious reactions or seizures, recurrent otherwise severe hypoglycemia, unstable cardiac status, end-stage renal disease, and the frail elderly warrant consideration of less tight glycemic control targets. For example, if a patient has unconscious hypoglycemic reactions, it may be quite appropriate to accept a target BG range of 140 to 200 in order to minimize risk of recurrences.

FSBG measurements will in general be checked a minimum of four times daily in patients being managed with intensive insulin therapy regimens, and not uncommonly even more frequently. The times of day that it is desirable to see representative BG values are those times that will enable meaningful adjustments in insulin doses or the lifestyle regimen. Typical times for checking are fasting and premeals to assess the appropriateness of basal insulin dosing, 60 to 90 minutes after a meal to assess the impact of premeal insulin doses, and 2 to 3 AM in order to assess the level of glycemic control overnight as it affects one's ability to move basal insulin doses up or down to optimize nocturnal BG control. Patients should be encouraged to gather sample BG readings from each of these time points when there is a question about the appropriateness of particular insulin doses and/or prior to office visits so that the health-care provider will have sufficient information to be able to assist in determining if the current insulin regimen is optimal. Those who will check less frequently should be advised to vary the times of day they are checking so that information from each of these times points is sampled.

In the initial stages of education, at a minimum, patients learning pattern management and self-titration of insulin doses should be encouraged to keep detailed records of BG results, meal content, meal timing, activity, and exercise, etc. This will allow the diabetes team and the patient to learn the impact of these elements on glycemic control and insulin requirements. The patient should record comments in the BG diary whenever BGs are above or below target at the time that the BG value is noted, so that recall of circumstances that may have made the sugar high or low will be accurate. Insulin doses will then be adjusted, as is appropriate, based on identified relationships amongst BG, food intake, and changes in activity.

Insulin Adjustment Guidelines

General Principles

Insulin adjustment is an art that should be guided by the science of what is known about how each component insulin of the total daily insulin requirement acts and how lifestyle and other variables impact BG levels. Insulin adjustment guidelines are grounded in a sound knowledge of the pharmacokinetics of insulin, as discussed earlier in this chapter. When BG levels are outside target ranges and it is determined that an adjustment in insulin dosing is necessary, knowledge of the action curves of the insulins that the patient is taking will guide the decision as to how to adjust the insulin regimen appropriately (Fig. 1). The information presented in the following section is a composite of published information on this topic and a consensus of the accumulated clinical experience of the authors in caring for adult patients with DM1. We have attempted in presenting this information to provide a practical framework upon which the reader may build and convey to one's patients the nuts and bolts of pattern management insulin adjustments.

For the patient with DM1 on an MDI regimen or using an insulin pump, the underlying principles for adjusting the insulin regimen are essentially the same. Fasting BGs that are not well-controlled will be corrected by adjusting the basal insulin dose(s), i.e., if the fasting BG is low, the basal insulin dose will be decreased and if the fasting BG is high, the basal insulin dose will be increased. Postmeal BGs that are not well-controlled will be corrected

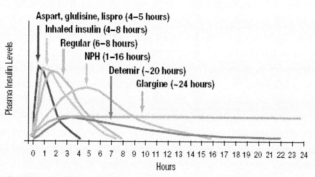

Hirsch IB. Medscape Gen Med. 2005;7:49. Plank J, et al. Diabetes Care. 2005;28:1107-1112. Rave K, et al. Diabetes Care. 2005;28:1099-1082. Used with permission from the Council for the Advancement of Diabetes Research and Education (CADRE).

Figure 1 Time–action profiles of available insulin preparations. *Source*: http://www.insulinideas. org/pdf/InsulinIDEASNewsV1N3Q7final_Oct2006.pdf (2/12/2007).

Table 3 General Principles for Adjusting the Insulin Regimen

	Fasting BG	Postmeal BG
BG < target	↓ Basal	↓ Premeal bolus
BG > target	↑ Basal	↑ Premeal bolus

If fasting BG erratic (alternates between highs and lows) have patient check 3 AM BG to exclude *somogyi effect vs. dawn phenomenon.*

by adjusting the premeal insulin dose. If the postmeal BG is low, then the bolus insulin dose given prior to the meal will be reduced; if the postmeal BG is high, then the bolus insulin dose given prior to the meal will be increased (Table 3). Insulin doses will be changed up or down by 10% to 20% or per a prespecified dose adjustment formula or algorithm whenever required, based on the presence of hyperglycemia or hypoglycemia, respectively. In the outpatient setting, it is typical to wait several days in order to determine trends and/or patterns in BGs by time of day before making changes to the prescribed insulin regimen. This practice is known as pattern management.

Guidelines for Basal Insulin Adjustment

In the MDI regimen when the basal insulin is once daily glargine or detemir, the dose will be adjusted based upon the fasting BG. When the basal insulin is twice daily detemir or NPH the evening dose will be adjusted if the fasting BG is not at target and if the predinner BG is not at target, the morning NPH dose will be changed.

In CSII, basal insulin rates are adjusted empirically based on glucose monitoring results. Certain time periods during the day may require higher, while other periods may require lower infusion rates depending on individual factors including lifestyle and the dawn phenomenon. Two to four basal rates are routinely applied to meet insulin requirements over the course of a 24-hour period. For example, patients often need a lower basal rate between bedtime and 3 AM and a higher basal rate between 3 AM and the time they get up in the morning to attenuate the dawn phenomenon. An intermediate basal rate may be needed during the rest of the day. Adjustments to the basal rate(s) are usually made in 10% to 20% increments in order to affect clinically meaningful changes in BG levels. Anticipatory changes in basal infusion rates should be made about 1 to 2 hours before a change in plasma BG level is required, e.g., prior to exercise.

Guidelines for Prandial-Bolus Insulin Adjustment

Rapid-acting insulin analogs are preferred for use as the meal-time bolus insulin in the intensive insulin regimen for the person with DM1 for several reasons. They may be given at the time that the meal will be eaten, rather than 30 to 45 minutes before the meal, as is necessary with regular insulin. The rapid-acting analogs may also be given at the end of or even up to 20 minutes after a meal, as discussed earlier in this chapter. This feature is particularly useful if the amount of food that will be eaten is uncertain. As the rapid-acting analogs peak 60 to 90 minutes after being taken, a FS BG is taken 60 to 90 minutes after the meal to assess the appropriateness of the bolus insulin dose that was delivered. The premeal insulin dose can then be adjusted to control postprandial glucose levels, i.e., if the postmeal BG is above the patient's postmeal BG goal, or rises by more than 25 to 50 mg/dL from the premeal value, the meal bolus can be increased and conversely, if the postmeal BG is lower than desired, the premeal bolus insulin dose will be reduced (Table 3).

Practically speaking, for the patient who is either not able, for example due to time constraints, or not willing to check postprandial BGs, one may adjust the premeal insulin dose based on the BG prior to the next meal, as has been done in some Exubera and Apidra trials with good results (51,57).

In the DM1 patient who is being treated with conventional mixed, split subcutaneous insulin therapy rather than MDI (e.g., two injections per day of mixed rapid-acting or regular and NPH insulin), adjustments in the prandial component of the prebreakfast dose are made based on the postbreakfast or prelunch BG, changes in the intermediate-acting insulin component of the AM dose will be based on the presupper BG. To make adjustments in the presupper doses of insulin, the prandial component of the presupper insulin dose will be determined by the postsupper or bedtime BG levels, whereas the NPH insulin component of the presupper dose is based on 3 AM and/or fasting BG levels.

GUIDELINES FOR DOSING CORRECTION/SUPPLEMENTAL INSULIN

Correction or supplemental doses of insulin (CDI) are administered to correct hyperglycemia that results in spite of the patient having taken the usual prescribed basal and prandial insulin doses. CDI is taken *in addition* to the usual basal and/or bolus insulin dose(s) to be administered at the time when the FS BG is checked and found to be high. The CDI should not be large enough to cause, nor taken so frequently that overlapping peaks (insulin stacking) will result in hypoglycemia. Typically, approximately 1 U of short- or rapid-acting insulin will lower BG by 40 to 50 mg/dL in the patient with DM1. The BG lowering response depends on the patient's insulin sensitivity and daily insulin requirements varying from 0.5 to 3 U of short- or rapid-acting insulin for every 50 mg/dL lowering of BG. If correction dose insulin is needed at bedtime, it should be administered at a reduced dose compared to other times of day in order to reduce risk of nocturnal hypoglycemia.

Several methods for determining CDI are in use; however, studies to determine their specific safety and efficacy are lacking. Each method will take into account the patient's relative sensitivity to insulin, either through an association with the known TDD of insulin being taken or the patient's body weight. A key point to make regarding any method whereby CDI of insulin are used is that the impact on BG for an individual must be carefully monitored and the CDI adjusted as necessary if it does not lower the BG as expected or if it leads to hypoglycemia. This will require monitoring before and after the initial CDI recommended is taken to allow determination of the most appropriate CDI for the individual patient.

One method for determining starting correction insulin doses is to determine the dose as a simple percentage of the total number of units of insulin (basal plus bolus) that makes up the patient's TDDI. Typically, the correction dose will be 10% of the TDDI. If marked hyperglycemia is present and/or urine ketones are positive, the correction dose will be 20% of the TDDI, rounded down to the nearest unit. For example, if the basal insulin dose is 14 U of glargine and the meal dose is 5 U of insulin aspart with breakfast, 3 U with lunch, and 4 U with dinner, the total daily dose of insulin is 26 U. A CDI for moderate elevation in BG would be 2 U of rapid-acting insulin and for more marked hyperglycemia, if urine ketones are present, would be 4 U of rapid-acting insulin. This correction dose will be taken in addition to a usual basal and/or bolus insulin dose to be taken whenever the FS BG is above a predesignated target value for that time of day.

A second method in widespread use was developed by Paul Davidson and applies an insulin correction factor. It is known as the rule of 1800 when a rapid-acting insulin analog is

Table 4 Sample Correction/Supplemental Dose Scale for Insulin Administration

For blood glucose (mg/dL)	Correction dose scale for insulin[a]			
	Low dose[b]	Medium dose[c]	High dose[d]	Personal dose scale
150–199	1 unit	1 unit	2 units	_____ units
200–249	2 units	3 units	4 units	_____ units
250–299	3 units	5 units	7 units	_____ units
300–349	4 units	7 units	10 units	_____ units
> 349	5 units	8 units	12 units	_____ units

At bedtime and/or overnight, *reduce* the correction dose by half (50%), or take _____ units. (If this amount of insulin is less than one unit, do not take a dose.)
[a] For fingerstick glucose that is over 150 mg/dL or over _____, take a correction insulin dose as shown on the selected scale *in addition to* your usual basal and meal insulin doses.
[b] Requires < 40 units insulin daily; or < 70 kg weight.
[c] Requires 40–99 units insulin daily; or 71–99 kg weight.
[d] Requires ≥ 100 units insulin daily; or > 100 kg weight.

used and the rule of 1500 when regular insulin is used as the CDI. The correction factor calculated will provide an estimation of the number of mg/dL that 1 U of the correction insulin will lower the BG. The CDI will be the same insulin being used as prandial insulin for the patient. To calculate the correction factor for rapid-acting insulin analogs, 1800 is divided by the TDDI (116). For example, if a patient has a TDDI of 45 U, then the insulin correction factor would be: 1800 divided by 45 = 40. And 1 U of rapid-acting insulin would be expected to lower the BG by 40 mg/dL. If the patient has a premeal blood sugar of 180 mg/dL and wants to correct to 100 mg/dL or cause the value to fall by 80 mg/dL, then the patient would take an extra 2 U of (80 mg/dL lowering divided by 40 mg/dL expected from 1 U correction dose) *added* to the number of units to be taken to cover the carbohydrates to be consumed in the meal.

Finally, a CDI scale may be prescribed for the patient. Such scales will provide incremental, discrete stepped doses of insulin to be taken in response to progressively higher BG levels, typically rising by 50 mg/dL/step on the scale. The correction dose scale differs from sliding scale insulin conceptually in two ways: (*i*) the selected dose of insulin will be given *in addition* to the prescribed basal plus prandial insulin doses to *correct* hyperglycemia and (*ii*) the correction dose scale will factor in a surrogate measure of the patient's known insulin sensitivity (i.e., TDDI or weight). CDI scales are stratified as low, medium, or high dose with the option to provide an individualized scale (as shown in Table 4).

SPECIFIC PRACTICAL GUIDELINES FOR PATTERN MANAGEMENT

Core Insulin Adjustment Guidelines

Core insulin adjustment guidelines will address basic recommendations for correction of hypoglycemia, hyperglycemia, variations in food intake or level of physical activity, and days when the patient is sick or stressed. When glycemic control is suboptimal and both hyperglycemia and hypoglycemia are present, one should first address hypoglycemia and correct it. This approach is recommended for several reasons. First and foremost, the short-term hypoglycemia is a safety issue. In addition, if hyperglycemia is due to rebound from hypoglycemic episodes, e.g., nocturnal hypoglycemia leading to high fasting BG or to sequential extra correction doses of insulin, then increasing the insulin dose to treat highs will only exacerbate the tendency for hypoglycemia, perpetuating a vicious cycle of lows and highs.

Adjusting for Hypoglycemia

In evaluating episodes of hypoglycemia, one must first establish whether the lows are explained or unexplained as this will impact whether or not insulin doses need to be adjusted as the corrective action of choice. An exploration of variables that may be causing the hypoglycemia should be undertaken. Is the hypoglycemia explained by a decreased food intake, e.g., skipped meal or bedtime snack; an increase in the number of insulin doses taken, e.g., serial correction doses to treat a high; an increase in the number of units of insulin taken in a dose, e.g., a large correction dose; or by an increase in physical activity? If the explanation was an isolated occurrence, then the corrective action is to try and avoid the circumstances that caused it, e.g., to carry a snack when it is likely a meal will be skipped. If it is known that the explanation is going to be an ongoing phenomenon, e.g., beginning of an effort to lose weight through a cut in caloric intake or initiation of a regular exercise program, then the responsible insulin is adjusted downward to avoid further recurrences, per the general guidelines for basal and bolus insulin adjustment discussed earlier in this section.

Guidelines for Treating Hypoglycemia

Simple carbohydrate is taken to treat hypoglycemia. The patient should be advised to avoid indiscriminately ingesting large quantities of food or calories-containing beverages (such as regular soda or juice) in response to symptoms of hypoglycemia, as this will contribute to subsequent hyperglycemia. In general for BG of 51 to 70 mg/dL, treatment with 10 to 15 g of fast-acting carbohydrate is recommended; BG less than or equal to 50 mg/dL is treated with 20 to 30 g. BG should be retested 15 minutes after carbohydrate ingestion and repeat treatment taken as needed, based upon the BG result. The patient should also be advised to eat a more substantial snack or a meal that was missed or is late following initial treatment of a hypoglycemic reaction. This will prevent a recurrence. Once BG is more than 70 to 80 mg/dL, the patient can generally safely take an appropriate prandial dose to cover carbohydrate intake with the next scheduled meal to be eaten.

Adjusting for Hyperglycemia

Insulin doses will be adjusted upward when a pattern demonstrating hyperglycemia at a given time of day is present for 2 to 3 days in a row at the same time of day *and* the hyperglycemia is unexplained by increased food intake, inactivity, or the somogyi phenomenon (rebound hyperglycemia).

If the hyperglycemia is explained by an increased food intake or a decline in physical activity, it is preferable to correct the underlying lifestyle indiscretion rather than to raise the insulin dose(s). If fasting hyperglycemia is present, and particularly if fasting hyperglycemia is seen in association with wide variation in BG values, including the presence of normal and/or lower values, one must exclude the possibility that the highs represent rebound in response to nocturnal hypoglycemia. This distinction is accomplished by asking the patient to check a BG reading between 2 and 3 AM to see if it is normal. If the overnight BG is high, then it is appropriate to adjust the basal insulin dose upward to move BG levels toward the desired target range. If this value is low, it demonstrates that nocturnal hypoglycemia with subsequent rebound is the likely cause of the fasting highs, and the appropriate insulin adjustment is a reduction by 10% to 20% in the basal insulin that is acting at this time of night, e.g., once daily glargine or detemir dose or the evening dose of twice daily dosed insulin NPH or detemir.

Adjusting Insulin for Variations in Food Intake

In order that postprandial BG levels will be optimized, it is necessary for the provider and the patient to have an understanding of the relationship between the caloric content, and in particular the carbohydrate content of the meal, as the latter is the major contributor to the postprandial glycemic excursion. Prandial insulin dose will be matched with the anticipated or actual carbohydrate content of the meal. In the consistent carbohydrate meal plan, the number of grams of carbohydrate included in a given meal from day to day will be kept constant, thus allowing a prespecified insulin dose prescribed to be taken with the meal to control the postmeal glucose excursion. The nutritionist diabetes educator will typically provide a meal plan that incorporates in the range of 30 to 45 g of carbohydrate with each of breakfast and lunch and 45 to 60g of carbohydrate daily with dinner, depending on the patient's total daily caloric intake. The bedtime snack will contain 15 or more grams of carbohydrate if it is to be taken with a dose of insulin.

The second method whereby insulin doses are matched to carbohydrate content of the meals is carbohydrate counting in which a predetermined insulin-to-carbohydrate ratio is matched to the premeal anticipated or postmeal known carbohydrate content. Carbohydrate counting requires the patient to count grams of carbohydrate and estimate insulin doses based on carbohydrate intake. An average of 1 U of short- or rapid-acting insulin will dispose off 10 to 15 g (one starch equivalent) of carbohydrate, with a range of 0.5 to 2.0 U. In the adult with DM1, where the total daily insulin requirement is typically not very high and insulin resistance is not present, it is generally safe to start with an insulin-to-carbohydrate ratio of 1 U of insulin for every 15 g of carbohydrate. This method allows flexibility in the content of each meal. The patient can increase the amount of insulin taken with the meal, e.g., if eating out, or to reduce it in the event that a meal will be small or one does not feel like eating.

The insulin-to-carbohydrate ratio will account for insulin sensitivity relative to the postprandial glycemic excursion. It is important to note that insulin-to-carbohydrate ratios can vary with time of day, and that they are affected by stress, illness, and variations in physical activity. One should also note that the dawn phenomenon often induces a state of relative insulin insensitivity in the early morning, in which case it may be necessary to provide one insulin-to-carbohydrate ratio for the patient to take with breakfast, e.g., 1/10 and another ratio for the other meals of the day, e.g., 1/12 or 1/15 to appropriately match each to individual requirements.

Several formulae may also be applied to calculate an individual insulin-to-carbohydrate ratio: the 450 or 500 rule and the weight method (120). The 500 or the 450 rule may be used when a dose of insulin given before a meal results in postprandial BG levels in the target range. The insulin-to-carbohydrate ratio by the 450 or 500 rule is calculated as follows:

- Rapid-acting insulin (aspart, glulisine, or lispro)-to-carbohydrate ratio = 500 divided by TDDI.
- Regular insulin-to-carbohydrate ratio = 450 divided by TDDI.

As an example, if the individual TDD is 50 U and the patient uses a regimen with prandial rapid-acting then the insulin-to-carbohydrate ratio would be 500 divided by 50 or 1 U of analog for 10 g of carbohydrate.

Table 5 Weight-Based Insulin
to Carbohydrate Ratios (117)

Weight (lbs)	Ratio
120–129	1:15
130–139	1:14
140–149	1:13
150–169	1:12
170–179	1:11
180–189	1:10
190–199	1:9
> 200	1:8

The weight method for determining the insulin-to-carbohydrate ratio uses assignment of a ratio from a table based upon the patient's weight (Table 5) to provide the insulin-to-carbohydrate ratio (117).

Whichever method of matching insulin-to-carbohydrate content of the meal is used, it is important to assess the impact of the dose on postmeal BG levels by checking a FS value 60 to 90 minutes after a dose of rapid-acting insulin analog has been given with a meal or 2 hours after the meal if regular insulin is provided as the prandial insulin. If this value is high, and a consistent carbohydrate diet is being used, the premeal insulin bolus dose will be raised by 10% to 20%. If the postmeal BG is above target and if an insulin-to-carbohydrate ratio is used to determine the premeal dose, the ratio will be increased, typically in 2 to 5 g increments, e.g., from 1/15 to 1/12 or 1/10, depending upon the rise in magnitude of the BG after the meal. Conversely, when BG following a meal is lower than desired, the number of units of insulin given per gram of carbohydrate prior to the meal will be reduced.

Adjusting Insulin for Changes in Activity/Exercise

Increased levels of physical activity, including formal exercise, impact BG control by promoting movement of glucose into glycogen stores in the peripheral tissues. The entry of glucose into skeletal muscle is increased during exercise via an insulin-independent increase in the number of GLUT 4 transporters in muscle cell membranes. This increase in glucose entry persists for several hours after exercise and regular exercise training can produce prolonged periods of time where insulin sensitivity is increased. Exercise can precipitate hypoglycemia in diabetes not only because of the increase in muscle uptake of glucose but also because absorption of injected insulin is more rapid during exercise. Patients with diabetes will often need to either take in extra calories or reduce their insulin dosage when they exercise (5). If body weight is a concern, it is preferable to lower insulin doses in anticipation of exercise rather than to ingest extra calories to prevent hypoglycemia. Determination of the optimum insulin regimen for the patient with DM1 for exercise will be facilitated by careful BG monitoring in the periexercise period until insulin requirements are determined and appropriate insulin doses for these times have been determined. BG testing is recommended before, during, and after the activity to monitor the patient's response to exercise (118,119). Exercise-induced hypoglycemia may occur many hours after the activity as glycogen stores are repleted. This is particularly true following intense exercise, such as weight lifting and/or prolonged periods of aerobic exercise such as long-distance running or biking.

If exercise is planned, insulin dosages will be adjusted in anticipatory fashion in order to decrease risk for hypoglycemia either during or following the period of increased physical activity. It is not uncommon for the patient with DM1 who exercises regularly to have one insulin regimen for exercise days and another for days on which exercise is not undertaken. Premeal rapid-acting or regular insulin can be reduced 25% to 50% for moderate levels of planned postprandial activity. If the activity is strenuous, the patient may need additional carbohydrate along with the reduction in premeal insulin (120). Patients using insulin pumps can temporarily lower the basal rate by 20% to 40% for sustained periods of exercise, particularly those lasting over 60 minutes. A reduction in the basal rate by 25% during postexercise hours may also be necessary to avoid postexercise hypoglycemia (121). Suspending the basal rate for more than one hour is *not* recommended in the insulin deficient patient who has DM1 as ketogenesis may develop.

If exercise is unplanned, ingestion of additional carbohydrate will be necessary (15–30 g of carbohydrate for every 30 to 45 minutes of moderate exercise). It is also important to note that it is always necessary for the patient with diabetes to maintain adequate hydration during exercise as dehydration has a negative impact on insulin sensitivity.

Adjusting Insulin for Illness or During Periods of Stress: Sick Day Rules

Stress and illness clearly impact glycemic control. In the patient with DM1, release of insulin counterregulatory hormones under such circumstances will typically lead to hyperglycemia. Indeed progressive development of hyperglycemia without other aggravating factors may indicate that an illness, e.g., urinary tract infection or viral syndrome is in its prodromal stages. Careful questioning of the patient about symptoms that suggest underlying illness is part of a thorough assessment under these circumstances. It is necessary for the patient to have a plan of action to enable glycemic control on sick days.

Diabetes education for the adult patient with DM1 should include a thorough grounding in the general principles of sick day management, (Table 6) which includes the following:

- Checking FS BGs every 4 hours if not eating, or before meals and bedtime if eating discrete meals.
- Check 2 to 3 AM BG if running high at bedtime or nocturnal hypoglycemia is suspected.
- Take all usual prescribed doses of basal insulin glargine or detemir, with adjustment in basal dose(s) as described below.
- Reduce NPH insulin doses by 1/3 to 1/2 if food intake curtailed (to prevent hypoglycemia when the NPH peaks).
- Take usual meal insulin doses if eating well with a correction insulin dose if premeal BG is high; if not eating well, decrease meal insulin dose by 50% and consider taking at the end of the meal after assuring that the food is eaten.
- Maintain hydration.
- Check urine for ketones.
- If vomiting and cannot keep food or liquids down, go to the emergency room.

Table 6 Practical Guidelines for Insulin Adjustment in Adults with Type 1 Diabetes Mellitus[a]

Clinical circumstance and/or glycemia pattern	Insulin adjustment	Comments
Hypoglycemia		
Unexplained	Decrease responsible insulin by 10–20% when *next* scheduled dose due, particularly if unexplained severe hypoglycemia or at high risk for severe hypoglycemia	When *both* lows *and* highs are present, adjust insulin to correct hypoglycemia *first*
e.g., by reduced food, increased activity, or excess insulin	Reduce insulin dose(s) responsible for the lows	
Pattern at given time of day	Do not make adjustment to insulin dose(s) for single event	
Explained	If it will recur, consider anticipatory insulin adjustment as below	
e.g., by transient/situational decrease in food intake or increase in physical activity that will not be sustained or recurrent		
Anticipatory	Make anticipatory downward adjustment in the insulin dose that will be acting during the activity period to prevent hypoglycemia from occurring	
If planned increase in activity or decrease in food intake		
Hyperglycemia		
Unexplained and sustained	Increase basal insulin *first* if all BGs running high, *then* increase prandial insulin.	In general, 10–20% increase in responsible insulin dose will be necessary to impact BGs; increase basal insulin if premeal and overnight BGs high; adjust prandial insulin if postmeal BG high;
Consider underlying early infection; stress; pump failure; missed basal insulin dose, premenstrual; insulin inactive/expired	Supplement with correction dose insulin as needed	Calculate correction dose of insulin by rule of 1800 for rapid-acting insulin analog as: 1800/TDDI = number of mg/dL one unit of insulin will drop BG
Pattern at given time of day	Increase responsible insulin unless sustainable reduction in food intake or increase in physical activity will correct hyperglycemia	
Explained and sporadic	Treat with correction dose of insulin, e.g., meal was larger than anticipated	If fasting hyperglycemia, check overnight (2–3 AM) BG to distinguish nocturnal hypoglycemia with early morning rebound (Smogyi effect), which requires reduction in basal insulin dose, from the dawn phenomenon, which requires increase in basal insulin that is active in early morning hours
Anticipatory	If planned decrease in activity or increase in food intake, e.g., large meal, adjust insulin dose upward to avoid hyperglycemia	
Variation in food intake		
Anticipated		
Increase in food intake	Raise prandial dose of insulin	Carbohydrate counting using individualized insulin-to-carbohydrate ratio will allow optimal matching of insulin to nutritional intake and control of postprandial BG
Decrease in food intake	Lower prandial dose of insulin	

Unanticipated Increase with resultant hyperglycemia Decrease with hypoglycemia	Give correction dose of insulin Treat hypoglycemia	Calculate correction insulin dose as for hyperglycemia above 15 g of rapid-acting carbohydrate, e.g., 4 oz of juice, followed by snack or missed meal
Variation in activity level		
Anticipated Increase in activity level	Lower insulin dose(s) that will be acting during period of increased activity; use temporary basal rate or suspend pump for high level of exertion	Adults with type 1 diabetes commonly require one set of insulin doses for exercise days and another slightly higher set of doses for non–exercise days. A snack may also be required before or during exercise to prevent hypoglycemia.
Decrease in usual activity level	Increase insulin dose(s)/basal that will be acting during period of decreased activity	
Unanticipated Increase in activity level	Take 15–30 g rapid-acting carbohydrate immediately prior to or during the activity	
Reduction in usual activity level	Correct hyperglycemia with correction dose(s) of insulin	
Sick day rules Hyperglycemia	Moderate illness or stress: – Check FSBG before meals and hs – Take correction dose(s) of insulin per BG results Severe illness or stress – Check finger-stick BG minimum of every 4 hr – MDI take correction dose(s) of insulin per BG results; if anticipate prolonged duration of illness or stress, increase basal insulin and use CDI as needed – Pump increase basal insulin rate by 50% and boluses by 20%; use CDI as needed	Sick day rules apply to any day where intercurrent illness or stress adversely impact BGs (may be high or low) The patient with DM Type 1 *always* requires basal insulin to prevent DKA due to unchecked gluconeogenesis and ketogenesis If appetite curtailed due to illness, it is key to maintain adequate hydration Take calorie-containing liquids, e.g., broth, regular soda, or bland foods, e.g., applesauce, regular jello, crackers, as able if not eating discrete meals. Check dip urine for ketones
Hypoglycemia Risk for hypoglycemia increases if po intake curtailed	MDI – Prandial insulin: Lower or withhold doses or give rapid acting insulin dose *at end* of food ingestion matched to grams of carbohydrate taken – Basal insulin: Reduce NPH dose to 1/2–2/3 to avoid hypoglycemia with peak; reduce glargine or detemir only if anticipate prolonged inability to eat and BGs low	When to call the doctor or go to the emergency room - Persistent nausea/vomiting; unable to maintain adequate hydration; recurrent hypoglycemia; hyperglycemia not responsive to insulin dose adjustments; recurrent persistence of urinary ketones greater than trace positive.

(Continued)

Table 6 Practical Guidelines for Insulin Adjustment in Adults with Type 1 Diabetes Mellitus[a] (*Continued*)

Clinical circumstance and/or glycemia pattern	Insulin adjustment	Comments
	Pump	
	– Decrease basal insulin rate(s)	
	– Withold prandial insulin if not eating	
	– Match insulin conservatively to carbohydrates ingested and deliver bolus at end of meal	
Perimenstrual		
Hyperglycemia prior to onset of menses	– Increase basal insulin for hyperglycemia pattern	Increase in BGs in days prior to onset of menses not uncommon;
	– Anticipate need to return to usual basal doses with onset of period	if this pattern identified, adjust basal insulin upward when trend for BG to rise
Dialysis		
Peritoneal	Regular insulin in dialysate to meet PD needs or adjust SQ insulin doses to control BGs based on anticipated total carbohydrate delivery (by PD and meals)	Increase in BG generally proportional to concentration of dextrose in dianeal and to dwell time. Use lowest feasible dextrose concentration to minimize hyperglycemia
Hemodialysis	Anticipatory increase in insulin dose(s) day prior to dialysis if needed. Resume usual insulin doses other days	Insulin resistance prior to dialysis often leads to increased total daily insulin requirement the day before procedure

[a]The practical guidelines set forward in this table are based upon the principles of an anticipatory physiologic basal-bolus insulin regimen, pattern management, and knowledge of the usual impact of various clinical circumstances and lifestyle changes on blood glucose levels and total daily insulin requirements. Frequent BG monitoring and individualization of insulin adjustment recommendations is *always* required to enable safe and effective insulin management.

MDI insulin dose adjustments are made to minimize hyperglycemia on sick days or during periods of stress.

- If all BGs are running high, basal insulin dose(s) will be adjusted upward by 20% increments.
- CDI will be given in addition to basal and prandial insulin doses when hyperglycemia is present. CDI will be determined by calculation of a correction dose based on the total daily insulin requirement, e.g., by the rule of 1800 or as 10% of the TDDI if urine is dip negative for ketones and as 20% of the total daily insulin requirement if there are ketones in the urine (as discussed earlier), or by use of a correction dose scale.
- As with all insulin doses prescribed, it is essential to review the impact of sick day doses given to an individual patient and to revise these doses per BGs obtained to assure that they lower BG appropriately while minimizing risk of hypoglycemia.

CSII dose adjustments

- When the patient is being treated with an insulin pump, the sick day insulin dose adjustments are to increase the basal insulin rate by about 50% and the bolus insulin doses by 20%.

HOSPITAL MANAGEMENT

The principles of using physiologic insulin replacement to mimic normal insulin secretion patterns that are used in the outpatient with DM1 generally are applied in hospital management of adults with DM1 as well (Fig. 2).

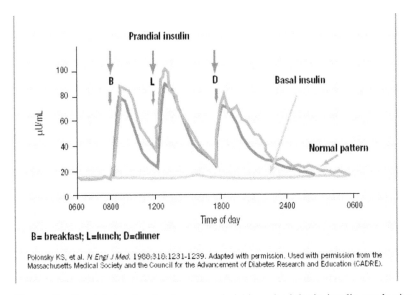

B= breakfast; L=lunch; D=dinner

Polonsky KS, et al. *N Engl J Med.* 1988;318:1231-1239. Adapted with permission. Used with permission from the Massachusetts Medical Society and the Council for the Advancement of Diabetes Research and Education (CADRE).

Figure 2 Basal–bolus insulin therapy: mimicking physiologic insulin production and release. *Source*: http://www.insulinideas.org/pdf/InsulinIDEASNewsV1N3Q7final_Oct2006.pdf (2/12/2007).

REFERENCES

1. Harris MI, Robbins DC. Prevalence of adult-onset IDDM in the US population. Diabetes Care 1994;17:1337.
2. The Diabetes Control and Complications Trial Research Group. The effect of intensive treatment of diabetes on the development and progression of long-term complications in insulin-dependent diabetes mellitus. N Engl J Med 1993;329:977.
3. Nathan DM, Cleary PA, Backlund JY, et al. Intensive diabetes treatment and cardiovascular disease in patients with type 1 diabetes. N Engl J Med 2005;353:2643.
4. The Diabetes Control and Complications Trial Research Group. Effect of intensive therapy on residual beta-cell function in patients with type 1 diabetes in the diabetes control and complications trial. A randomized, controlled trial. Ann Intern Med 1998;128:517.
5. William F. Ganong. Review of Medical Physiology, 22 nd edn. New York: Lange Medical Books/McGraw-Hill, 2005.
6. Bertram G. Katzung. Basic and Clinical Pharmacology, 9th edn. New York: Lange Medical Books/McGraw-Hill, 2004.
7. Goodner CJ, Walike BC, Koerker DJ, et al. Insulin, glucagon, and glucose exhibit synchronous, sustained oscillations in fasting monkeys. Science 1977;195:177.
8. Ferrannini E, Pilo A. Pattern of insulin delivery after intravenous glucose injection in man and its relation to plasma glucose disappearance. J Clin Invest 1979;64:243.
9. McCulloch DK, Bingley PJ, Colman PG, et al. Comparison of bolus and infusion protocols for determining acute insulin response to intravenous glucose in normal humans. The ICARUS group. Islet cell antibody register user's study. Diabetes Care 1993;16:911.
10. Bingley PJ, Matthews DR, Williams AJ, et al. Loss of regular oscillatory insulin secretion in islet cell antibody positive non-diabetic subjects. Diabetologia 1992;35:32.
11. Nosek L, Becker RHA, Frick AD, et al. Prandial blood glucose control with pre- and post-meal insulin glulisine versus regular human insulin. Diabetes 2004;53(Suppl 2):A139–A140.
12. Garg S, Rosenstock J, Ways K. Efficacy and safety of post-meal insulin glulisine (GLU) compared with pre-meal regular human insulin (RHI) in a basal-bolus regimen with insulin glargine. Diabetes 2004;53(Suppl 2):A125.
13. Clement S, Braithwaite S, Magee MF, et al. Management of diabetes and hyperglycemia in hospitals: American diabetes association technical review. Diabetes Care 2004;27:553–587.
14. Magee MF, Clement S. Subcutaneous insulin therapy in the hospital setting: Issues, concerns, and implementation. Endocr Pract 2004;10(Suppl 2):81–88.
15. Campbell KB, Braithwaite SS. Hospital management of hyperglycemia. Clin Diabetes 2004;22:81–88.
16. Beylot M, Sautot G, Dechaud H, et al. Lack of beta-adrenergic role for catecholamines in the development of hyperglycemia and ketonaemia following acute insulin withdrawal in type I diabetic patients. Diabete Metab 1985;11(2):111–117.
17. McKeage K, Goa KL. Insulin glargine: A review of its therapeutic use as a long-acting agent for the management of type 1 and type 2 diabetes mellitus. Drugs 2001;61:1599–1624.
18. LaGow B, Kerolus M. Physician's Desk Reference (PDR). Thomson PDR, 2007.
19. Hamann A, Matthaei S, Rosak C, et al. A randomized clinical trial comparing breakfast, dinner, or bedtime administration of insulin glargine in patients with type 1 diabetes. Diabetes Care 2003;26:1738.
20. Raskin P, Chaykin L, Mak C, et al. Comparison of insulin detemir and glargine using a basal-bolus regimen in a Treat-To-Target Study in Patients with Type 2 Diabetes. IDF 2006 Abstract.
21. Havelund S, Plum A, Ribel U, et al. The mechanism of protraction of insulin detemir, a long-acting, acylated analog of human insulin. Pharm Res 2004;21:1498.
22. Chapman TM, Perry CM. Insulin detemir: A review of its use in the management of type 1 and type 2 diabetes mellitus. Drugs 2004;64:2577–2595.
23. Plank J, Bodenlenz M, Sinner F, et al. A double-blind, randomized, dose-response study investigating the pharmacodynamic and pharmacokinetic properties of the long-acting insulin analog detemir. Diabetes Care 2005;28:1107.

24. Pieber TR, Draeger E, Kristensen A, et al. Comparison of three multiple injection regimens for type 1 diabetes: Morning plus dinner or bedtime administration of insulin detemir vs. morning plus bedtime NPH insulin. Diabet Med 2005;22:850.

25. Hermansen K, Fontaine P, Kukolja KK, et al. Insulin analogues (insulin detemir and insulin aspart) versus traditional human insulins (NPH insulin and regular human insulin) in basal-bolus therapy for patients with type 1 diabetes. Diabetologia 2004;47:622.

26. Home P, Bartley P, Russell-Jones DL. Insulin detemir offers improved glycemic control compared with NPH insulin in people with type 1 diabetes: A randomized clinical trial. Diabetes Care 2004;27:1081–1087.

27. Russell-Jones DL, Simpson R, Hylleberg B, et al. Effects of QD insulin detemir or NPH on blood glucose control in patients with type 1 diabetes mellitus using a basal-bolus regimen. Clin Ther 2004;26:724–736.

28. De Leeuw I, Vague P, Selam JL, et al. Insulin detemir used in basal-bolus therapy in people with type 1 diabetes is associated with a lower risk of nocturnal hypoglycaemia and less weight gain over 12 months in comparison to NPH insulin. Diabetes Obes Metab 2005;7:73.

29. Meneghini LF, Rosenberg KH, Koenen C, et al. Insulin detemir improves glycaemic control with less hypoglycemia and no weight gain in patients with type 2 diabetes who were insulin naïve or treated with NPH or insulin glargine: Clinical practice experience from a German subgroup of the PREDICTIVE study. Diabetes, Obesity and Metab. Oxford: Blackwell Publishers, 2006.

30. Hennige AM, Sartorius T, Tschritter O. Tissue selectivity of insulin detemir action in vivo. Diabetologia 2006;49:1274–1282.

31. Hordern SVM, Wright JE, Umpleby AM, et al. Comparison of the effects on glucose and lipid metabolism of equipotent doses of insulin determir and NPH insulin with a 16-h euglycemic clamp. Diabetologia 2005;48:420–426.

32. Barnett AH. A review of basal insulins. Diabet Med 2003;20:873–885.

33. Plank J, Siebenhofer A, Berghold A, et al. Systematic review and meta-analysis of short-acting insulin analogues in patients with diabetes mellitus. Arch Intern Med 2005;165:1337.

34. Hirsch IB. Insulin analogues. N Engl J Med 2005;352:174–183.

35. Holleman F, Van Den Brand JJG, Hoven RA, et al. Comparison of LysB28, ProB29 – human insulin analog and regular human insulin in the correction of incidental hyperglycemia. Diabetes Care 1996;19:1426.

36. Raskin P, Guthrie RA, Leiter L, et al. Use of insulin aspart, a fast-acting insulin analog, as the mealtime insulin in the management of patients with type 1 diabetes. Diabetes Care 2000;23:583.

37. Becker RHA, Frick AD, Kapitza C, et al. Pharmacodynamics (PD) and pharmacokinetics (PK) of insulin glulisine compared with insulin lispro (IL) and regular human insulin (RHI) in patients with type 2 diabetes. Diabetes 2004;53(Suppl 2):A119.

38. Available at www.medscape.com/viewarticle/551560?sssdmh=dml.246187&src=ddd#2. Accessed on February 12, 2007.

39. Anderson JH Jr, Brunelle RL, Koivisto VA, et al. Reduction of postprandial hyperglycemia and frequency of hypoglycemia in IDDM patients on insulin-analog treatment. Diabetes 1997;46:265.

40. Joseph SE, Korzon-Burakowska A, Woodworth JR, et al. The action profile of lispro is not blunted by mixing in the syringe with NPH insulin. Diabetes Care 1998;21:2098.

41. Brunelle RL, Llewelyn J, Anderson JH, et al. Meta-analysis of the effect of insulin lispro on severe hypoglycemia in patients with type 1 diabetes. Diabetes Care 1998;21:1726–1731.

42. Hirsch IB. Intensive treatment of type 1 diabetes. Med Clin North Am 1998;82:689–719.

43. Simon C, Follenius M, Brandenberger G. Postprandial oscillations of plasma glucose, insulin and C-peptide in man. Diabetologia 1987;30:769.

44. Madsbad S. Insulin analogues: Have they changed insulin treatment and improved glycaemic control? Diabetes Metab Res Rev 2002;18 (Suppl 1):S21–S28.

45. Gerich JE. Novel insulins: Expanding options in diabetes management. Am J Med 2002;113:308–316.

46. Skyler JS, Cefalu WT, Kourides IA, et al. Efficacy of inhaled human insulin in type 1 diabetes mellitus: A randomized proof-of-concept study. Lancet 2001;357:331.

47. Laube BL, Benedict GW, Dobs AS. The lung as an alternative route of delivery for insulin in controlling postprandial glucose levels in patients with diabetes. Chest 1998;114:1734.
48. Cefalu WT, Skyler JS, Kourides IA, et al. Inhaled human insulin treatment in patients with type 2 diabetes mellitus. Ann Intern Med 2001;134:203.
49. Gerber RA, Cappelleri JC, Kourides IA, et al. Treatment satisfaction with inhaled insulin in patients with type 1 diabetes: A randomized controlled trial. Diabetes Care 2001;24:1556.
50. Royle P, Waugh N, McAuley L, et al. Inhaled insulin in diabetes mellitus. Cochrane Database Syst Rev 2003;CD003890.
51. Hollander PA, Blonde L, Rowe R, et al. Efficacy and safety of inhaled insulin (Exubera) compared with subcutaneous insulin therapy in patients with type 2 diabetes: Results of a 6-month, randomized, comparative trial. Diabetes Care 2004;27:2356–2362.
52. Weiss SR, Cheng SL, Kourides IA, et al. Inhaled insulin provides improved glycemic control in patients with type 2 diabetes mellitus inadequately controlled with oral agents: A randomized controlled trial. Arch Intern Med 2003;163:2277.
53. Rave KM, Nosek L, Heinemann L, et al. Inhaled micronized crystalline human insulin using a dry powder inhaler: Dose-response and time-action profiles. Diabet Med 2004;21:763–768.
54. Rave KM, Nosek L, de la Pena A, et al. Dose response of inhaled dry-powder insulin and dose equivalence to subcutaneous insulin lispro. Diabetes Care 2005;28:2400–2405.
55. Heinemann L, Traut T, Heise T. Time-action profile of inhaled insulin. Diabet Med 1997;14: 63–72.
56. Kapitza C, Hompesch M, Scharling B, et al. Intrasubject variability of inhaled insulin in type 1 diabetes: A comparison with subcutaneous insulin. Diabetes Technol Ther 2004;6:466–472.
57. Skyler JS, Weinstock RS, Raskin P, et al. Use of inhaled insulin in a basal/bolus insulin regimen in type 1 diabetic subjects: A 6-month, randomized, comparative trial. Diabetes Care 2005;28:1630.
58. Royle P, Waugh N, McAuley L, et al. Inhaled insulin in diabetes mellitus (review). Cochrane Database Syst Rev 2003;CD003890.
59. Garg S, Rosenstock J, Silverman BL, et al. Efficacy and safety of preprandial human insulin inhalation powder versus injectable insulin in patients with type 1 diabetes. Diabetologia 2006.
60. Heise T, Bott S, Tusek C, et al. The effect of insulin antibodies on the metabolic action of inhaled and subcutaneous insulin: A prospective randomized pharmacodynamic study. Diabetes Care 2005;28:2161.
61. Quattrin T, Belanger A, Bohannon NJ, et al. Exubera phase III study group. Efficacy and safety of inhaled insulin (Exubera) compared with subcutaneous insulin therapy in patients with type 1 diabetes: Results of a 6-month, randomized, comparative trial. Diabetes Care 2004;27: 2622–2627.
62. Skyler JS, Cefalu WT, Kourides IA, et al. Efficacy of inhaled human insulin in type 1 diabetes mellitus: A randomized proof-of-concept study. Lancet 2001;357:331–335.
63. DeFronzo RA, Bergenstal RM, Cefalu WT, et al. Exubera phase III study group. Efficacy of inhaled insulin in patients with type 2 diabetes not controlled with diet and exercise: A 12-week, randomized, comparative trial. Diabetes Care 2005;28:1922–1928.
64. Weiss SR, Cheng SL, Kourides IA, et al. Inhaled insulin phase II study group. Inhaled insulin provides improved glycemic control in patients with type 2 diabetes mellitus inadequeately controlled with oral agents: A randomized controlled trial. Arch Intern Med 2003;163: 2277–2282.
65. Fineberg SE, Kawabata T, Finco-Kent D, et al. Antibody response to inhaled insulin in patients with type 1 or type 2 diabetes. An analysis of initial phase II and III inhaled insulin (Exubera) trials and a two-year extension trial. J Clin Endocrinology Metab 2005;90:3287–3294.
66. Heise T, Bott S, Tusek C, et al. The effect of insulin antibodies on the metabolic action of inhaled and subcutaneous insulin: A prospective randomized pharmacodynamic study. Diabetes Care 2005;28:2161–2169.
67. Ceglia L, Lau J, Pittas AG. Meta-analysis: Efficacy and safety of inhaled insulin therapy in adults with diabetes mellitus. Ann Intern Med 2006;145(9):665–75.
68. Cefalu WT. Evolving strategies for insulin delivery and therapy. Drugs 2004;64:1149.

69. Mann JL. Function and diabetes. Pract Diabetol 2006.
70. Bloomgarden ZT. American diabetes association annual meeting,1999: More on cardiovascular disease. Diabetes Care 2000;23:845–852.
71. Arnalich F, Hernanz A, Lopez-Maderuelo D, et al. Enhaced acute-phase response and oxidative stress in older adults with type II diabetes. Horm Metab Res 2000;32:407–412.
72. Gumieniczek A, Hopkala H, Wojtowicz Z, et al. Changes in antioxidant status of lung tissue in experimental diabetes in rabbits. Clin Biochem 2002;35:147–149.
73. Davis TM, Knuiman M, Kendall P, et al. Reduced pulmonary function and its associations in type 2 diabetes: The Fremantle Diabetes Study. Diabetes Res Clin Pract 2000;50:153–159.
74. Sandler M, Bunn AE, Stewart RI. Cross-section study of pulmonary function in patients with insulin-dependent diabetes mellitus. Am Rev Respir Dis 1987;135:223–229. Erratum in: Am Rev Respir Dis 1987;135:1223.
75. Hilmmelmann A, Jendle J, Mellen A, et al. The impact of smoking on inhaled insulin. Diabetes Care 2003;26:677–682.
76. Binder C, Lauritzen T, Faber O, et al. Insulin pharmacokinetics. Diabetes Care 1984;7:188.
77. Sindelka G, Heinemann L, Berger M, et al. Effect of insulin concentration, subcutaneous fat thickness and skin temperature on subcutaneous insulin absorption in healthy subjects. Diabetologia 1994;37:377.
78. Heise T, Nosek L, Ronn BB, et al. Lower within-subject variability of insulin detemir in comparison to NPH insulin and insulin glargine in people with type 1 diabetes. Diabetes 2004;53:1614.
79. Galloway JA, Spradlin CT, Nelson RL, et al. Factors influencing the absorption, serum insulin concentration, and blood glucose responses after injections of regular insulin and various insulin mixtures. Diabetes Care 1981;4:366.
80. Micossi P, Cristallo M, Librenti MC, et al. Free-insulin profiles after intraperitoneal, intramuscular, and subcutaneous insulin administration. Diabetes Care 1986;9:575.
81. Koivisto VA, Felig P. Alterations in insulin absorption and in blood glucose control associated with varying insulin injection sites in diabetic patients. Ann Intern Med 1980;92:59.
82. Klemp P, Staberg B, Madsbad S, et al. Smoking reduces insulin absorption from subcutaneous tissue. Br Med J (Clin Res Ed) 1982;284:237.
83. Koivisto, VA, Felig, P. Effects of leg exercise on insulin absorption in diabetic patients. N Engl J Med 1978;298:79.
84. Koivisto VA. Sauna-induced acceleration in insulin absorption from subcutaneous injection site. Br Med J 1980;280:1411.
85. Linde B. Dissociation of insulin absorption and blood flow during massage of a subcutaneous injection site. Diabetes Care 1986;9:570.
86. Berger M, Cüppers HJ, Hegner H, et al. Absorption kinetics and biologic effects of subcutaneously injected insulin preparations. Diabetes Care 1982;5:77.
87. Skyler JS, Weinstock RS, Raskin P, et al. Inhaled insulin phase III type 1 diabetes study group. Use of inhaled insulin in a basal/bolus insulin regimen in type 1 diabetic subjects: A 6-month, randomized, comparative trial. Diabetes Care 2005;28:1630–1635.
88. Fritsche A, Haring H. At last, a weight neutral insulin? Int J Obes Relat Metab Disrod 2004;28(Suppl 2):S41–S46.
89. Wang PH, Lau J, Chalmers TC. Meta-analysis of effects of intensive blood glucose control on later complications of type I diabetes. Lancet 1993;341:1306.
90. Smith LE, Shen W, Perruzzi C, et al. Regulation of vascular endothelial growth factor-dependent retinal neovascularization by insulin-like growth factor-1 receptor. Nat Med 1999;5:1390.
91. Schernthaner G. Immunogenicity and allergenic potential of animal and human insulins. Diabetes Care 1993;16(Suppl 3):155–165.
92. Bodtger U, Wittrup M. A rational clinical approach to suspected insulin allergy: Status after five years and 22 cases. Diabet Med 2005;22 (1):102–106.
93. Hirsch IB, Bode BW, Garg S, et al. Continuous subcutaneous insulin infusion (CSII) of insulin aspart versus multiple daily injection of insulin aspart/insulin glargine in type 1 diabetic patients previously treated with CSSI. Diabetes Care 2005;28(3).

94. Egger M, Davey SG, Stettler C, et al. Risk of adverse effects of intensified treatment in insulin-dependent diabetes mellitus: A meta-analysis. Diabet Med 1997;14:919.

95. Lifetime benefits and costs of intensive therapy as practiced in the diabetes control and complications trial. The diabetes control and complications trial research group. JAMA 1996;276:1409.

96. Herman WH, Dasbach EJ, Songer TJ, et al. The cost-effectiveness of intensive therapy for diabetes mellitus. Endocrinol Metab Clin North Am 1997;26(3):679–695.

97. Hirsch IB, Farkas-Hirsch R, Skyler JS. Intensive insulin therapy for treatment of type 1 diabetes. Diabetes Care 1990;13:1265.

98. Lougheed WD, Zinman B, Strack TR, et al. Stability of insulin lispro in insulin infusion systems. Diabetes Care 1997;20:1061–1065.

99. Bode BW, Steed RD, Davidson PC. Reduction in severe hypoglycemia with long-term continuous subcutaneous insulin infusion in type I diabetes. Diabetes Care 1996;19:324–327.

100. Clement S, Braithwaite SS, Magee MF, et al. Management of diabetes and hyperglycemia in hospitals. American diabetes association diabetes in hospitals writing committee. Diabetes Care 2004;27:553–591.

101. Campbell KB, Braithwaite SS. Hospital management of hyperglycemia. American diabetes association. Clin Diabetes 2004;22:81–88.

102. Magee MF, Clement S. Subcutaneous insulin therapy in the hospital setting: Issues, concerns, and implementation. Endocr Pract 2004;10(Suppl 2):81–88.

103. Strowig SM. Initiation and management of insulin pump therapy. Diabetes Educ 1993;19:50.

104. American Diabetes Association. Continuous subcutaneous insulin infusion. Diabetes Care2002;25(Suppl 1):116.

105. Dunn FL, Nathan DM, Scavini M, et al. Long-term therapy of IDDM with an implantable insulin pump. Diabetes Care 1997;20:59.

106. Saudek CD, Duckworth WC, Giobbie-Hurder A, et al. Implantable insulin pump versus multiple dose insulin for non-insulin-dependent diabetes mellitus. A randomized controlled trial. JAMA 1996;276:1322.

107. Gin H, Melki V, Guerci B, et al. Clinical evaluation of a newly designed compliant side port catheter for an insulin implantable pump: the EVADIAC experience. Evaluation dans le diabete du traitement par implants actifs. Diabetes Care 2001;24:175.

108. Kessler L, Tritschler S, Bohbot A, et al. Macrophage activation in type 1 diabetic patients with catheter obstruction during peritoneal insulin delivery with an implantable pump. Diabetes Care 2001;24:302.

109. Renard E, Raingeard I, Costalat G, et al. Aseptic peritonitis revealed through recurrent catheter obstructions in type 1 diabetic patients treated with continuous peritoneal insulin infusion. Diabetes Care 2004;27:276.

110. Jeandidier N, Boullu S, Busch-Brafin MS, et al. Comparison of antigenicity of Hoechst 21PH insulin using either implantable intraperitoneal pump or subcutaneous external pump infusion in type 1 diabetic patients. Diabetes Care 2002;25:84.

111. Riddle MC, Rosenstock J, Gerich J. The treat-to-target trial. Randomized addition of glargine or human NPH insulin to oral therapy of type 2 diabetic patients. Diabetes Care 2003;26: 3080–3086.

112. Garber AJ, Wahlen J, Wahl T, et al. Attainment of glycaemic goals in type 2 diabetes with once-, twice- or thrice-daily dosing with biphasic insulin aspart 70/30 (the 1–2–3 study). Diabetes Obes Metab 2006;8:58–66.

113. Monnier L, Mas E, Ginet C, et al. Activation of oxidative stress by acute glucose fluctuations compared with sustained chronic hyperglycemia in patients with type 2 diabetes. JAMA 2006;295:1681–1687.

114. Brownlee M, Hirsch IB. Glycemic variability: A hemoglobin A1 C-independent risk factor for diabetic complications. JAMA 2006;295: 1707–1708.

115. Hirsch IB. Blood glucose monitoring technology: Translating data into practice. Endocr Pract 2004;10:67–76.

116. Stoller WA. Individualizing insulin management: Three practical cases, rules for regimen adjustment. Postgrad Med 2002;111(5):51–66.

117. Pastors JG, Waslaski J, Gunderson H. Diabetes meal-planning strategies. In: Ross TA, Boucher JL, O'Connell BS, eds. Diabetes Medical Nutrition Therapy and Education. Chicago, IL: American Diebetic Association, 2005.
118. Horton ES. Role and management of exercise in diabetes mellitus. Diabetes Care 1988;11:201.
119. Kemmer FW. Prevention of hypoglycemia during exercise in type I diabetes. Diabetes Care 1992;15:1732.
120. Schiffrin A, Parikh S. Accommodating planned exercise in type I diabetic patients on intensive treatment. Diabetes Care 1985;8:337.
121. Sonnenberg GE, Kemmer FW, Berger M. Exercise in type I (insulin-dependent) diabetic patients treated with continuous subcutaneous insulin infusion. Diabetologia 1990;33:696.
122. Davidson MB, Mehta AE, Siraj ES. Inhaled human insulin: An inspiration for patients with diabetes mellitus? Cleve Clin J Med. 2006;73:569–578.
123. Standards of medical care in diabetes mellitus. Diabetes Care 2007;30:S4–S41.
124. American college of endocrinology consensus statement on guidelines for glycemic control. Endocr Pract 2002;8(Suppl 1):5–11.

6
Pramlintide and Other Adjunctive Therapies

C. H. Wysham
Washington State University, Spokane, Washington, U.S.A.

INTRODUCTION

The Diabetes Control and Complications Trial (DCCT) definitely proved that the microvascular complications of type 1 diabetes mellitus could be prevented or delayed by improving glucose control (1). Since the publication of this study, the aim for therapy of individuals with type 1 diabetes has been to achieve glucose and A1c values as close to normal as safely possible (2). However, the DCCT and follow-up study, Epidemiology of Diabetes Interventions and Complications (EDIC), also proved how difficult it was to attain and maintain normoglycemia (1,3). Despite considerable support from diabetologists, diabetes educators and registered dieticians, the average A1c in the subjects randomized to the intensive group of the DCCT was 7.2%, far above the goal A1c of less than or equal to 6.05%. Moreover, less than 5% of the intensive cohort was able to maintain average A1c at or below target (1). One year after the end of the intensive intervention of the DCCT study, the average A1c in the intensive group rose to 7.7%, approaching the level of 8.1% in the conventional group. The differences between the groups continued to narrow over the next 5 years (3). One decade after the publication of the DCCT study results, glycemic control, as measured by A1c, has improved in people with type 1 diabetes. An Australian study of 1335 children with type 1 diabetes reported improvement in average A1c from 10.9% in 1992 to 8.1% in 2002 (4). Several recent studies report similar findings, with average A1c levels ranging between 8.2% and 9.0% (5–7), far higher than the targets set by the American Diabetes Association.

CLINICAL BARRIERS TO OPTIMAL GLYCEMIC CONTROL

Maintenance of near-normal glucose levels is demanding, in that it requires an educated and motivated patient to coordinate the complex task of adjusting insulin doses based upon ambient glucose levels, dietary intake, activity, illness, or stress. Although psychosocial barriers such as lack of economic or social support, poor access to specialized centers, eating disorders, and other psychological problems are associated with poor control (6), factors inherent in insulin therapy contribute to the challenge of keeping glucose levels in the near-normal range (Table 1).

Table 1 Clinical Barriers Associated with Insulin Therapy

Increased risk of hypoglycemia	Risk increases exponentially as patients approach normoglycemia
	Risk sustained over years
Failure to normalize postprandial glycemia	Insulin replacement is still not physiological (peripheral vs. portal)
	Insulin is only one of the hormonal regulators of postprandial glucose homeostasis
Excessive diurnal glucose fluctuations	Make it difficult for patients to predict glucose levels and adjust insulin therapy
	New glucose-sensing technology has highlighted the magnitude of this barrier
Excessive weight gain	Underappreciated in patients with type 1 diabetes
	Cosmetic concern of many patients
	Negative effects on lipids and blood pressure

Source: Adapted from Ref. 27.

Hypoglycemia

Hypoglycemia, particularly severe hypoglycemia, represents the major limiting factor in achieving good glycemic control in patients with type 1 diabetes. People with diabetes are fearful of the risk for acute injury or death due to severe hypoglycemia and often alter their food and/or insulin regimen so as to avoid it. An inverse relationship between glycemic control and risk of hypoglycemia was demonstrated in the DCCT, with a frequency threefold higher in the intensive versus conventional group (0.61 vs. 0.18 events per patient-year) (1). In a study of children with type 1 diabetes, those with average A1c less than 7% experienced a 4.3-fold increased risk of severe hypoglycemia when compared with those who had A1c levels greater than 10%. Fortunately, cognition and quality of life were not impaired in the intensively treated patients (4). The risk for hypoglycemia is reduced by the use of optimal basal–bolus therapy, using insulin analogues in multiple daily injection or insulin pump therapy but the rate of severe hypoglycemia remains high, occurring at a rate of approximately one per patient per year in those attempting to attain recommended targets for A1c (8). This leaves people with type 1 diabetes with a difficult dilemma: How to balance the need for good glucose control to avoid the long-term complications of diabetes against the persistent risk of severe hypoglycemia.

Weight Gain

Patients with type 1 diabetes will generally gain weight with intensive insulin therapy, the extent of which correlates with improvement in hemoglobin A1c levels. At the end of DCCT study, the average weight gain by the subjects in the intensive arm was 4.5 kg more than the conventionally treated group. An almost twofold higher increase in the rate of obesity was seen in the intensively treated group (9). Mechanisms behind the weight gain in intensively treated patients are not completely understood, but probably include reduction of glycosuria, increased appetite, hypoglycemia (defensive eating), and the anabolic effect of insulin on the adipocyte (10). Weight gain in people with type 1 diabetes is not innocuous. As occurs in the general public, metabolic syndrome and associated cardiovascular risk factors often complicate weight gain in people with type 1 diabetes. In subjects with type 1 diabetes, impaired glucose response to intravenous (IV) insulin was significantly associated with increased risk for death from vascular disease (11). In the intensive group of the DCCT study, excessive weight gain occurred in about 25% of the subjects and was associated with higher total cholesterol, LDL-C, apo-B levels and systolic blood pressure, despite roughly equivalent glycemic control across the weight gain spectrum (12). Furthermore, there was a strong correlation between weight gain and the levels of the inflammatory marker hsCRP in the intensively treated subjects who gained weight (13). Epidemiology studies suggest that risk for cardiovascular disease in type 1 diabetes is more strongly correlated with determinants of the metabolic syndrome than with degree of glycemic control (14).

The association of weight gain with insulin therapy can be a barrier to adherence to prescribed insulin regimen, leading to poor glycemic control (10). Eating disorders occur in up to one-third of females with type 1 diabetes, with intentional omission of insulin representing the predominant weight-control behavior. Compared to females with type 1 diabetes without disordered eating, those inflicted with disordered eating have higher glycosylated hemoglobin levels and are at significantly higher risk for microvascular complications (15).

Postprandial Hypoglycemia

Despite careful calculation of carbohydrate intake and insulin doses, continuous glucose sensing reveals that most people with type 1 diabetes experience large glucose fluxes (16), especially in the postprandial period. Growing evidence suggests that the risk for long-term vascular complications of diabetes may not be entirely explained by average glucose levels, as measured by the A1c (17). Glycemic exposure, as measured by A1c, age at diagnosis and duration of diabetes explains as little as one-third of the variability in the development of microvascular complications (18). Rather, the metabolic milieu associated with glycemic excursions may be additive to the effects of chronic hyperglycemia (17,19,20). Although hyperglycemia is associated with activation of many biochemical pathways known to have deleterious effects upon the endothelium, an imbalance between free radical production and antioxidant consumption (oxidative stress) appears to activate many of these pathways (20). If studies can confirm the benefit of minimizing glycemic excursions and oxidative stress for reducing the vascular risk in diabetes, different treatment strategies to minimize glycemic excursions will need to be explored.

NORMAL GLUCOSE HOMEOSTASIS

The inability of subcutaneous (SC) insulin to control glucose levels in the postprandial period is due, in part, to its failure to replicate normal concentrations of insulin in the portal and system circulations. However, it has become increasingly apparent that, in addition to insulin secretion, normal postprandial glucose regulation involves interactions of several hormones: insulin, glucagon, amylin, GLP-1, GIP as well as other pancreatic and gut-derived hormones (21). As illustrated in Figure 1, these hormones work in concert to balance the appearance of glucose into the plasma with the insulin-mediated disappearance of glucose into the peripheral tissues.

In people with type 1 diabetes, glucose influx exceeds glucose efflux for several hours after eating due to the combined defects of severe insulin deficiency, elevated post-prandial glucagon levels and accelerated gastric emptying. Optimal SC insulin therapy cannot correct the defects of glucagon regulation and gastric motility in people with type 1 diabetes.

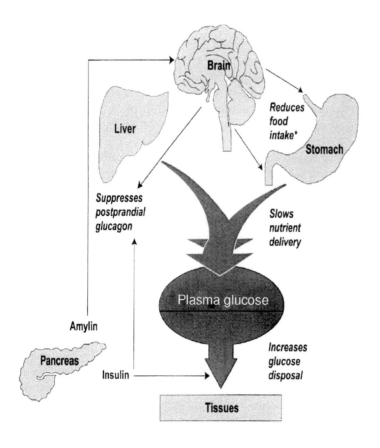

'Reported in rodents

Figure 1   Hormonal regulation of postprandial glucose. *Source*: Adapted from Ref. 27.

Amylin Physiology

The explanation for the abnormal postprandial glucagon secretion in people with type 1 diabetes was unidentified until the discovery of the beta cell product, amylin, in 1987. Amylin, a 37 amino acid peptide, is coproduced and cosecreted with insulin by the beta cell of the pancreas in response to nutritional stimuli, glucagon, GLP-1, and cholinergic agonists. Its secretion is inhibited by somatostatin (21). The normal plasma concentration of amylin parallels that of insulin, with low levels in the fasting state and a marked increase in secretion in response to meals (22). The physiologic action of amylin is to reduce the rate and amount of glucose entering the circulation through several mechanisms: slowing of gastric emptying, suppressing postprandial glucagon secretion and reducing food intake (23). Most of the actions of amylin can be explained by effects on the central nervous system, as suggested by the high concentration of amylin binding sites in the brain. In rats, receptors for amylin are found in the area postrema, dorsal raphe, and the nucleus accumbens. In particular, the area postrema, with its location outside of the blood–brain barrier and its close proximity to the central chemoreceptor trigger zone for nausea, appears to be an important site of action for amylin (24,25). The effects of amylin on food intake and gastric emptying are abolished when lesions are placed in the area postrema or with bilateral vagotomy. With its multiple effects on glucose regulation, amylin acts as a partner hormone to insulin to help maintain normal glucose levels, especially in the postprandial state.

Table 2 Potential Targets/Mechanisms for Adjunctive Agents in Patients with Type 1 Diabetes Mellitus

Adjunctive therapy	Agent	Main mechanism(s) of action
Enhancement of insulin action	Metformin	Reduces hepatic glucose production
	Thiazolidinediones	Activate PPARγ receptor
Alteration of gastrointestinal nutrient delivery	Pramlintide	Slows nutrient delivery to the small intestine and suppresses glucagon secretion
	Incretin therapies	
	Alpha-glucosidase inhibitors	Delays carbohydrate digestion

PPARγ = peroxisome proliferator-activated receptor
Source: Adapted from Ref. 67.

POTENTIAL TREATMENTS FOR ADJUNCTIVE THERAPY IN TYPE 1 DIABETES

It is nearly impossible to normalize postprandial glucose excursions with SC insulin alone, without causing hypoglycemia. Given the limitations of insulin therapy, there is a need for adjunctive therapies to safely improve glycemic control in people with type 1 diabetes. An ideal adjunctive agent would minimize postprandial glucose excursions, without increasing the risks for hypoglycemia and weight gain. Potential targets for pharmacologic intervention are listed in Table 2.

Of the compounds listed, only pramlintide has been approved by the United States Food and Drug Administration (FDA) as adjunctive therapy in patients with type 1 diabetes.

PRAMLINTIDE

Background

In theory, through its multiple mechanisms to control postprandial glucose excursions, the physiologic replacement of amylin might address many of the shortcomings of insulin therapy. However, amylin is unsuitable as a pharmacologic intervention due to its tendency to precipitate from solution. To overcome this limitation, an analog to amylin, Pramlintide, was developed by substituting proline for the amino acid residues at 25 (alanine), 28 (serine), and 29 (serine) (26). In animal and human studies, pramlintide mimics the actions of amylin to blunt postprandial glucose excursions by slowing gastric emptying, suppressing postprandial glucagon secretion, and by decreasing food intake (27). In March 2005, pramlintide was approved by the US FDA as an adjunctive therapy in people with type 1 or type 2 diabetes and who fail to attain adequate glycemic control despite optimal insulin therapy.

Studies in Type 1 Diabetes

When administered in physiologic doses to people with type 1 diabetes, injections of pramlintide result in sustained reductions in A1c associated with significant blunting of the glucose response to a standardized meal. In addition, significant reductions in the postprandial concentrations of triglycerides, and of several measures of oxidative stress:

nitrotyrosine, oxidated-LDL, and total radical-trapping antioxidant parameter have been reported (28–30).

Several long-term, randomized, placebo-controlled trials of pramlintide in people with type 1 diabetes have shown consistent reductions in A1c accompanied by modest weight loss. In all of the studies, patients treated with pramlintide experienced a two- to threefold higher rate of nausea than those in the placebo group. Most of the nausea was described as mild to moderate and tended to decrease in frequency and severity with time (31–33). In one study, only 7.4% of subjects on pramlintide discontinued the study due to nausea (33). In a large 52-week trial, the SC administration of 60 μg of pramlintide three or four times per day led to a reduction in A1c of 0.29% and 0.34%, respectively. Both groups treated with pramlintide experienced a modest weight loss of 0.4 kg, compared to weight gain of 0.8 kg in the placebo group. Those treated with pramlintide experienced a fourfold higher rate of severe hypoglycemia, the frequency of which decreased to levels below that of the placebo group after the first 4 weeks. Investigators were asked to maintain constant insulin doses, unless hypoglycemia occurred (32). In contrast, the SC administration of 30 and 60 μg of pramlintide in another trial resulted in a placebo-adjusted 0.27% reduction in A1c and 1.5 kg weight loss without an increase in risk of severe hypoglycemia. The lower rate of severe hypoglycemia in this study is likely due to the protocol allowance of investigator-initiated reductions in the dose of insulin at the initiation of study drug.

Analysis of the results of these trials prompted the manufacturer to recommend aggressive reduction in prandial insulin doses upon the introduction of pramlintide. A recent study, comparing the addition of pramlintide or placebo to maximized insulin therapy, showed that a prospective 30% to 50% reduction in prandial insulin dose resulted in a marked reduction in the risk of severe hypoglycemia in both groups. Starting at a baseline average 8%, A1c was reduced by 0.5% in both groups, but those on pramlintide experienced weight loss, lower postprandial glucose levels and lower triglyceride levels (31). Subjects treated with continuous SC insulin infusion were evaluated with continuous glucose monitoring before, during, and after 30 μg pramlintide t.i.d. was added to their preexisting regimen. To avoid hypoglycemia, the baseline insulin dosage was reduced by at least 10% at the initiation of pramlintide therapy. Compared to baseline measures, mean 24-hour glucose concentration was significantly reduced by the addition of 30 μg pramlintide t.i.d. to preexisting continuous SC insulin infusion. The number of glucose measurements above 140 mg/dL decreased from 59% to 48%, without an increase in those below 80 mg/dL (29).

The optimal timing of pramlintide was studied in 38 subjects with type 1 diabetes given a standardized mixed meal. Insulin doses were adjusted before the study, but kept constant for each of the five meal tests. Relative to the meal, the subjects were given regular insulin at −30 minutes or insulin lispro at 0 minute in addition to either placebo at −15 minutes or pramlintide 60 μg at −15, 0, +15, and +30 minutes. Glucose area under the curve was significantly lower after each pramlintide treatment, but only preprandial pramlintide dosing blunted the immediate postprandial rise. Those receiving insulin lispro and pramlintide immediately before meals had a reduction in glucose at 60 minutes but experienced a gradual rise in glucose for the remainder of the 6-hour study. Postprandial glucose levels appeared to be more stable in those treated with regular insulin. There were no episodes of severe hypoglycemia in this study (34) (Fig. 2).

Clinical Use of Pramlintide in Type 1 Diabetes

Patients with type 1 diabetes who have failed to achieve adequate glycemic control despite optimal insulin therapy are candidates for therapy with pramlintide. For optimal response

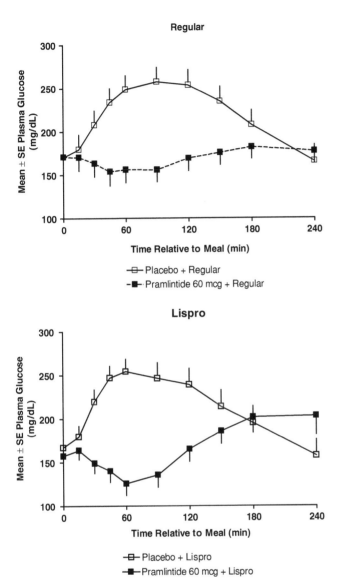

Figure 2 Comparison of regular insulin versus insulin lispro on postprandial glucose profiles following pramlintide versus placebo injections. *Source*: Data from Ref. 34.

and safety, care should be taken to select appropriate patients. Certain clinical features predict either a poor response to or an increased risk with pramlintide therapy. It should not be used in patients who fail to keep appointments with the diabetes care team, have demonstrated poor adherence to their insulin regimen or glucose monitoring schedule, and in those with hypoglycemia unawareness or recurrent severe hypoglycemia. People with a confirmed diagnosis of gastroparesis or severe renal failure are unlikely to tolerate pramlintide, due to gastrointestinal side effects (35). In the prescribing information, the manufacturer suggests that pramlintide should not be used when A1c > 9.0%, however a consensus of diabetes experts agreed that an A1c > 10% may be more reflective of problematic adherence issues.

If the patient appears to be a good candidate for pramlintide, they should be counseled to help them balance realistic expectations for the benefits with the cost, the side effects, and the risk for hypoglycemia. If they wish to proceed, the patient should be asked to perform pre- and postprandial glucose measurements and to keep a detailed dietary and exercise log for at least 1 week prior to initiation of pramlintide therapy. Most patients will benefit from at least one visit to a diabetes educator who is experienced in the use of pramlintide. Many diabetes educators have training and experience to counsel the patient on appropriate adjustments in diet and insulin doses that might be needed when pramlintide in started. Prior to starting pramlintide, insulin therapy should be optimized with a physiologic regimen using basal–bolus insulin replacement via multiple daily injections or an insulin pump. In the event that basal insulin dose exceeds 50% of the total daily dose of insulin, additional office visits may be needed to optimize their baseline insulin regimen prior to the addition of pramlintide therapy.

The excess risk for insulin-induced severe hypoglycemia, reported in the early pramlintide clinical trials, can be minimized by reducing the dose of prandial insulin by as much as 50% prior to the initiation of pramlintide (35). If patients are counting carbohydrates, their insulin to carbohydrate ratio should be reduced. For example, if the patient is using a ratio of 1 U per 15 g of carbohydrate, it should be reduced to 1 U per 20 to 30 g of carbohydrate. Patients should be cautioned about using correction insulin, but if used, the correction factor should also be doubled. While a 50% reduction will likely eliminate any increase in risk for hypoglycemia, it often frustrates the patient due to the frequent occurrence of marked hyperglycemia. The expert members of the consensus panel agreed that, in many cases, a reduction of prandial insulin in the range of 25% to 50% may be more appropriate (36). Furthermore, if basal insulin represents more than 50% of the total daily dose, it should be decreased by 50% (37).

Because pramlintide induces satiety, postmeal administration of the rapid acting analog will ensure appropriate insulin dosing for the actual amount of carbohydrate ingested. For patients using insulin pumps, the prandial insulin can either be given after the meal or premeal, as a 1-hour extended bolus. Premeal regular insulin is an option for those on multiple daily injections who have difficulty remembering a postmeal injection.

To minimize gastrointestinal side effects, pramlintide should be started at a low dose and increased as tolerated. As recommended by the manufacturer, an initial dose of 15 µg (2.5 U) should be given immediately before carbohydrate-containing meals at least 2 inches away the site of the insulin injection. After at least 3 days without clinically significant nausea or hypoglycemia, the dose should be titrated at 15 µg (2.5 U) increments to a maintenance dose of 30 µg (5.0 U) or 60 µg (10 U), as tolerated. If a patient is unable to tolerate the 15 µg starting dose, it may be reasonable to reduce the starting dose to as low as 6 µg (1 U) and titrate using smaller increments. Those unable to titrate to the full dose of 60 µg t.i.d. should be encouraged to increase their dose slowly to the maximally tolerated dose. An alternative protocol is reported to be easier to implement. Pramlintide can be started at a dose of 12 µg (2 U) t.i.d., increasing by increments of 6 µg (1 U) every other day until reaching the target dose of 60 µg (10 U) (38). At the same time, mealtime insulin should be decreased by 25%.

It is recommended that pramlintide and insulin be given at different injections sites, however, no significant effects were seen when pramlintide was mixed with human regular, NPH or 70/30 insulins (39). Although far from uniform, obese patients with type 1 diabetes often experience fewer gastrointestinal side effects from pramlintide and may tolerate, and benefit, from increasing the dose beyond the recommended dose of 60 µg.

Within the first week after starting pramlintide, patient contact in the form of an office visit, phone call or email is encouraged. There is considerable variation in the length of time it takes for patients to reach stable glucose levels, but it may take 1 to 2 months after the addition of pramlintide. During that time, frequent contacts with the health-care team will likely be needed. Patients should be encouraged to contact the health-care team in the event of intolerable side effects, severe hypoglycemia, or marked fluctuations in blood glucose levels. A referral to an experienced diabetes educator to supervise the initiation of pramlintide therapy will often ease the transition for patient and for their provider.

An individual's response to therapy can be quite variable, but is best be evaluated by frequent self-monitoring of blood glucose or continuous glucose monitoring. Once stabilized, most patients will note a decrease in their average blood sugar accompanied by an improvement in the variability of their blood sugars. While weight loss is a goal for many who decide to start pramlintide, the effects are generally modest, averaging 1 to 2 kg (32,33). To avoid disappointment, realistic expectations must be presented at the outset. Although no studies have reported data about changes in quality of life with pramlintide therapy, patients frequently report an improvement in overall sense of well-being as a benefit of the use of pramlintide. The mechanism for this is unknown, but may be due to blunted glycemic excursions (37).

METFORMIN

Background

Metformin, an oral antihyperglycemic agent, has been used in the therapy of type 2 diabetes for over 40 years. Through mechanisms that have been incompletely defined, metformin lowers fasting glucose by 25% to 30%, primarily by reducing the excessive hepatic gluconeogenesis that characterizes type 2 diabetes. Studies also point to the contribution of improved insulin-stimulated glucose uptake by peripheral tissues to metformin's effects on glycemic control (40). When added to insulin therapy in patients with type 2 diabetes, metformin is associated with an improved in glycemic control and up to a 50% reduction in insulin requirements (41). Therapy with metformin is also associated with improved lipoprotein profile, increased fibrinolysis, and a modest weight loss, all of which may contribute to the 39% reduction in risk for myocardial infarction that was seen in the UKPDS 34 study.

Studies of Metformin in Type 1 Diabetes

Theoretically, metformin, through its effects on hepatic glucose output, might improve glycemic control in people with type 1 diabetes who fail to reach glycemic targets despite optimal insulin and dietary therapies. When metformin 850 mg t.i.d. was added to insulin in 15 subjects with type 1 diabetes, insulin requirements, as measured by an artificial pancreas, decreased by 25.8% (42). Several small studies have assessed the effects of the addition of metformin to background insulin therapy in type 1 diabetes: a placebo corrected reduction in A1c of 0.6% to 1.1%, a reduction in insulin dose, but variable effects on weight were demonstrated (43–46). In the studies that included measures on insulin sensitivity, an inverse relationship between baseline insulin sensitivity and reduction in A1c was evident (44). The largest study evaluated the addition of metformin to continuous SC insulin infusion in 62 c-peptide negative adolescents with average BMI of 26 kg/m^2. There was no apparent improvement in glucose control, as measured by A1c. However, the mean baseline A1c level of 7.4% was much lower than was reported in the other studies. A 7.9% reduction in the requirement for basal insulin was noted with metformin treatment, compared with an increase of 2.8% with placebo. Metformin also exerted a beneficial effect on LDL cholesterol (201 ± 27 vs. 185 ± 26 mg/dL). There was no significant difference in weight or rate of hypoglycemia between the treatment groups. Overall, the safety profile of metformin treatment was excellent. However, 5% of the metformin-treated group was unable to complete the study due to mild to moderate gastrointestinal side effects (47). The authors report that a subset of their study subjects experienced 20% or greater reduction in insulin requirements with stable and satisfactory glucose control, but they were unable to identify criteria that might predict response (48). In contrast, in a 16-week study of 15 of overweight adults with type 1 diabetes with a mean BMI of 31 kg/m^2, treatment with metformin 850 mg t.i.d. was associated with a fall in A1c from 8.5% to 7.8%, compared to no change in the placebo group. Fasting glucose levels fell by 56 mg/dL and insulin requirements were 16% lower in the metformin group at the end of the study. The improvement in glucose control with metformin occurred without an increased risk for hypoglycemia. Like previous studies, weight did not change with metformin treatment in this study (43).

Clinical Use of Metformin in Type 1 Diabetes

There is little data to guide the clinician on the use of metformin in patients with type 1 diabetes. Given the data above, metformin may improve glucose control in overweight patients with type 1 diabetes without increasing the risk for hypoglycemia. It is contraindicated in chronic renal failure, congestive heart failure, and severe hepatic disease. Although gastrointestinal side effects occur in up to 30% of treated patients, only 5% of subjects with type 2 diabetes rated them as severe enough to stop treatment (41). If a trial of therapy with metformin is appropriate, it is reasonable to use current recommendations for people with type 2 diabetes: start metformin at 500 mg once or twice daily and gradually increase the dose up to 2000 mg per day or to the maximum tolerated dose. Due to its insulin sparing effect, when metformin is added to insulin therapy in patients with type 1 diabetes, basal insulin dose should be reduced by 10% to 20%. Metformin therapy should be discontinued if glucose control fails to improve, when measured by A1c, frequency of hypoglycemia or by glucose excursions. Metformin should not be used in people at high risk for lactic acidosis, especially those with significant renal or hepatic disease.

THIAZOLIDINEDIONES

Background

Thiazolidinediones (TZDs), through stimulation of the peroxisome-proliferator-activated receptor gamma (PPARγ), improve glucose control in type 2 diabetes by enhancing insulin-mediated glucose uptake. In animal and human subjects, insulin resistance contributes to the risk for cardiovascular disease, through its association with several key risk factors for cardiovascular disease: hyperglycemia, hypertension, dyslipidemia, abnormal fibrinolysis, and inflammation. The most important site of action of TZDs is in the adipose tissue, where these medications have been shown to regulate the secretion of several adipocyte products (adipokines) that play a major role in insulin sensitivity, endothelial dysfunction, and atherosclerosis (49). In addition to lowering the concentrations of free fatty acids, insulin and glucose, therapy with TZD's have been shown to improve many of the traditional and nontraditional risk factors for cardiovascular disease (50). The addition of the TZD, rosiglitazone, to insulin therapy in subjects with type 2 diabetes, resulted in a reduction of A1c from a baseline value of 9.0% to 7.9%, accompanied by a 12% reduction in insulin requirements after 26 weeks (51). Additionally, subjects with type 2 diabetes and cardiovascular disease had a 16% reduction in the secondary composite endpoint of all-cause mortality, myocardial infarcts, and stroke when pioglitazone (vs. placebo) was added to their glycemic regimen (52), suggesting a cardiovascular benefit of specifically treating insulin resistance in this population. When a TZD is added to insulin in subjects with type 2 diabetes, significant edema occurs in about 15%, sometimes precipitating congestive heart failure. Other common side effects include mild anemia and weight gain.

Studies of Thiazolidinediones in Type 1 Diabetes

Given that intensive control of type 1 diabetes is associated with a very high prevalence of obesity and metabolic syndrome, it seems reasonable to consider using these agents in those who have not achieved adequate glycemic control on intensive insulin regimens.

However, only one study testing the effects of the addition of a TZD to insulin therapy in type 1 diabetes has been published. Fifty adult subjects with type 1 diabetes and a BMI ≥ 27 kg/m^2 were randomized to receive either rosiglitazone 4 mg twice daily or placebo for 8 months. Changes in the insulin regimen were encouraged in both groups. Patients in both treatment arms experienced a reduction in A1c of approximately 1%, without a significant differences between the groups. Total daily insulin dose decreased by an average of 2 U in the subjects taking rosiglitazone, but increased by an average of 8 U in the subjects taking placebo. The average weight increased by approximately 3 kg in both groups. In the subset of subjects with BMI ≥ 30 kg/m^2, those treated with rosiglitazone experienced a significantly greater reduction in A1c of 1.4% compared to a reduction of 0.64% in those receiving placebo (53). The change in A1c in the rosiglitazone arm correlated inversely with an estimate of insulin sensitivity (54). Another study suggests that early introduction of TZD therapy in patients with latent autoimmune diabetes of the adult (LADA) may help to preserve islet beta cell function. In a small study, the addition of rosiglitazone to SC insulin therapy in patients with LADA appeared to preserve c-peptide response to glucose when compared to those treated with insulin alone (55). Pioglitazone is another thizaolidinedione approved for treatment of type 2 diabetes, however no clinical studies using this agent in type 1 diabetes have been published to date.

Clinical Use of Thiazolidinediones in Type 1 Diabetes

Although there is very little data to guide the use of TZDs in type 1 diabetes, it appears that a subset of obese subjects might benefit with improvement in glycemic control and decrease in insulin requirements and may also benefit from their putative cardioprotective actions. If, after carefully weighing the risks and benefits, a trial of a TZD is deemed to be worthwhile, insulin doses should be decreased by about 10% upon initiation of the thiazolidinedione. Close follow-up is essential to evaluate insulin therapy, determine effectiveness, and to watch for side effects. If no clinical response is evident by 3 to 6 months, therapy should be discontinued. TZDs should not be used in people with stage III or IV congestive heart failure or severe liver disease.

ALPHA-GLUCOSIDASE INHIBITORS

Background

Acarbose, through the inhibition of intestinal alpha-glucosidase enzyme, delays the absorption of ingested carbohydrates.

Studies of Alpha-Glucosidase Inhibitors in Type 1 Diabetes

Although only approved in the United States for management of type 2 diabetes, the results of several small studies in type 1 diabetes have been reported. The acute administration of up to 200 mg of acarbose, with a test meal, to subjects with type 1 diabetes is associated with a 20% to 30% reduction in postprandial glucose levels and a 40% reduction in insulin requirements as compared to placebo treatment (56,57). The chronic administration of acarbose also lowers postprandial glucose levels, but has a variable effect on A1c levels. In an open-label 16 week study of 62 adults with type 1 diabetes, given acarbose at daily dose of 75 to 300 mg, A1c fell from 8.5% to 8.2%. Compared to baseline, only the postlunch glucose levels were significantly lower with acarbose treatment (58). In contrast, a 24-week double-blind, placebo-controlled multicenter trial of acarbose in 121 subjects with type 1 diabetes demonstrated no difference in A1c, despite a 47 mg/dL average reduction of postprandial glucose levels (59). When acarbose 300 mg t.i.d. was compared to placebo as adjunctive therapy to insulin in 264 subjects with type 1 diabetes, a reduction in postmeal glucose of 59 mg/dL was accompanied by a 0.48% improvement in A1c after 36 weeks (60). Dose-dependent side effects of flatulence and diarrhea occurred in up to 75% of patients treated with acarbose, approximately double that of the placebo-treated subjects (59). Two other alpha-glucosidase inhibitors have been marketed. However, these agents have not been specifically studied in type 1 diabetes.

Clinical Use of Alpha-Glucosidase Inhibitors in Type 1 Diabetes

Very limited guidance exists for the use of these agents in type 1 diabetes. Based upon the clinical trial results, these agents may be helpful to decrease postprandial glucose levels in patients with poorly controlled type 1 diabetes. If used, they should be initiated at the usual starting dose of 25 mg with the first bite of each carbohydrate-containing meal and titrated up according to response and tolerability. The maximum dose of acarbose is 100 mg t.i.d with meals, though doses above 50 mg t.i.d. are not recommended for those weighing less than 60 kg. They should not be used in patients with liver disease. Adjustment in insulin doses should be based upon the evaluation of postprandial glucose levels before and after the initiation of therapy. Therapy should be discontinued if postprandial glucose levels or A1c do not improve within 3 months. Obviously the side effect profile may limit the widespread application of these medications in type 1 diabetes.

INCRETIN THERAPIES

Background

Through multiple mechanisms, the intestinal hormones, glucagon-like intestinal peptide-1 (GLP-1), and gastric inhibitory polypeptide (GIP) pay an important role in the regulation of the glycemic response to carbohydrate ingestion. Both GLP-1 and GIP stimulate insulin secretion in response to food. GLP-1, but not GIP, has other important glycemic actions including suppression of the secretion of glucagon by the pancreatic alpha cell, slowing of gastric emptying and suppression of food intake. The combined actions of the incretins contribute to limit the rise in glucose in the postprandial state in individuals with normal glucose metabolism (21). Meal tolerance tests indicate that postprandial GLP-1 secretion is deficient in type 2 diabetes. Acutely, treatment with IV infusions of GLP-1 nearly normalizes blood glucose levels and leads to weight loss in subjects with type 2 diabetes (61). Studies also suggest that GLP-1 may increase the number of beta cells in animal models of diabetes by increasing beta cell proliferation and neogenesis and by reducing the rate of apoptosis (62). GLP-1 receptor agonists and inhibitors of the enzymatic inactivation of GLP-1 have been developed for the treatment of type 2 diabetes.

Studies in Type 1 Diabetes

In c-peptide positive type 1 diabetes, the administration of IV infusion of GLP-1, in place of prandial insulin, prevented the rise in glucose level after a carbohydrate-containing meal. Supression of postprandial glucagon secretion and slowing of the delivery of gastric contents to the small intestine likely contributed to the blunting of the glycemic excursion in this study. The effect of GLP-1 on insulin secretion in this population was not reported (63). When given to subjects with c-peptide negative type 1 diabetes, a SC injection of GLP-1 along with usual doses of preprandial insulin blunted the rise in postprandial glucose levels. Not surprisingly, there was no demonstrable increase in insulin levels (64). Similar effects were seen when the GLP-1 receptor agonist, Exenatide-4 was given subcutaneously at a dose of 0.03 μg/kg 15 minutes before a test meal along with usual prandial insulin dose to subjects with c-peptide negative type 1 diabetes. It effectively reduced the postprandial excursion of glucose 15 to 60 minute delay in gastric emptying was demonstrated by measuring the rate of appearance of a dose of acetaminophen given concurrently with the meal (65).

The results of several small studies suggest that incretin therapies may have a role to improve the outcomes of islet cell transplants. When exenatide was given to patients with secondary islet cell graft failure, glucose levels normalized, preventing the need for insulin therapy in two patients. An additional eight patients, already on insulin therapy, had a significant reduction in their insulin requirements (28). When given at the time of islet transplantation, exenatide decreased the number of islet cell transplantations needed for insulin independence (66).

SUMMARY

Optimal insulin therapy, using insulin analogues and modern patient self-management techniques, is not sufficient to achieve near-normoglycemia in the majority of our patients. Several classes of therapeutic agents look promising as adjunctive therapy for patients with type 1 diabetes, including pramlintide, metformin, thiazolidinediones, alpha glucosidase inhibitors, and incretin therapies. Of these, only pramlintide is approved to be used in this setting. When pramlintide is added to an optimal insulin regimen, it helps to meet the goals of many patients by improving control of postprandial glucose levels, reducing glycemic variability, and inducing satiety and modest weight loss. However, in the obese patient with suboptimally controlled type 1 diabetes, therapy with metformin or a thiazolidinedione appears to be safe and may be helpful to improve glycemic control. Weight gain, however, is a complication of thiazolidinedione therapy. Whatever adjunctive therapy is used, careful selection of patients with good self-management skills will be necessary to minimize the occurrence of severe hypoglycemia that might result. During the transition, patients should be advised of the potential risk of hypoglycemia and should be encouraged to test pre- and postprandial blood glucose levels, particularly when using agents with predominant postprandial effects such as pramlintide and alpha-glucosidase inhibitors. At present, the use of incretin mimetics in type 1 diabetes should be limited to clinical trials to better understand their role, if any in this patient population. The data suggesting that thiazolidinediones and incretin therapies may slow the loss of beta cells warrants further study in newly diagnosed patients with type 1 diabetes or with latent autoimmune diabetes of the adult.

REFERENCES

1. The Diabetes Control and Complications Trial Research Group. The effect of intensive treatment of diabetes on the development and progression of long-term complications in insulin-dependent diabetes mellitus. N Engl J Med 1993;329(14):977–986.
2. American Diabetes Association. Standards of medical care in diabetes—2006. Diabetes Care 2006;29(suppl 1):S4–S42.
3. The Diabetes Control and Complications Trial/Epidemiology of Diabetes Interventions and Complications Research Group. Retinopathy and nephropathy in patients with type 1 diabetes four years after a trial of intensive therapy. N Engl J Med 2000;342(6):381–389.
4. Bulsara MK, Holman CD, Davis EA, Jones TW. The impact of a decade of changing treatment on rates of severe hypoglycemia in a population-based cohort of children with type 1 diabetes. Diabetes Care 2004;27(10):2293–2298.
5. Scottish Study Group for the Care of the Young. Factors influencing glycemic control in young people with type 1 diabetes in Scotland: A population-based study (DIABAUD2). Diabetes Care 2001;24(2):239–244.
6. The French Pediatric Diabetes Group: Rosilio M, Cotton JB, Wieliczko MC, et al. Factors associated with glycemic control. A cross-sectional nationwide study in 2,579 French children with type 1 diabetes. The French Pediatric Diabetes Group. Diabetes Care 1998;21(7):1146–1153.
7. Danne T, Morensen HB, Hougaard P, et al. Persistent differences among centers over 3 years in glycemic control and hypoglycemia in a study of 3,805 children and adolescents with type 1 diabetes from the Hvidore study group. Diabetes Care 2001;24(8):132–1347.
8. Cryer PE. Hypoglycaemia: The limiting factor in glycaemic management of type 1 and type 2 diabetes. Diabetologia 2002;45:937–948.
9. The Diabetes Control and Complications Trial Research Group. Influence of intensive diabetes treatment on body weight and composition of adults with type 1 diabetes in the Diabetes Control and Complications Trial. Diabetes Care 2001;24(10):1711–1721.
10. Kaufman F. Consequences of weight gain associated with insulin therapy in adolescents. Endocrinologist 2006;16(3):155–162.
11. Martin FIR, Hopper JL. The relationship of acute insulin sensitivity to the porgression of vascular disease in long-term type 1 (insulin-dependent) diabetes mellitus. Diabetologia 1987;30(3):149–153.
12. Purnell JQ, Hokanson JE, Santica M, et al. Effect of excessive weight gain with intensive therapy of type 1 diabetes on lipid levels and blood pressure: Results From the DCCT. JAMA 1998;280(2):140–146.
13. Schaumberg DA, Glynn RJ, Jenkins AJ, et al. Effect of intensive glycemic control on levels of markers of inflammation in type 1 diabetes mellitus in the Diabetes Control and Complications Trial. Circulation 2005;111(19):2446–2453.
14. Orchard TJ, Olson JC, Erbey JR, et al. Insulin resistance-related factors, but not glycemia, predict coronary artery disease in type 1 diabetes: 10-year follow-up data from the Pittsburgh Epidemiology of Diabetes Complications Study. Diabetes Care 2003;26(5):1374–1379.
15. Rydall AC, Rodin GM, Olmsted MP, et al. Disodered eating behavior and microvascular complications in young women wtih insulin-dependent diabetes mellitus. N Engl J Med 1997;336:1849–1854.
16. Boland E, Monsod T, Delucia M, et al. Limitations of conventional methods of self-monitoring of blood glucose: Lessons learned from 3 days of continuous glucose sensing in pediatric patients with type 1 diabetes. Diabetes Care 2001;24(11):1858–1862.
17. The Diabetes Control and Complication Research. The relationship of glycemic exposure (HbA1c) to the risk of development and progression of retinopathy in the diabetes control and complications trial. Diabetes 1995;44(8):968–983.

18. Dyck PJ, Davies JL, Clark VM, et al. Modeling chronic glycemic exposure variables as correlates and predictors of microvascular complications of diabetes. Diabetes Care 2006;29(10):2282–2288.
19. The Diabetes Control and Complication Research. The absence of a glycemic threshold for the development of long-term complications: The perspective of the Diabetes Control and Complications Trial. Diabetes 1996;45(10):1289–1298.
20. Ceriello A. Postprandial hyperglycemia and diabetes complications: Is it time to treat? Diabetes 2005;54(1):1–7.
21. Riddle MC, Drucker DJ. Emerging therapies mimicking the effects of amylin and glucagon-like peptide 1. Diabetes Care 2006;29(2):435–449.
22. Koda JE, Fineman M, Rink TJ, et al. Amylin concentrations and glucose control. Lancet 1992;339(8802):1179–1180.
23. Brownlee M, Hirsch IB. Glycemic variability: A hemoglobin A1c-independent risk factor for diabetic complications. JAMA 2006;295(14):1707–1708.
24. Beaumont K, Kenney MA, Young AA, Rink TJ. High affinity amylin binding sites in rat brain. Mol Pharmacol 1993;44(3):493–497.
25. Rushing P. Central amylin signaling and the regulation of energy homeostasis. Curr Pharm Des 2003;9(10):819–827.
26. Kruger DF, Gloster MA. Pramlintide for the treatment of insulin-requiring diabetes mellitus: Rationale and review of clinical data. Drugs 2004;64(13):1419–1432.
27. Edelman SV, Weyer C. Unresolved challenges with insulin therapy in type 1 and type 2 diabetes: Potential benefit of replacing amylin, a second beta-cell hormone. Diabetes Technol Ther 2002;4(2):175–189.
28. Thompson RG, Peterson J, Gottlieb A, Mullane J. Effects of pramlintide, an analog of human amylin, on plasma glucose profiles in patients with IDDM: Results of a multicenter trial. Diabetes 1997;46(4):632–636.
29. Levetan C, Want LL, Weyer C, et al. Impact of pramlintide on glucose fluctuations and postprandial glucose, glucagon, and triglyceride excursions among patients with type 1 diabetes intensively treated with insulin pumps. Diabetes Care 2003;26(1):1–8.
30. Ceriello A, Piconi L, Quagliaro L, et al. Effects of pramlintide on postprandial glucose excursions and measures of oxidative stress in patients with type 1 diabetes. Diabetes Care 2005;28(3):632–627.
31. Edelman S, Garg S, Frias J, et al. A double-blind, placebo-controlled trial assessing pramlintide treatment in the setting of intensive insulin therapy in type1 diabetes. Diabetes Care 2006;29(10):2189–2195.
32. Ratner RE, Dickey R, Fineman M, et al. Amylin replacement with pramlintide as an adjunct to insulin therapy improves long-term glycaemic and weight control in type 1 diabetes mellitus: A 1-year, randomized controlled trial. Diabet Med 2004;21(11):1204–1212.
33. Whitehouse F, Kruger DF, Fineman M, et al. A randomized study and open-label extension evaluating the long-term efficacy of pramlintide as an adjunct to insulin therapy in type 1 diabetes. Diabetes Care 2002;25(4):724–730.
34. Weyer C, Gottlieb A, Kim DD, et al. Pramlintide reduces postprandial glucose excursions when added to regular insulin or insulin lispro in subjects with type 1 diabetes: A dose-timing study. Diabetes Care 2003;26(11):3074–3079.
35. Symlin, (pramlintide acetate) injection (package insert). San Diego, California: Amylin Pharmaceuticals, Inc. 2005.
36. Hirsch IB, et al. Consensus Development Conference on Pramlintide in the Management of Type 1 and Type 2 Diabetes. The Diabetes Education Group, Lakeville, CT, 2006.
37. Want L, Ratner R. Pramlintide: A new tool in diabetes management. Curr Diab Rep 2006;(6):344–349.
38. Want L. Use of pramlintide: The patient's perspective. Diabetes Educ 2006;32(Suppl 3):111S–118S.
39. Weyer C, Fineman MS, Strobel S, et al. Properties of pramlintide and insulin upon mixing. Am J Health Syst Pharm 2005;62(8):816–822.

40. Kirpichnikov D, McFarlane SI, Sowers JR. Metformin: An Update. Ann Intern Med 2002; 137(1):25–33.

41. DeFronzo RA. Pharmacologic therapy for type 2 diabetes mellitus. Ann Intern Med 1999;131(4): 281–303.

42. Pagano G, Tagliaferro V, Carta Q, et al. Metformin reduces insulin requirement in type 1(insulin-dependent) diabetes. Diabetologia 1983;24(5):351–354.

43. Khan AS, McLoughney CR, Ahmed AB. The effect of metformin on blood glucose control in overweight patients with type 1 diabetes. Diabet Med 2006;23(10):1079–1084.

44. Sarnblad S, Kroon M, Aman J. Metformin as additional therapy in adolescents with poorly controlled type 1 diabetes: Randomised placebo-controlled trial with aspects on insulin sensitivity. Eur J Endocrinol 2003;149(4):323–329.

45. Urakami T, Morimoto S, Owada M, Harada K. Usefulness of the addition of metformin to insulin in pediatric patients with type 1 diabetes mellitus. Pediatr Int 2005;47(4):430–433.

46. Hamilton J, Cummings E, Zdravkovic V, et al. Metformin as an adjunct therapy in adolescents with type 1 diabetes and insulin resistance: A randomized controlled trial. Diabetes Care 2003;26(1):138–143.

47. Meyer L, Bohme P, Delbachian I, et al. The benefits of metformin therapy during continuous subcutaneous insulin infusion treatment of type 1 diabetic patients. Diabetes Care 2002;25(12):2153–2158.

48. Meyer L, Guerci B. Metformin and insulin in type 1 diabetes: The first step. Diabetes Care 2003;26(5):1655–1666.

49. Yki-Jarvinen H. Thiazolidinediones. N Engl J Med 2004;351(11):1106–1118.

50. Kunhiraman BP, Jawa A, Fonseca VA. Potential cardiovascular benefits of insulin sensitizers. Endocrin Metabol Clin N Am 2005;34(1):117–135.

51. Raskin P, Rendell M, Riddle MC, et al. A randomized trial of rosiglitazone therapy in patients with inadequately controlled insulin-treated type 2 diabetes. Diabetes Care 2001;24(7):1226–1232.

52. Dormandy JA, Charbonnel B, Eckland DJA, et al. Secondary prevention of macrovascular events in patients with type 2 diabetes in the PROactive study (PROspective pioglitAzone Clinical Trial In macroVascular Events): A randomised cotnrolled trial. Lancet 2005;366(9493):1279–1289.

53. Strowig SM, Raskin P. The effect of rosiglitazone on overweight subjects with type 1 diabetes. Diabetes Care 2005;28(7):1562–1567.

54. Strowig SM, Raskin P. The effect of rosiglitazone on overweight subjects with type 1 diabetes. Response to Orchard. Diabetes Care 2006;29(3):747.

55. Zhou Z, Li X, Huang G, et al. Rosiglitazone combined with insulin preserves islet beta cell function in adult-onset latent autoimmune diabetes (LADA). Diabetes Metab Res Rev 2005;21(2):203–208.

56. Dimitriadis G, Karaiskos C, Raptis S. Effects of prolonged (6 months) alpha-glucosidase inhibition on blood glucose control and insulin requirements in patients with insulin-dependent diabetes mellitus. Horm Metab Res 1986;18(4):253–255.

57. Lecavalier L, Hamet P, Chiasson JL. The effects of sucrose meal on insulin requirement in IDDM and its modulation by acarbose. Diabetes Metab 1986;12(3):156–161.

58. Sels JP, Verdonk HE, Wolffenbuttel BH. Effects of acarbose (Glucobay) in persons with type 1 diabetes: A multicentre study. Diabetes Res Clin Pract 1998;41(2):139–145.

59. Riccardi G, Giacco R, Parillo M, et al. Efficacy and safety of acarbose in the treatment of type 1 diabetes mellitus: A placebo-controlled, double-blind, multicentre study. Diabet Med 1999;16(3):228–32.

60. Hollander P, Pi-Sunyer X, Coniff RF, Acarbose in the treatment of type I diabetes. Diabetes Care 1997;20(3):248–253.

61. Drucker DJ. Enhancing incretin action for the treatment of type 2 diabetes. Diabetes Care 2003;26:2929–2940.

62. Li Y, Hansotia T, Yusta B, et al. Glucagon-like peptide-1 receptor signaling modulates beta cell apoptosis. J Biol Chem 2003;278:471–478.

63. Dupre J, Behme MT, Hramiak, et al. Glucagon-like peptide 1 reduces postprandial glycemic excursions in IDDM. Diabetes 1995;44:626–630.

64. Behme MT, Dupre J, McDonald TJ. Glucagon-like peptide-1 improved glycaemic control in type 1 diabetes. BMC Endocr Disord 2002;3:3.
65. Dupre J, Behme MT, McDonald TJ. Exendin-4 normalized postcibal glycemic excursions in type 11 diabetes. J Clin Endocrinol Metab 2004;89(7):3469–3473.
66. Hatipoglu B, Avilla J, Benedetti E, et al. Exenatide combined with islet transplantation for the treatment of type i diabetes. Abstract 256-OR. In: 66th Scientific Sessions of the American Diabetes Association, Washington DC, 2006.
67. Jeffries CA, Hamilton J, Daneman D. Potential adjunctive therapies in adolescents with type 1 diabetes mellitus. Treat Endocrinol. 2004;3:337–343.

7
Hyperglycemia-Induced Tissue Damage: Pathways and Causes

K. K. Hood
Section on Behavioral and Mental Health Research, Section on Genetics and Epidemiology, Joslin Diabetes Center, Harvard Medical School, Boston, Massachusetts, U.S.A.

H. A. Keenan
Section on Vascular Cell Biology, Joslin Diabetes Center, Harvard Medical School, Boston, Massachusetts, U.S.A.

A. M. Jacobson
Section on Behavioral and Mental Health Research, Joslin Diabetes Center, Harvard Medical School, Boston, Massachusetts, U.S.A.

Since the initial findings from the Diabetes Control and Complications Trial (DCCT) were published in 1993 (1), the intensification of diabetes management to prevent or slow the onset of the complications associated with type 1 diabetes (T1D) has been a hallmark of diabetes treatment. The DCCT findings confirmed the strong link between hyperglycemia and the complications and put to rest a debate about the necessity of tight glycemic control [see (2) and (3) for the history of this debate]. During the past two decades, much attention has been paid to the mechanisms that promote hyperglycemia-induced tissue damage and to the potential ways to modify this process (4–6). The targeted population for intensified diabetes management may well be 2 million adults with T1D in the United States—based on the estimate of 10% of the 20.6 million diabetes patients (7). Further, the incidence of T1D appears to be increasing with a tendency toward younger age at onset (8–10). Taken together, there is a large population of individuals at risk for complications due to T1D with the likelihood of growing numbers in the future.

In this chapter, we discuss the evidence for hyperglycemia-induced tissue damage that results in the occurrence of complications and also address five topic areas: (*i*) complications that result from T1D, focusing on retinopathy and nephropathy as examples of microvascular complications and noting specific aspects of macrovascular complications, (*ii*) findings from the DCCT and several epidemiologic studies (11), as they directly relate to complications from T1D, (*iii*) findings concerning the pathways from hyperglycemia to tissue damage at the molecular level, highlighting the most accepted pathways and common links between them, (*iv*) the genetic and environmental factors that contribute to chronic hyperglycemia and eventually to long-term complications, and (*v*) the current momentum and

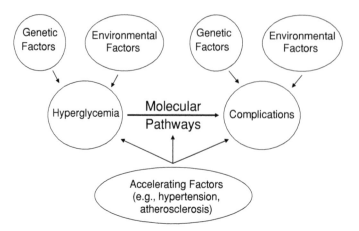

Figure 1 Pathways and mechanisms of hyperglycemia-induced tissue damage.

the potential future work for finding effective treatments and interventions for preventing or slowing the complications associated with T1D. The conceptual framework that illustrates these associated topic areas is depicted in Figure 1. There are genetic and environmental influences that promote both the occurrence of hyperglycemia as well as the progression to complications. Further, the link between hyperglycemia and complications occurs through several pathways that may be moderated by various accelerating factors.

COMPLICATIONS ASSOCIATED WITH T1D

T1D places demands on the individuals as well as their support system (i.e., spouses or partners, children); however, the physical consequences of T1D specifically affect the individuals. Many adults with T1D end up facing complications as the result of long-term exposure to fluctuations in glucose levels. Indeed, complications associated with T1D are typically initiated by chronic hyperglycemia (1). The most common microvascular complication of T1D is retinopathy; however, other common microvascular complications include nephropathy and neuropathy. Large-scale epidemiologic studies have found that nearly three-quarters of their samples with 20 years of T1D have retinopathy [e.g., Wisconsin data (12) and Pittsburgh data (13)] and rates of retinopathy are high in racial and ethnic minority groups (e.g., African-American) as evidenced by a 6-year progression to nonproliferative retinopathy of 56% and progression to proliferative retinopathy of 15% (14).

Much of what we know about the occurrence of complications associated with diabetes has developed from the DCCT and the Epidemiology of Diabetes Interventions and Complications (EDIC) study (11). The DCCT and EDIC data reflect a consistent and escalating relationship between glycemic levels and the occurrence of complications (Fig. 2). In other words, as glycemic control worsens, the risk of complications continuously increases. Recently, both Nathan (3) and Genuth (15) reviewed the DCCT and EDIC studies and highlighted the findings as they related to long-term complications. The main conclusions of the DCCT and EDIC studies include (*i*) the risks of three main microvascular complications (retinopathy, nephropathy, neuropathy) and the development of atherosclerosis are reduced by intensive treatment; (*ii*) intensive treatment should be implemented as early as possible; (*iii*) near-normoglycemia should be the target and efforts should be made to keep hemoglobin A1C as close to the normal range as possible; and (*iv*) the benefits of

A

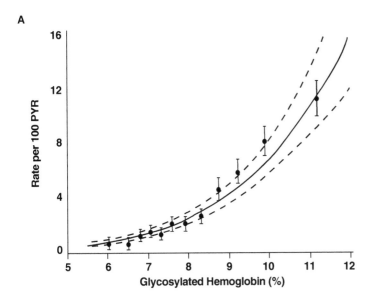

B

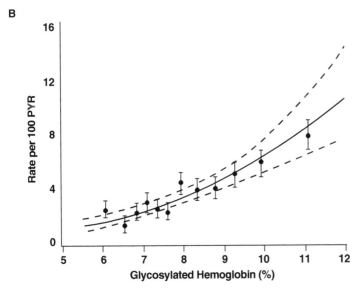

Figure 2 Glycemic control and complications (from DCCT/EDIC findings).

near-normoglycemia persist well after the start of intensive insulin therapy, as captured in the concept of "metabolic memory."

Participants in the DCCT were either part of a primary prevention cohort with no complications and 1 to 5 years of T1D or a secondary intervention cohort with mild microalbuminuria and 1 to 15 years of T1D. The benefits of intensive treatment were found in both groups; however, the benefit was stronger in the primary prevention cohort (1). For example, with regard to the incidence of retinopathy, there was a 76% reduction in the primary prevention group and 54% reduction in the secondary cohort as compared to those in the standard treatment arm. This supports the suggestion that early intervention, prior to the onset of complications, is beneficial and that tight control after developing complications can slow progression. Moreover, the intensively treated group continued to show sustained benefit, in comparison to the conventionally treated group, from prior tight control (16–18). The findings of similar A1C levels for both the intensively and conventionally treated groups during the EDIC follow-up further illustrates this notion of "metabolic memory" (18). In addition, as with other studies (12–14,19,20), there appears to be a "momentum" of retinopathy that becomes difficult to slow, even with intensive treatment. This is evidenced by the DCCT findings that those who entered the study with the highest baseline A1C values and the longest duration of diabetes were most resistant to changing the course of retinopathy development (1).

Nephropathy is another major microvascular complication associated with T1D and has the highest mortality rate of the complications. Rates of nephropathy in individuals with T1D can be best classified by rates of each of the various stages (i.e., microalbuminuria, proteinuria, and end-stage renal disease). Specific rates of microalbuminuria are highest, nearly reaching 60%, by 20 years (21,22). Proteinuria rates climb to nearly 30% by 20 years and end-stage renal disease occurs in nearly a quarter of patients by 35 years (23). However, DCCT and EDIC data show a clear benefit in terms of reduced nephropathy through intensive insulin therapy. After approximately 8 years, there was a sustained 59% reduction in rates of microalbuminuria and 84% reduction in frank albuminuria for the DCCT intensively treated cohort in comparison to the conventionally treated controls (18). Nephropathy is often initially detected as microalbuminuria and can proceed to proteinuria and end-stage renal disease; however, recent findings suggest that it is reversible at the microalbuminuria stage. Specifically, there was regression to normal albumin secretion in a large sample of T1D patients when there was a shorter duration of microalbuminuria and in the context of tightened glycemic control and other health-related factors (e.g., low systolic blood pressure, low serum cholesterol and triglycerides) (24).

Another class of complications associated with T1D affects the nervous system. Neuropathy often manifests as polyneuropathy, with the most common symptomatic form being distal symmetric polyneuropathy. Rates of neuropathy approach 70% after 30 years of T1D (13). Like nephropathy and retinopathy, the development and course of neuropathy was significantly impacted in the DCCT, with a 60% reduction of clinically detected neuropathy in the intensively treated group (1). Recent findings from the EDIC study reveal long-term benefit (8.5-years post-DCCT close out) for those in the intensively treated group, further illustrating the benefit of earlier tight glycemic control (25).

There is far less research on the effects of T1D on the central nervous system (CNS); however, some studies show changes in brain structure in T1D patients (26–29). Recently, Musen and colleagues (30) found differences between T1D patients and controls in terms of gray matter density. Lower levels of gray matter density in the T1D patients were found and this diminished density was associated with both persistent hyperglycemia and the occurrence of severe hypoglycemic events. The brain regions implicated in this study include those areas important to attention, memory, and language processing. Figure 3 provides a depiction of those findings. Of note, this was one of the few studies to use participants without diabetes as controls and to elucidate structural changes associated with T1D using these brain-imaging techniques.

Other researches have examined the effects of T1D on changes in white matter; these studies reveal mixed results (26–29). In separate studies of modestly sized samples of type 1 and type 2 diabetes patients, Brands and colleagues found increased rates of white matter hyperinsensitivities in type 2 diabetes patients, but not in type 1 diabetes patients (31,32). Changes in the CNS, if confirmed by further research, could reflect the impact of recurrent severe hypoglycemia and/or hyperglycemia. These changes could lead to cognitive changes when they occur in younger patients with longer durations of diabetes than seen in the DCCT or EDIC studies or in elderly patients with type 1 or type 2 diabetes.

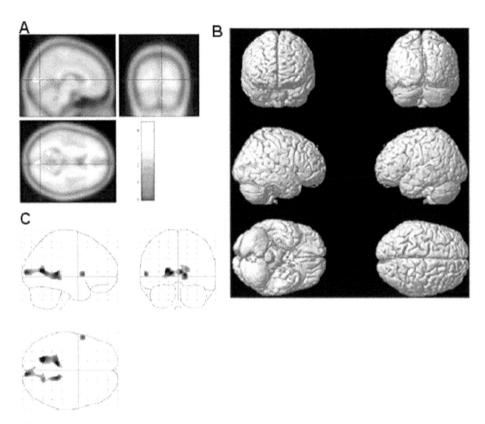

Figure 3 CNS-related complications from diabetes. *Source*: Adapted with permission from Ref. 30.

Moreover, they could lead to other behavioral consequences known to be associated with diabetes (i.e., the increased prevalence of affective and anxiety disorders) if the changes occur in the brain regions involved in emotion regulation.

Neurocognitive function may also be impaired in individuals with diabetes, as evidenced by mental slowing, and there are indications that this may be associated with both hypo- and hyperglycemia (33,34). As part of the DCCT and EDIC studies, participants' cognitive functioning was assessed across several areas such as memory and processing speed. In a recent report on EDIC participants by Jacobson and colleagues (35), individuals with a mean follow-up of 18.5 years (range 15–22 years) showed no cognitive declines associated with prior intensive treatment or history of severe hypoglycemia—one of the major risks of intensive insulin therapy. With regard to glycemic control, it appeared that lower A1C levels exerted a mild protective benefit on two domains of cognitive functioning— motor speed and psychomotor efficiency. These results belie the suggestion that increased hypoglycemia with intensive therapy adversely affects long-term cognitive function, and further support the benefit of improved glycemic control.

Macrovascular complications generally include cardiovascular disease (CVD) with specific conditions such as hypertension and atherosclerosis as the primary forms of these complications. It was traditionally thought that macrovascular complications were the result of long-term exposure to diabetes, but were linked less strongly to glycemic control than microvascular complications (36). However, long-term follow-up of the DCCT cohorts demonstrated a reduced risk for macrovascular events in the intensively treated group (37) as well as the risk factors for atherosclerosis (i.e., carotid intima-media thickening)

(38). Moreover, a recent meta-analysis showed evidence of reduction in the incidence of macrovascular events in the presence of improved glycemic control (39). A combined National Institutes of Health working group, representing the National Heart, Lung, and Blood Institute and National Institute of Diabetes and Digestive and Kidney Diseases, recently reported on the relationship between glycemic variations in T1D and CVD (40). In addition, macrovascular events, in the form of hypertension and atherosclerosis, are associated with the progression of certain microvascular complications associated with T1D, particularly nephropathy (39,40), and inflammatory markers and insulin resistance have also been associated with the progression of nephropathy (41–43). Taken together, the accumulating data on the development of macrovascular complications and their association with glycemic control seem to suggest that hyperglycemia can (*i*) induce macrovascular events that produce complications associated with T1D and (*ii*) set into motion a cascade of factors that may produce an acceleration of mechanisms associated with microvascular complications of T1D (e.g., hypertension and nephropathy).

Summary

In sum, the effect of chronic hyperglycemia on the classic microvascular complications is now extremely well documented. There are also suggestions of hyperglycemia-induced damage to the CNS. Moreover, mounting evidence suggests hyperglycemia-induced macrovascular damage (e.g., CVD). Treatment that lowers hemoglobin A1C can delay the onset and progression of microvascular and macrovascular complications (1,3,15,39). These effects have been shown to persist well after the application of such therapies. Taken together, these findings emphasize the value of early application of therapies that promote glycemic control close to the normal range.

PATHWAYS OF HYPERGLYCEMIA-INDUCED DAMAGE

As glucose is metabolized, both intra- and extracellular environments are affected by hyperglycemia and endothelial damage can occur. There is a debate (4,6,44) over the pathways through which these hyperglycemia-induced changes in cellular conditions lead to complications. We focus on four major pathways that have been implicated in the process leading to microvascular complications: (*i*) increased polyol pathway flux, (*ii*) increased advanced glycation end product (AGE) formation, (*iii*) activation of protein kinase C (PKC) isoforms, and (*iv*) increased hexosamine pathway flux. While we will focus on these pathways and their association with microvascular complications, these pathways may be implicated in macrovascular complications as well. Further, these pathways are not mutually exclusive. One or more of the pathways may be operating at a given time, and the progression toward complications may require an interaction among them.

(*i*) In the presence of a hyperglycemic environment, there is an overproduction of the polyalcohol sorbitol and a decrease in NADPH (used by aldose reductase to reduce glucose to sorbitol). This change in the intracellular environment results in a build up of sorbitol in the cell, which is toxic and alters the redox balance (6). Another result of decreased NADPH is an accumulation of free radicals, which interfere with the mitochondrial production of energy, potentially leading to the formation of AGEs (45).

(*ii*) AGEs cause tissue damage and have been used to detect damage due to hyperglycemia (46). AGEs are disruptive to the overall process of glucose metabolism in that these end products tend to accumulate on proteins and modify their functions. Increased levels of AGEs due to hyperglycemia leads to a rise in the RAGE and AGE complex, which

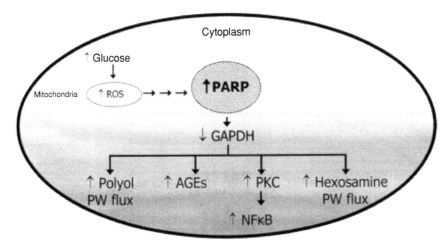

Figure 4 Brownlee's depiction of the four mechanisms and unifying principle. *Source*: Adapted with permission from Ref. 44.

is a catalyst for an inflammatory process involving activation and production of cytokines and vascular growth factors, contributing to overall vascular pathology (47,48). The AGE pathway from hyperglycemia to microvascular complications is also supported by the findings that an AGE inhibitor, aminoguanidine, slowed the progression of nephropathy in patients with T1D (51,52).

(*iii*) PKC is a group of proteins with important roles in cell signaling, expression of genes, and control over cell division and differentiation (51). There are at least 12 proteins of the PKC family and 9 have a domain that binds phospholipid diacylglycerol. The majority of PKC are classic forms and in the presence of calcium and diacylglycerol, these forms activate vascular growth and apoptotic processes (51). Hyperglycemia increases the amount of diacylglycerol, thus promoting the activation of PKC (52). With the increased activation of PKC, this signaling pathway between hyperglycemia and tissue damage may occur through several mechanisms (e.g., inhibiting the expression of endothelial nitric oxide synthetase, expression of vascular endothelial growth factor) with resulting vascular damage (53). Use of ruboxistaurin to significantly inhibit PKC activity has been shown to mediate abnormalities in the retinal and renal blood flow in animal models (53). Further, use of this PKC-β inhibitor has been shown to reduce proteinuria and macular edema (54), illustrating a promising approach to the treatment and prevention of microvascular complications associated with T1D (6).

(*iv*) Hyperglycemia has also been linked to tissue damage, especially in the mesangial cells of the kidney, through hexosamine pathway flux. In general, this process may allow the cell to determine the level of glucose in its extracellular environment. Activation of this pathway increases the activity of transforming growth factor-β1, vascular adhesion molecule-1, and necrosis factor kappa B (NF-κB) enhancer. These proteins are associated with inflammation, which leads to vascular damage. Systematically, the activation of NF-κB in macrophages increases the production of inflammatory factors such as vascular adhesion molecule-1, interleukin-6, and tumor necrosis factor-alpha, furthering possible vascular damage (4,5). It is hypothesized that as the concentration of glucose increases in the extracellular area, the amount of glucose shunted through the glucosamine pathway is increased, thus activating NF-κB and the associated inflammatory processes such as increased expression of the PAI-1 gene (55).

UNIFYING MECHANISM

These four pathways have garnered the most attention when considering the molecular link between hyperglycemia and tissue damage. However, there is still an uncertainty whether a unifying hypothesis links all of these pathways into a single mechanism. Brownlee and colleagues (4,44,56) advocate that the common process linking these four pathways of hyperglycemia-induced damage is the overproduction of superoxide in the mitochondrial electron-transport chain (Fig. 4). Oxygen free radicals may cause tissue damage in individuals with diabetes. Evidence for the overproduction of superoxide by the mitochondria and its impact on microvascular complications appears to be accumulating (44). Sheetz and King (6) suggest that this unifying hypothesis does not fully capture all of the possible ways by which hyperglycemia leads to complications. They point to mixed findings in antioxidant trials as an illustration of two conclusions: (*i*) there is a potential for these treatments, but the dosing and specific targeting of the antioxidants is yet to be worked out and (*ii*) there is not enough attention on the signaling pathways when simply focusing on removing the intracellular glucotoxins (i.e., substances formed by hyperglycemia). Considering the first point, this thought is echoed in a report by Ceriello (57) noting that antioxidant therapy is promising, yet the specific doses and appropriate target populations have yet to be ascertained. To the second point, they highlight the signaling pathways (through PKC and mitogen-activated protein kinase) as mediators between hyperglycemia and the effects of the glucotoxins (6). For example, PKC inhibitors have been shown to reduce glucotoxins' effects on the cellular damage of AGEs (58), the production of oxidants (59), and the vascular endothelial growth factor (60).

Summary

In sum, there is considerable research supporting several potential pathways of hyperglycemia-induced tissue damage leading to complications. Coupling the work aimed at specifically targeting the effects of glucotoxins with the research on approaches to inhibiting signaling pathways that promote the glucotoxins' effects (e.g., PKC) may be the best way to understand this process. Further, it is possible that once the effects of hyperglycemia are neutralized through either of these pathways, there is a potential for long-term benefit as the momentum toward complications is slowed.

CAUSES OF HYPERGLYCEMIA

Genetic Factors

The examination of the genetic factors associated with T1D reveal indicators of susceptibility to the development of T1D (61–63) as well as the development of complications (64). The most significant findings regarding the risk for T1D are polymorphisms located in the human leukocyte antigen region. Certain polymorphisms in this region have been associated with a ten-fold increase in the risk for developing the disease (63). Several studies, both by candidate gene approach and by genome wide scan, have been done to understand the vascular complications of retinopathy (65,66) and nephropathy (24). Recently, a study has been published that identified a genetic variation in the HTRA1 gene that may be responsible for 49% of the retinopathy experienced by T1D patients (66). This supports the findings of large epidemiologic studies (e.g., DCCT), which found familial clustering of retinopathy (67).

Epidemiologic studies (both family-based and population-based) show a similar, familial clustering of nephropathy. These studies and others (68,69) indicate that the initiation and progression of renal disease is in part, genetically determined (70,71). Moreover, candidate gene analysis has revealed a significant marker of nephropathy on chromosome 10 (72), providing further evidence of genetic factors in the development of nephropathy. One example of genetic variation playing a role in the risk for nephropathy comes from an examination of the role of the angiotensin converting enzyme (ACE) gene in the development of nephropathy. In this study (73), there was a protective effect for certain ACE genotypes in that they reduced the risk of persistent microalbuminuria and severe nephropathy. The power of the large EDIC sample likely aided in the identification of this three-marker haplotype as only a small proportion of the prevalence of nephropathy was explained by these variations, 0.5% to 0.8%. Moreover, in a recent paper, presenting data from the Pittsburgh Epidemiology of Diabetes Complications Study, examination of individuals who did not show evidence of common complications (possibly a "protected group") found that the deletion of the ACE polymorphism was associated with an increased risk of nephropathy (74). Thus, ACE genotypes may be implicated in nephropathy risk; however, as the authors of the study note, these investigations are preliminary but they do offer a promising avenue of research aimed at further elucidating the genetic factors associated with the development of complications.

Environmental Factors

The environmental factors associated with the onset and progression of complications include physiologic characteristics influenced by lifestyle (dietary intake, participation in unhealthy behaviors such as smoking) as well as other behaviors (e.g., adherence to the diabetes management regimen) and emotional conditions (e.g., depression). In the post-DCCT era, much attention is paid to the intensification of diabetes management (75). This places new demands on adults with T1D and the promotion of self-management adherence is a major aim of clinicians and clinical researchers. Adherence is not a univariate construct, but one that is influenced by more specific areas—adherence to blood glucose monitoring, taking prescribed medication, following treatment recommendations—and a construct that is influenced by lifestyle, educational, and motivational barriers (76–79). There is evidence that adherence is linked with glycemic control, with indicators such as less frequent blood glucose monitoring associated with suboptimal glycemic control (80).

Emotional conditions also may contribute to the occurrence of hyperglycemia. For example, stress—associated with physiologic alterations such as increased levels of glucocorticoids—has been linked with both protective and damaging effects on the immune system (81). Indeed, in both animal and human models, stress has been shown to be a factor in the expression of T1D (82) as well as in conditions likely to progress to diabetes (83). Further, recent reports examining the epidemiology of diabetes in the United States suggest that stress and depression, along with socioeconomic variables, are related to the incidence of diabetes (both type 1 and type 2) (84,85). Another recently reported study from Sweden implicated a pattern of life conflict and symptoms of depression in the onset of T1D in young adults (86). Given that these factors are linked with the onset of T1D, their continued presence may further contribute to hyperglycemia and eventual complications.

Depression has been examined with regard to its link to diabetes (87). A meta-analysis of the prevalence of depression in adults with diabetes (88), including 48 studies totaling nearly 22,000 adults, found the overall prevalence of depression in adults with diabetes was 25.3%, in contrast to the rate found in control participants in these studies (11.4%). Further, calculations of the odds ratios for developing depression in adults with diabetes showed that the odds were slightly greater than two to one for adults with diabetes compared to adults without diabetes. There were slightly higher rates of depression in women than in men, but no difference between the rates of depression in adults with type 1 versus type 2 diabetes.

In a meta-analysis of depression and glycemic control, 26 studies were reviewed and a positive association existed between the presence of depression and poor glycemic control (89). The mechanisms underlying this connection between depression and diabetes may not be fully delineated (90), but one avenue may be adherence as a mediating variable between depression and health outcomes (80) or as noted earlier, a direct link due to stress hormones. Further, some of the factors that appear to be associated with depression in adults with diabetes include female gender, low income (an indicator of socioeconomic status), and poor social support (91). Depression has also been linked to complications associated with T1D (92). An increase in depression was associated with severity or number of complications in this meta-analysis. The authors highlighted the possibility that depression may precede or follow complications. Future studies are needed to clarify the direction of this relationship.

Recently, Lustman and colleagues (93) found that while depression and adherence were both associated with hyperglycemia directly, a mediational path indicated previously (94) was not confirmed. In other words, depression was directly associated with hyper-glycemia, but not indirectly through adherence. This suggests that there may be a different mechanism between depression and adherence, one that is not fully elucidated at this point. In another recent study by Lustman and colleagues (95), individuals recovering from depression were either exposed to sertraline (an antidepressant in the serotonin-specific reuptake inhibitor class) or placebo. Approximately half of the 152 patients (both type 1 and type 2 diabetes) received the antidepressant and reduced their risk of recurrence of depression by half and experienced a four-fold increase in time to recurrence, as compared to the placebo group. During that time, these individuals also experienced an improvement in glycemic control. Whether these glycemic improvements are attributable to depression in unclear, but these results show promise for future work in treating depression to improve the glycemic outcomes associated with T1D.

Summary

Genetic and environmental factors are associated with various aspects of diabetes (e.g., hyperglycemia) and the development of complications, either directly through biologic mechanisms or indirectly through such factors as behavior or emotional conditions. In large part, these areas need further support, but offer a promising perspective on ways to prevent hyperglycemia and long-term complications associated with T1D. In the following section, we discuss approaches to modify the effects of hyperglycemia on complications, whatever the specific biologic pathways and genetic influences.

PREVENTION OF TISSUE DAMAGE AND COMPLICATIONS

There appear to be several approaches to preventing or slowing the progression of com-plications associated with T1D. In this chapter, we have highlighted the research on hy-perglycemia as the number one culprit in the development of long-term complications. However, as we have demonstrated, the etiology of hyperglycemia is multifactorial. In addition, once hyperglycemia is present, the molecular pathways that ultimately lead to complications are varied and may or may not rest on a unifying link. Taken together, our chapter highlights that multiple methods are necessary in order to prevent the long-term complications commonly associated with T1D. One method concerns a focus on stopping hyperglycemia before it happens by identifying the risk across multiple factors (e.g., genetics, lifestyle, and emotional factors) and intervening early, before these factors can cause prolonged hyperglycemia. A second method is aimed at attacking hyperglycemia on the molecular level through novel pharmacologic approaches.

The attainment of near-normoglycemia from very early on in the onset of the disease to protect or delay complications was illustrated in the DCCT and confirmed with long-term data from the EDIC study and other epidemiologic studies (1,11,13,18,19). If the knowledge of such findings was enough, clinical investigators would no longer search for ways to promote near-normoglycemia. For example, less than two-thirds of a large sample of adults with T1D monitor blood glucose levels at the rate prescribed by the American Diabetes Association (79). Various psychological programs have attempted to improve monitoring as well as co-occurring areas of poor adherence, showing promise for the promotion of self-management (96,97). However, the direct link with glycemic control is not always apparent. Thus, while there are established programs that promote diabetes and other health-related outcomes, work remains in order to reduce the exposure to hyperglycemia that many individuals with T1D experience.

Researchers examining the molecular pathways between hyperglycemia and tissue damage have proposed several methods for both the prevention of the adverse effects of hyperglycemia and its prevention. Sheetz and King (6) offer a selection of approaches to prevent complications resulting from hyperglycemia. They describe the first approach as a "classic" one in which the glucotoxins are neutralized, thus protecting the cell from the destruction commonly associated with hyperglycemia. As noted earlier, Ceriello (57) merges several avenues of current and potential work on antioxidants to suggest several methods for the role of reactive oxygen species. In the second approach, the one they refer to as a "promising" approach, the activity within the common signaling pathways are identified and normalized to counter the effects of glucose and glucotoxins created by hyperglycemia (6). Certainly, there is mounting evidence that PKC plays a pivotal role in this approach.

Brownlee (44) also advocates several therapeutic approaches on the molecular level. For example, one approach stems from the overproduction of superoxide (56) and includes transketolase activators. A simplistic description of this complex process is that transketolase is activated and the concentration of problematic metabolites is decreased, thus reducing the flux across the hyperglycemia-induced pathways (98). Through the administration of a thiamine derivative, Brownlee and colleagues were able to activate transketolase and decrease activation in the hexosamine pathway, decrease AGE formation and PKC activation (98). In animal studies, they have demonstrated beneficial effects from this novel therapy. Likewise, Brownlee (44) highlights promising work around poly(ADP-ribose) polymerase inhibitors and certain catalytic antioxidants such as endothelial nitric oxide synthetase.

In sum, we have described a multifactorial view of hyperglycemia-induced tissue damage. The pathways leading to the occurrence of hyperglycemia due to a number of relevant factors are just as important as the molecular pathways that cause the tissue damage ultimately leading to complications. Our review of the current state of the field suggests that many investigators are conducting promising work aimed at changing the causes of hyperglycemia and diminishing the effects of long-term exposure to high blood glucose values. The accumulation of research findings in some areas is substantial compared to others, but targeting both the causes and molecular pathways of vascular damage will ultimately lead to methods to prevent the onset of complications associated with T1D.

REFERENCES

1. The DCCT Research Group. The effect of intensive treatment of diabetes on the development and progression of long-term complications in insulin-dependent diabetes mellitus. N Engl J Med 1993;329:977–986.
2. Barnett DM, Krall LP. The history of diabetes. In: Kahn CR, Weir GC, King GL, et al., eds. Joslin's Diabetes Mellitus, 14th edn. Philadelphia, PA: Lippincott Williams & Wilkins, 2005, pp. 1–18.
3. Nathan DM. Relationship between metabolic control and long-term complications of diabetes. In: Kahn CR, Weir GC, King GL, et al., eds. Joslin's Diabetes Mellitus, 14th edn. Philadelphia, PA: Lippincott Williams & Wilkins, 2005, pp. 809–822.
4. Brownlee M. Biochemistry and molecular cell biology of diabetic complications. Nature 2001;414:813–820.
5. Rolo AP, Palmeira CM. Diabetes and mitochondrial function: Role of hyperglycemia and oxidative stress. Toxicol Appl Pharmacol 2006;212:167–178.
6. Sheetz MJ, King GL. Molecular understanding of hyperglycemia's adverse effects for diabetic complications. JAMA 2002;288:2579–2588.
7. American Diabetes Association. Diagnosis and classification of diabetes mellitus. Diabetes Care 2006;29(Suppl 1):S43–S48.
8. EURODIAB ACE study group. Variation and trends in incidence of childhood diabetes in Europe. EURODIAB ACE Study Group. Lancet 2000;355:873–876.
9. Feltbower RG, McKinney PA, Parslow RC, et al. Type 1 diabetes in Yorkshire, UK: Time trends in 0–14 and 15–29-year-olds, age at onset and age-period-cohort modelling. Diabet Med 2003;20:437–441.
10. Gale EA. The rise of childhood type 1 diabetes in the 20th century. Diabetes 2002;51:3353–3361.
11. Epidemiology of Diabetes Interventions and Complications (EDIC) Research Group. Epidemiology of diabetes interventions and complications (EDIC). Design, implementation, and preliminary results of a long-term follow-up of the Diabetes Control and Complications Trial cohort. Diabetes Care 1999;22:99–111.
12. Klein R, Klein BEK, Moss SE. The Wisconsin epidemiological study of diabetic retinopathy: A review. Diabetes Metab Rev 1989;5:559–570.
13. Orchard TJ, Dorman JS, Maser RE, et al. Prevalence of complications in IDDM by sex and duration. Pittsburgh Epidemiology of Diabetes Complications Study II. Diabetes 1990;39:1116–1124.
14. Roy MS, Affouf M. Six-year progression of retinopathy and associated risk factors in African American patients with type 1 diabetes mellitus. The New Jersey 725. Arch Opthalmol 2006;124:1297–1306.
15. Genuth S. Insights from the Diabetes Control and Complications Trial/Epidemiology of Diabetes Interventions and Complications Study on the use of intensive glycemic treatment to reduce the risk of complications of type 1 diabetes. Endocr Pract 2006;12:34–41.
16. The DCCT/EDIC Research Group. Retinopathy and nephropathy in patients with type 1 diabetes four years after a trial of intensive therapy. The Diabetes Control and Complications Trial/Epidemiology of Diabetes Interventions and Complications Research Group. N Engl J Med 2000;342:381–389.
17. White NH, Cleary PA, Dahms W, et al. Effect of intensive therapy on the microvascular complications of type 1 diabetes mellitus. JAMA 2002;287:2563–2569.
18. DCCT/EDIC Research Group. Sustained effect of intensive treatment of type 1 diabetes mellitus on development and progression of diabetic nephropathy: The Epidemiology of Diabetes Interventions and Complications (EDIC) study. JAMA 2003;290:2159–2167.

19. Klein R, Klein BEK, Moss SE, et al. The Wisconsin epidemiologic study of diabetic retinopathy. II. Prevalence and risk of diabetic retinopathy when age at diagnosis is less than 30 years. Arch Opthalmol 1984;102:520–526.
20. Krolewski AS, Warram JH, Rand LI, et al. Risk of proliferative diabetic retinopathy in juvenile-onset type 1 diabetes A 40-yr follow-up study. Diabetes Care 1986;9:443–452.
21. Stephenson JM, Fuller JH. Microalbuminuria is not rare before 5 years of IDDM. J Diabetes Complications 1994;8:166–173.
22. Warram JH, Gearin G, Laffel L, et al. Effect of duration of type I diabetes on the prevalence of stages of diabetic nephropathy defined by urinary albumin/creatinine ratio. J. Am.Soc.Nephrol 1996;7:930–937.
23. Krolewski AS, Eggers PW, Warram JH. Magnitude of end-stage renal disease in type 1 diabetes: A 35-year follow-up study. Kidney Int 1996;50:2041–2046.
24. Perkins BA, Ficociello LH, Silva KH, et al. Regression of microalbuminuria in type 1 diabetes. N Engl J Med 2003;348:2285–2293.
25. Martin CL, Albers J, Herman WH, et al. Neuropathy among the Diabetes Control and Complications Trial cohort 8 years after trial completion. Diabetes Care 2006;29:340–344.
26. Perros P, Deary IJ, Sellar RJ, et al. Brain abnormalities demonstrated by magnetic resonance imaging in adult IDDM patients with and without a history of recurrent severe hypoglycemia. Diabetes Care 1997;20:1013–1018.
27. Lunetta M, Damanti AR, Fabbri G, et al. Evidence by magnetic resonance imaging of cerebral alterations of atrophy type in young insulin-dependent diabetic patients. J Endocrinol Invest 1994;17:241–245.
28. Makimattila S, Malmber-Ceder K, Hakkinen AM, et al. Brain metabolic alterations in patients with type 1 diabetes-hyperglycemia-induced injury. J Cereb Blood Flow Metab 2004;24:1393–1399.
29. Dejgaard A, Gade A, Larsson H, et al. Evidence for diabetic encephalopathy. Diabet Med 1991;8:162–167.
30. Musen G, Lyoo IK, Sparks CR, et al. Effects of type 1 diabetes on gray matter density as measured by voxel-based morphometry. Diabetes 2006;55:326–333.
31. Brands AM, Kessels RP, Hoogma RP, et al. Cognitive performance, psychological well-being, and brain magnetic resonance imaging in older patients with type 1 diabetes. Diabetes 2006;55:1800–1806.
32. Manschot SM, Brands AM, van der Grond J, et al. Brain magnetic resonance imaging correlates of impaired cognition in patients with type 2 diabetes. Diabetes 2006;55:1106–1113.
33. Ryan CM. Diabetes and brain damage: More (or less) than meets the eye? Diabetologia 2006;49:2229–2233.
34. Brands AMA, Biessels GJ, de Haan EHF, et al. The effects of type 1 diabetes on cognitive performance. Diabetes Care 2005;28:726–735.
35. Jacobson AM, Ryan CM, Cleary PA, et al. for the DCCT/EDIC Research Group. The impact of diabetes and its treatment on cognitive function: an eighteen year follow-up of the DCCT cohort. N Engl J Med 2007;356(18):1842–1852.
36. UK Prospective Diabetes Study (UKPDS) Group. Intensive blood-glucose control with sulphonylureas or insulin compared with conventional treatment and risk of complications in patients with type 2 diabetes (UKPDS 33). Lancet 1998;352:837–853.
37. Nathan DM, Cleary PA, Backlund JY, et al. Intensive diabetes treatment and cardiovascular disease in patients with type 1 diabetes. N Engl J Med 2005;353:2643–2653.
38. Nathan DM, Lachin J, Cleary P, et al. Intensive diabetes therapy and carotid intima-media thickness in type 1 diabetes mellitus. N Engl J Med 2003;348:2294–2303.
39. Stettler C, Allemann S, Juni P, et al. Glycemic control and macrovascular disease in types 1 and 2 diabetes mellitus: Meta-analysis of randomized trials. Am Heart J 2006;152:27–38.
40. Libby P, Nathan DM, Abraham K, et al. Report of the National Heart, Lung, and Blood Institute–National Institute of Diabetes and Digestive and Kidney Diseases Working Group on Cardiovascular Complications of Type 1 Diabetes Mellitus. Circulation 2005;111:3489–3493.

41. Tesfaye S, Chaturvedi N, Eaton SE, et al. Vascular risk factors and diabetic nephropathy. N Engl J Med 2005;352:341–350.
42. Schram MT, Chaturvedi N, Schalkwijk CG. Markers of inflammation are cross-sectionally associated with microvascular complications and cardiovascular disease in type 1 diabetes—The EURODIAB Prosepctive Complications Study. Diabetologia 2005;48:370–378.
43. Orchard TJ, Chang YF, Ferrell RE. Nephropathy in type 1 diabetes: A manifestation of insulin resistance and multiple genetic susceptibilities? Further evidence from the Pittsburgh Epidemiology of Diabetes Complications Study. Kidney Int 2002;62:963–970.
44. Brownlee M. The pathobiology of diabetic complications. Diabetes 2005;54:1615–1625.
45. Wolin MS, Gupte SA, Oeckler RA. Superoxide in the vascular system. J Vasc Res 2002;39: 191–207.
46. Monnier VM, Bautista O, Kenny D, et al. Skin collagen glycation, glycoxidation, and crosslinking are lower in subjects with long-term intensive versus conventional therapy of type 1 diabetes: Relevance of glycated collagen products versus HbA1C as markers of diabetic complications. Diabetes 1999;48:870–880.
47. Li YM, Mitsuhashi T, Wojciechowicz D, Shimizu N, et al. Molecular identity and cellular distribution of advanced glycation endproduct receptors: Relationship of p60 to OST-48 and p90 to 80 K-H membrane proteins. Proc Natl Acad Sci USA 1996;93:11047–11052.
48. Schmidt AM, Stern DM: RAGE: A new target for the prevention and treatment of the vascular and inflammatory complications of diabetes. Trends Endocrinol Metab 2000;11:368–375.
49. Hammes HP, Martin S, Federlin K, et al. Aminoguanidine treatment inhibits the development of experimental diabetic retinopathy. Proc Natl Acad Sci USA 1991;88:11555–11558.
50. Friedman E. Advanced glycosylated end products and hyperglycemia in the pathogenesis of diabetic complications. Diabetes Care 1999;22(Suppl 2):B65–B71.
51. Newton A. Regulation of the ABC kinases by phosphorylation: Protein kinase C as a paradigm. Biochem J 2003;370:361–371.
52. Nishizuka Y. Intracellular signaling by hydrolysis of phospholipids and activiation of protein kinase C. Science 1992;258:607–614.
53. Ishii H, Koya D, King GL. Protein kinase C activation and its role in the development of vascular complications in diabetes mellitus. J Mol Med 1998;76:21–31.
54. PKC-DRS Study Group. The Effect of Ruboxistaurin on Visual Loss in Patients With Moderately Severe to Very Severe Nonproliferative Diabetic Retinopathy: Initial Results of the Protein Kinase C ß Inhibitor Diabetic Retinopathy Study (PKC-DRS) Multicenter Randomized Clinical Trial. Diabetes 2005;54:2188–2197.
55. Leighton JR, Tang D, Ingram A, et al. Flux through the hexosamine pathway is a determinant of nuclear factor B–dependent promoter activation. Diabetes 2002;51:1146–1156.
56. Nishikawa T, Edelstein D, Du XL, et al. Normalizing mitochondrial superoxide production blocks three pathways of hyperglycaemic damage. Nature 2000;404:787–790.
57. Ceriello A. New insights on oxidative stress and diabetic complications may lead to a "causal" antioxidant therapy. Diabetes Care 2003;26:1589–1596.
58. Ido Y, Chang KC, Lejenue WS, et al. Vascular dysfunction induced by AGE is mediated by VEGF via mechanisms involving reactive oxygen species, guanylate cyclase, and protein kinase C. Microcirculation 2001;8:251–263.
59. Dekker LV, Leitges M, Altschuler G, et al. Protein kinase C-beta contributes to NADPH-oxidase activiation in neutrophils. Biochem J 2000;347(pt 1):285–289.
60. Xia P, Aiello LP, Ishii H, et al. Characterization of vascular endothelial growth factor's effect on the activation of protein kinase C, its isoforms, and endothelial cell growth. J Clin Invest 1996;98:2018–2026.
61. Morales AE, She JX, Schatz DA. Prediction and prevention of type 1 diabetes. Curr Diab Rep 2001;1(1):28–32.
62. Knip M. Prediction and prevention of type 1 diabetes. Acta Paediatr. Suppl 1998;425:54–62.
63. Atkinson MA, Eisenbarth GS. Type 1 diabetes: New perspectives on disease pathogenesis and treatment. Lancet 2001;358:221–229.

64. Rich SS, Freedman BI, Bowden DW. Genetic epidemiology of diabetic complications. Diabetes Review 1997;5:165–173.
65. Klein RJ, Zeiss C, Chew EY, et al. Complement factor H polymorphism in age-related macular degeneration. Science 2005;308:385–388.
66. Yang Z, Camp NJ, Sun H, et al. A variant of the HTRA1 gene increases susceptibility to age-related macular degeneration. Science 2006;314:992–993.
67. Hallman DM, Gonzalez VH, Klein BE, et al. Familial aggregation of severity of diabetic retinopathy in Mexican Americans from Starr County, Texas. Diabetes Care 2005;28:1163–1168.
68. Quinn M, Angelico MC, Warram JH, et al. Familial factors determine the development of diabetic nephropathy in patients with IDDM. Diabetologia 1996;39:940–945.
69. Borch-Johnsen K, Norgaard K, Hommel E, et al. Is diabetic nephropathy an inherited complication? Kidney Int 1992;41:719–722.
70. Freedman BI, Bowden DW, Rich SS, et al. Genetic initiation of hypertensive and diabetic nephropathy. Am J Hypertens 1998;11:251–257.
71. Krolewski AS, Ng DP, Canani LH, et al. Genetics of diabetic nepropathy: How far are we from finding susceptibility genes? Adv Nephrol Necker Hosp 2001;31:295–315.
72. Iyengar SK, Fox KA, Schachere M, et al. Linkage analysis of candidate loci for end-stage renal disease due to diabetic nephropathy. J Am Soc Nephrol 2003;14:S195–S201.
73. Boright AP, Paterson AD, Mirea L, et al. Genetic variation at the ACE gene is associated with persistent microalbuminuria and severe nephropathy in type 1 diabetes. Diabetes 2005;54: 1238–1244.
74. Costacou T, Chang Y, Ferrell RE, et al. Identifying genetic susceptibilities to diabetes-related complications among individuals at low risk of complications: An application of tree-structured survival analysis. Am J Epidemiol 2006;164:862–872.
75. American Diabetes Association: Standards of medical care in diabetes—2006. Diabetes Care 2006;29(Suppl 1):S4–S42.
76. Glasgow RE, McCaul KD, Schafer LC. Self-care behaviors and glycemic control in type 1 diabetes. J Chronic Dis 1987;40:399–412.
77. Vincze G, Barner JC, Lopez D. Factors associated with adherence to self-monitoring of blood glucose among persons with diabetes. Diabetes Educ 2004;30:112–125.
78. Peyrot M, Rubin RR, Lauritzen T, et al. Psychosocial problems and barriers to improved diabetes management: Results of the cross-sectional Diabetes Attitudes, Wishes and Needs (DAWN) study. Diabet Med 2005;22:1379–1385.
79. Karter AJ, Ferrara A, Darbinian JA, et al. Self-monitoring of blood glucose: Language and financial barriers in a managed care population with diabetes. Diabetes Care 2000;23:477–483.
80. Wing RR, Phelan S, Tate D. The role of adherence in mediating the relationship between depression and health outcomes. J Psychosom Res 2002;53:877–881.
81. McEwen BS. Protective and damaging effects of stress mediators. N Engl J Med 1998;338: 171–179.
82. Lehman C, Rodin J, McEwen BS, et al. Impact of environmental stress of the expression of insulin-dependent diabetes mellitus. Behav Neurosci 1991;105:241–245.
83. Raikkonen K, Keltikangas-Jarvinen L, Adlercreutz H, et al. Psychosocial stress and the insulin resistance syndrome. Metabolism 1996;45:1533–1538.
84. Carnethon MR, Kinder LS, Fair JM, et al. Symptoms of depression as a risk factor for incident diabetes: Findings from the National Health and Nutrition Examination Epidemiologic Follow-up Study, 1971–1992. Am J Epidemiol 2003;158:416–423.
85. Eaton WW, Armenian H, Gallo J, et al. Depression and risk for onset of type II diabetes: A prospective population based-study. Diabetes Care 1996;19:1097–1102.
86. Bengt L, Sundkvist G, Nystrom L, et al. Family characteristics and life events before the onset of autoimmune type 1 diabetes in young adults: A nationwide study. Diabetes Care 2001;24: 1033–1037.
87. Jacobson AM. Depression and diabetes. Diabetes Care 1993;16:1621–1623.
88. Anderson RJ, Freedland KE, Clouse RE, et al. The prevalence of comorbid depression in adults with diabetes: A meta-analysis. Diabetes Care 2001;24:1069–1078.

89. Lustman PJ, Anderson RJ, Freedland KE, et al. Depression and poor glycemic control: A meta-analytic review of the literature. Diabetes Care 2000;23:934–942.
90. Katon W, Ciechanowski P. Impact of major depression on chronic medical illness. J Psychosom Res 2002;53:859–863.
91. Goldney RD, Phillips PJ, Fisher LJ, et al. Diabetes, depression, and quality of life: A population study. Diabetes Care 2004;27:1066–1070.
92. de Groot M, Anderson R, Freedland KE, et al. Association of depression and diabetes complications: A meta-analysis. Psychosom Med 2001;63:619–630.
93. Lustman PJ, Clouse RE, Ciechanowski PS, et al. Depression-related hyperglycemia in type 1 diabetes: A mediational approach. Psychosom Med 2005;67:195–199.
94. Peyrot M, McMurry JF, Jr., Kruger DF. A biopsychosocial model of glycemic control in diabetes: Stress, coping and regimen adherence. J Health Soc Behav 1999;40:141–158.
95. Lustman PJ, Clouse RE, Nix BD, et al. Sertraline for prevention of depression recurrence in diabetes mellitus. Arch Gen Psychiatry 2006;63:521–529.
96. Steed L, Cooke D, Newman S. A systematic review of psychosocial outcomes following education, self-management and psychological interventions in diabetes mellitus. Patient Educ Couns 2003;51:5–15.
97. Winkley, K, Ismail, K, Landau, S, et al. Psychological interventions to improve glycaemic control in patients with type 1 diabetes: Systematic review and meta-analysis of randomised controlled trials. BMJ 2006;333:65–69.
98. Hammes HP, Du X, Edelstein D, et al. Benfotiamine blocks three major pathways of hyperglycemic damage and prevents experimental diabetic retinopathy. Nat Med 2003;9:294–299.

8
Diabetic Retinopathy

J. M. Cropsey and M. S. Fineman
Wills Eye Institute, Philadelphia, Pennsylvania, U.S.A.

INTRODUCTION

Diabetic retinopathy (DR) is the leading cause of blindness in people aged 20 to 74 in industrialized nations (1). The vast majority of this blindness (95%) is preventable with the use of routine screening and the application of evidence-based therapy (2). Consequently, ophthalmologic screening in diabetics is absolutely critical.

DEFINITION, INCIDENCE, PREVALENCE, AND NATURAL HISTORY

DR is a progressive retinal microvascular dysfunction and its sequelae are caused by chronic hyperglycemia (2). Type 1 diabetes has a prevalence of approximately 2 per 1000 school-aged children in the United States, and both prevalence and incidence increase with age (3). The Wisconsin Epidemiologic Study of Diabetic Retinopathy found that the duration of type 1 diabetes is the best predictor of developing DR (4–6). This natural history study involved over 10,000 patients beginning in the early 1980s and found that retinopathy began to occur in type 1 diabetic patients between 3 and 5 years after diagnosis, and by 15 to 20 years, virtually all patients were affected. In contrast, only 50% to 80% of type 2 diabetics have DR at 20 years (7).

PATHOGENESIS

Evidence from the Diabetes Control and Complications Trial (DCCT) suggests that hyperglycemia is the primary cause of DR (8). In this study, 1441 patients with type 1 diabetes were randomly assigned to either conventional or intensive insulin treatment. The study was divided into a primary prevention arm (726 patients with no known DR) and a secondary intervention arm (715 patients with mild DR) with a mean patient follow-up time of 6.5 years. Intensive therapy reduced the risk of developing retinopathy by 76% and impeded the progression of retinopathy by 54% (9). This reduction in development and progression was directly correlated with glycemic control as measured by HbA1c (7.9 in the intensive therapy group vs. 9.9 in the conventional therapy group) (7). Similar reductions in microalbuminuria, albuminuria, and neuropathy were found. The most important negative consequence of intensive insulin treatment in the DCCT was a two- to threefold increase in severe hypoglycemia (9).

Exactly how hyperglycemia leads to DR is not completely understood. Three main hypotheses include: the accumulation of advanced glycosylation end products (AGEs); the accumulation of sorbital within retinal cells; and impaired autoregulation of retinal blood flow (7).

Chronic hyperglycemia leads to the glycosylation of proteins. Initially the glycosylation is reversible, but with time becomes irreversible and leads to AGEs through Amadori rearrangements (10,11). These AGEs then accumulate in vessel walls and cross-link with collagen causing microvascular damage (12). Compounds that inhibit the development of AGE formation have been shown to prevent chronic diabetic complications in animal models; therefore, further investigation is warranted for clinical application (12).

Aldose reductase metabolizes glucose to sorbitol intracellularly. Chronic hyperglycemia leads to intracellular elevations in sorbitol causing increased osmolality, which interferes with cellular metabolism (13). Exactly how this leads to microvascular damage is incompletely understood (10). In addition to sorbitol's effects on osmolality, it is also believed that its metabolism causes increased oxidative stress through free radical formation. Recent attempts to use aldose reductase inhibitors clinically have met with limited success (14). Sorbital's role in diabetic cataract formation has been attributed to osmotic rupture of lens fiber cells and oxidative damage leading to apoptosis (15).

Normally, autoregulation allows retinal blood flow to remain constant until mean arterial pressure rises above 40% of baseline (7). Hyperglycemia impairs autoregulation of retinal blood flow and leads to increased shear stress that stimulates the production of vasoactive substances (16). These vasoactive substances include vascular endothelial growth factor (VEGF), insulin-like growth factor-1, erythropoietin, fibroblastic growth factor, and hepatocyte growth factor and result in proliferative neovascularization (7).

Abnormalities in platelets and coagulation pathways have also been implicated in DR as increased blood viscosity and thrombosis cause focal capillary occlusion and ischemia in the retina contributing to DR (2,17).

Genetic and racial factors also influence the likelihood of developing severe DR. In the DCCT, patients with a relative with DR were three times more likely to develop severe DR. In multiple studies, African-Americans and Hispanics had an elevated risk for developing DR (7).

CLASSIFICATION

Early Nonproliferative Diabetic Retinopathy

The retina is particularly sensitive to the metabolic changes and ischemia seen in diabetes because it is one of the most metabolically active tissues in the body (8). Even before clinical or histological evidence of DR begins, retinal pericytes and vascular endothelial cells have already begun to die at an accelerated rate (18).

The first clinically detectable change is microaneurysm formation (Fig. 1). This occurs as capillary walls weaken secondary to pericyte loss. Hypercellular outpouchings form, and vascular integrity becomes increasingly compromised with lipid and proteinacious material leaking and accumulating as "hard" exudates (Fig. 2) (7). As weakening continues, capillaries begin to rupture. If they bleed deep in the retina, "dot and blot" hemorrhages are seen, whereas, superficial bleeds are seen as "splinter-" or "flame-"shaped hemorrhages

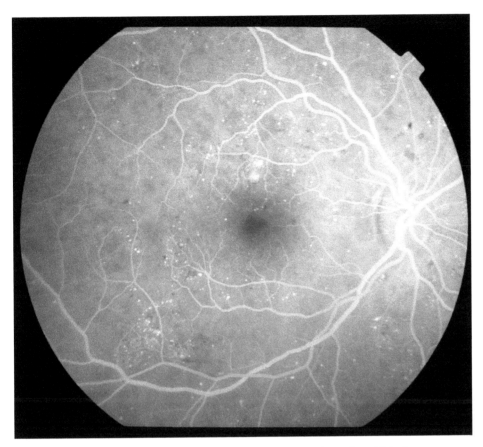

Figure 1   Fluorescein angiogram demonstrating microaneurysm formation with leakage.

(Fig. 2). These latter bleeds are identical to those seen in systemic hypertension, and consequently, blood pressure should be measured if present.

As the capillaries continue to leak and hemorrhage, retinal thickening in the form of macular edema can manifest as decreased vision (Fig. 3). The edema scatters light and opacifies the retina. It is the leading cause of legal blindness in diabetics, and it is important to note that it can occur in the early stages of nonproliferative diabetic retinopathy (NPDR) and can only be seen with a slit lamp in conjunction with high-power lenses.

Advanced NPDR

Once retinal microvascular disease progresses to the point of causing inner retinal hypoxia, signs of advanced NPDR begin to appear in the form of cotton-wool spots, venous beading and loops, intraretinal microvascular abnormalities (IRMA), and areas of capillary nonperfusion on fluorescein angiography (FA). Cotton-wool spots, also called "soft" exudates, are actually nerve fiber layer infarcts. As hypoxia develops in the nerve fiber layer, axoplasmic flow is halted and leads to swelling giving a white, fluffy appearance. Venous beading and looping are the result of sluggish circulation and exuberant endothelial replacement of previously damaged vascular endothelium (Fig. 4) (7). IRMAs are dilated capillaries that seem to function as collaterals. They do not leak and therefore can be distinguished from neovascularization using FA.

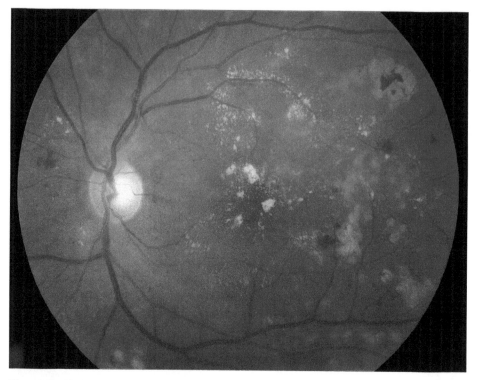

Figure 2 Hard exudates ring the fovea.

The Early Treatment Diabetic Retinopathy Study (ETDRS) found that multiple retinal hemorrhages, venous beading, and looping, IRMA, widespread capillary nonperfusion, and leakage on FA were all significant risk factors for progressing to proliferative DR; however, cotton-wool spots were not (19,20). Roughly half of patients with advanced NPDR develop proliferative diabetic retinopathy (PDR) within 1 year (21).

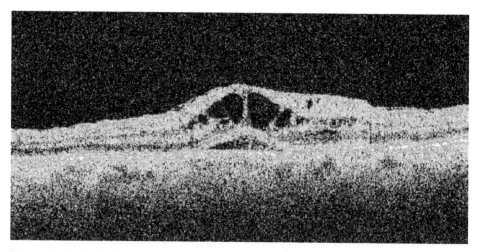

Figure 3 Optical coherence tomography demonstrating diabetic macular edema.

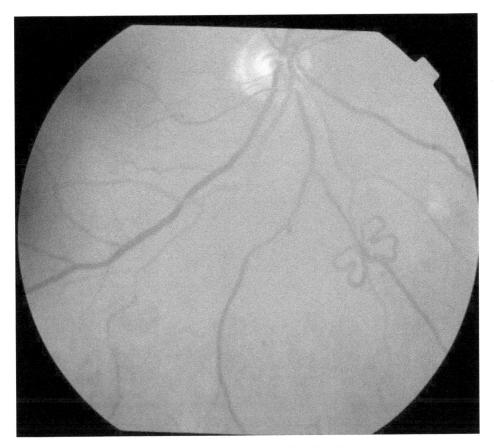

Figure 4   Venous loop in an eye with early proliferative diabetic retinopathy.

PDR

NPDR often causes legal blindness with significant residual vision, but PDR can produce rapid, disabling loss of sight. As the retinal environment becomes increasingly hypoxic, the ischemic tissues produce vasoproliferative agents such as vascular endothelial growth factor (VEGF) in an attempt to attract oxygen-laden blood flow. Lacy, delicate vessels referred to as neovascariztion begin to proliferate in response (Fig. 5). This often occurs at the optic disc, near ischemic zones of the retina, and, in severe cases, as anterior as the iris. These fragile vessels leak fluorescein on FA. The neovascularization tends to grow along the path of least resistance along the posterior vitreous (gel-like material filling the posterior chamber of the eye) face (Fig. 6). As the neovascular stalks mature, they become increasingly fibrous and can create bands of tension on the retina (Fig. 7). Many of the complications of PDR occur as the vitreous begins to contract and pull away from the retina with the stalks stretching between the two. This can lead to vitreous hemorrhage, retinal detachment, retinal breaks, retinal striae, dragging of the macula, and retinoschisis (22).

Other Ocular Complications

Corneal: decreased sensitivity, susceptible to abrasions and erosions.
Glaucoma: neovascular angle closure glaucoma, possible increase of primary open
angle glaucoma.

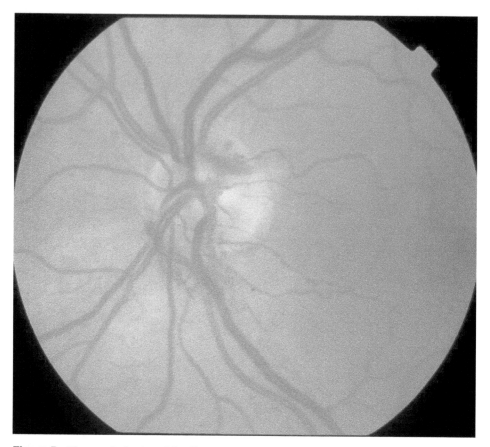

Figure 5   Neovascularization of the disc.

Lens: accelerated cataract formation with significantly increased risk of postoperative cataract extraction complications in the setting of DR, especially PDR, including macular and cystoid edema, PDR, vitreous hemorrhage, retinal detachment, pupillary block, posterior synechiae, severe iritis, and pigment deposition on the lens implant.

Cranial nerves: optic neuropathy and/or disc edema (often bilateral), pupil sparing 3rd, 4th, and 6th nerve palsy. Prognosis is generally good with recovery within 1 to 3 months.

TREATMENT TO REDUCE RISK AND PROGRESSION

The importance of early glucose control was demonstrated by the DCCT, which found that intensive insulin therapy reduces the risk of developing retinopathy by 76% and impedes the progression of retinopathy by 54% with progression being directly correlated with glycemic control as measured by HbA1c (9). This remains the mainstay of prevention and treatment in patients with mild to moderate NPDR. However, its benefit in advanced DR appears to be limited, if present (23,24).

Control of blood pressure slows the rate of progression of DR and reduces the risk of vitreous hemorrhage (25). The United Kingdom Prospective Diabetes Study (UKPDS)

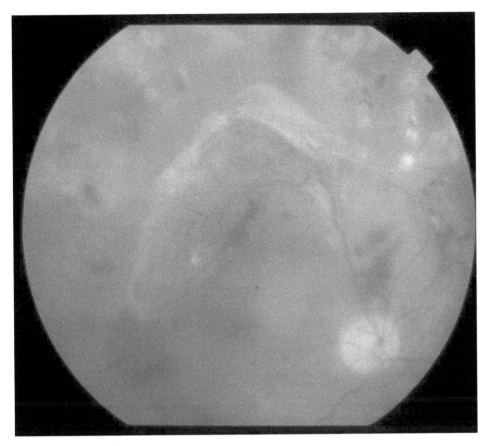

Figure 6 Neovascularization grows into the vitreous cavity.

found that in 1148 type 2 diabetic patients, there was a 34% and 47% reduction in progression of DR and deterioration of visual acuity, respectively in patients with tight blood pressure control (26). Angiotensin-converting enzyme inhibitors may have a similar benefit in DR as they do in nephropathy, and their protective benefit is still being evaluated (25).

Interestingly, it appears that antiplatelet therapy with aspirin has no positive or negative effect on the progression of PDR, vitreous or preretinal bleeding, or visual loss (27,28). This was observed in the ETDRS, a multicenter randomized clinical trial designed to assess the effect of photocoagulation and aspirin on 3711 patients with mild to severe NPDR or early PDR. Accordingly, there is no contraindication of aspirin therapy in patients with DR who require antiplatelet therapy for cardiovascular risk reduction (28,29).

TREATMENT OF ESTABLISHED DISEASE

Laser panretinal photocoagulation (PRP) of the retina is the primary treatment for PDR (Fig. 8). Its value was proven in the Diabetic Retinopathy Study (DRS), which randomly assigned PRP to one eye of 1758 diabetic patients with advanced retinopathy. The DRS found that photocoagulation reduces the risk of severe visual loss by 50% or more (30). The question of when to apply PRP was further delineated by the ETDRS. One eye of each patient was assigned randomly to early photocoagulation and the other to deferral of

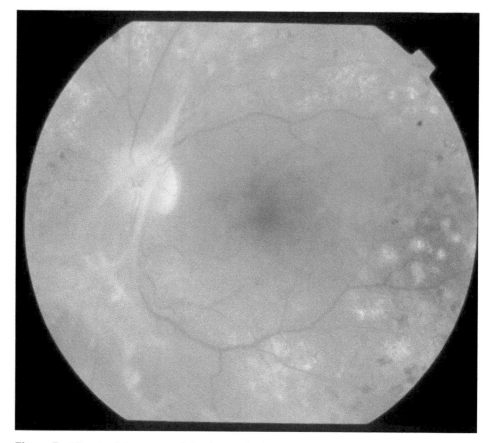

Figure 7   Fibrosis of the neovascularization results in traction on the retina.

photocoagulation (21). Based on the ETDRS, early photocoagulation is not recommended because severe visual loss is uncommon in treated and untreated eyes; moreover, PRP is associated with significant loss of visual acuity and peripheral vision, especially in the first few months after treatment (25). The DRS did identify high-risk characteristics for which PRP is clearly beneficial: (*i*) eyes with neovascularization and preretinal or vitreous hemorrhage and (*ii*) eyes with neovascularization on or within one disc diameter of the optic disc equaling or exceeding 1/4 to 1/3 disc area in extent even in the absence of preretinal or vitreous hemorrhage (30).

Early laser therapy has been found to be helpful in one exception, macular edema. In this setting, the ETDRS found early focal photocoagulation increased the chance of visual improvement, decreased the frequency of persistent macular edema, and caused only minor visual field loss. Therefore, focal laser treatment should be considered for eyes with macular edema that involves or threatens the fovea (21).

Anecdotal reports suggest intraocular injection of triamcinolone acetate into the vitreous is helpful in eyes with macular edema; however, there are no randomized clinical trials proving its efficacy in diabetic patients (25,31,32). In addition, it has been associated with elevations in intraocular pressure leading to glaucoma, cataract formation, endophthalmitis, vitreous hemorrhage, and retinal detachment (33,34). Despite these risks, the anecdotal evidence of its efficacy has made it a valuable option for the treatment of refractory macular edema.

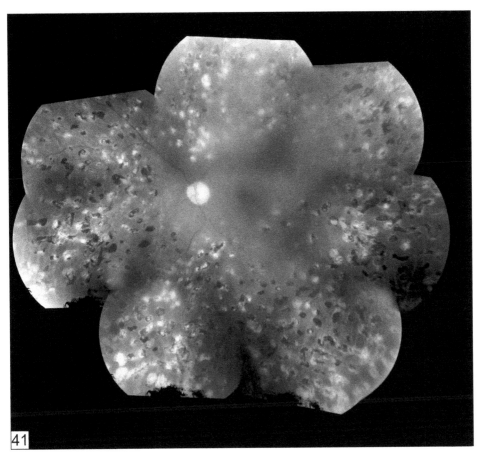

Figure 8   Panretinal photocoagulation is present in the retinal periphery for 360 degrees.

Laser therapy, unfortunately, is at times unable to deter the progression of neovascularization and secondary vitreous hemorrhage and traction retinal detachment. In these cases, the risk of severe visual disability rises dramatically and surgical intervention is necessary with vitrectomy. The timing of vitrectomy is important as found in the Diabetic Retinopathy Vitrectomy Study (DRVS). The DRVS enrolled 370 eyes with advanced, active PDR and visual acuities of 10/200 or better and randomly assigned the eyes to either early vitrectomy or conventional management. It found that if vitrectomy was delayed until central retinal detachment occurred, only 28% of eyes had a visual acuity of 10/20 or better at 4 years; whereas, 44% had a 10/20 visual acuity or better if vitrectomy was preformed early (25,35). The major indications for vitrectomy are macular-involving/threatening traction retinal detachment, combined traction-rhegmatogenous (i.e., torn) retinal detachment, and nonclearing vitreous hemorrhage (2).

If vitreous hemorrhage occurs, it can be managed conservatively with observation and laser treatment, surgical vitrectomy, or pharmacologic vitrectomy. Pharmacologic vitrectomy can be preformed with hyaluronidase (Vitrase) injection, which has shown therapeutic utility in clinical trials (36). A recent case report found that the anti-VEGF antibody bevacizumab (Avastin) caused marked regression of neovascularization and rapid resolution of vitreous hemorrhage (37) (Fig. 9).

A

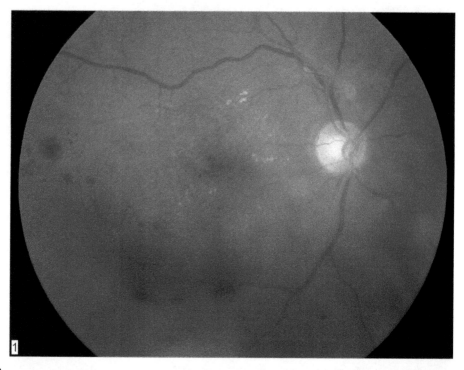

B

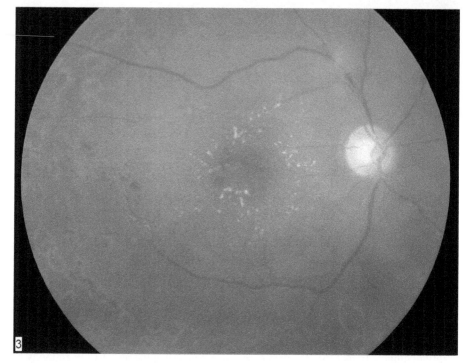

Figure 9 (**A**) Proliferative diabetic retinopathy with vitreous hemorrhage and tractional retinal detachment prior to vitrectomy surgery. (**B**) Same eye following vitrectomy surgery with excision of the fibrotic neovascularization and removal of the hemorrhage.

Recently, the use of anti-VEGF therapies has shown great promise in treating multiple manifestations of DR. Bevacizumab (Avastin), a monoclonal anti-VEGF antibody, was originally developed as an anti-angiogenic agent for the treatment of metastatic colorectal cancer. It did not take long before its antiangiogenic properties were considered for use in ocular, neovascular disease. In a series of 45 treated eyes with PDR, bevacizumab showed astonishing, rapid regression of retinal and iris neovascularization (38).

Recently, two other anti-VEGF agents, pegaptanib (Macugen) and ranibizumab (Lucentis), have been approved by the Food and Drug Administration (FDA) for the treatment of age-related macular degeneration.

Pegaptanib is an RNA oligonucleotide of 28 bases in length with extremely high affinity for the human $VEGF_{165}$ peptide (39). In a recent randomized, double-masked, controlled trial, 172 diabetic patients with a best-corrected visual acuity between 20/50 and 20/320 with macular edema involving the center of the macula where randomized to intraocular pegaptanib injections (0.3 mg) versus sham injections. The median visual acuity at 3 months was 20/50 in the pegaptanib group versus 20/63 in the sham group. The pegaptanib arm had a measurable decrease in macular edema versus an increase in the sham group. The pegaptanib arm also required less photocoagulation (40), and in eyes with neovasularization, 62% in the treatment arm had regression versus none in the sham arm (41). Ranibizumab, a recombinant humanized monoclonal antibody fragment with specificity for all isoforms of human VEGF, may have even greater potential as seen in the ARMD trials. One advantage it has over pegaptanib is that it is a fragment and not a whole antibody. In monkeys, it can penetrate the internal limiting membrane and reach the subretinal space after intravitreal injection (39). In an early pilot study of 10 patients, ranibizumab's use in diabetic macular edema had impressive results (42). Currently, anti-VEGF therapies are only approved to treat the wet variant of age-related macular degeneration, but with further investigation, it is hoped their approval for use within DR will be forthcoming.

SCREENING GUIDELINES (43)

The American Diabetes Association has set forth the following guidelines for screening patients with diabetes:

Type 1:
- ❖ Comprehensive eye exam (dilated exam by an ophthalmologist or optometrist) within 3 to 5 years after the onset of diabetes, but no need before age 10 in most cases
- ❖ Annual comprehensive eye exam thereafter

Type 2:
- ❖ Comprehensive eye exam at the time of diagnosis
- ❖ Annual comprehensive eye exam thereafter

Pregnancy (type 1 or type 2):
- ❖ Prepregnancy comprehensive eye exam and counseling regarding risks of development/progression of DR during pregnancy
- ❖ Comprehensive eye exam during first trimester with a close follow-up
- ❖ Note: these recommendation do not apply to gestational diabetes as it confers no increased risk of developing DR.

In 1990, the Dana Center for Preventive Ophthalmology calculated that the federal government would save $62.1 to $108.6 million annually if the above type 1 guidelines were followed (44). Once DR is diagnosed, screening intervals will vary based upon the severity of the disease. A knowledgeable ophthalmologist or optometrist is essential for appropriate care at this time.

CONCLUSION

Diabetes remains the leading cause of blindness in the working aged in industrialized nations largely because of poor screening. With intense blood sugar control, type 1 diabetic patients can significantly delay the onset and slow the progression of DR. Once DR is diagnosed, timely focal and panretinal photocoagulation can preserve the majority of patients' vision. If DR progresses despite these measures, vitrectomy can be used to prevent and manage devastating complications. Promising new drugs offer hope in the future for the most severe disease. Annual screening is cost-effective and is the key to preventing diabetes-related vision loss.

REFERENCES

1. Fong DS, Aiello L, Gardner TW, et al. Retinopathy in diabetes. Diabetes Care 2004;27(Suppl1): S84–S87.
2. Yanoff M, Duker JS. Ophthalmology (textbook). 2004;2nd:1652.
3. Lueder GT, Silverstein J. Screening for Retinopathy in the Pediatric Patient With Type 1 Diabetes Mellitus. Pediatrics 2005;116(1):270–273.
4. Klein R, Klein BE, Moss SE. Epidemiology of proliferative diabetic retinopathy. Diabetes Care 1992;15(12):1875–1891.
5. Klein R, Klein BE, Moss SE, et al. The wisconsin epidemiologic study of diabetic retinopathy. XIV. Ten-year incidence and progression of diabetic retinopathy. Arch Ophthalmol 1994; 112(9):1217–1228.
6. Klein R, Klein BE, Moss SE, et al. The wisconsin epidemiologic study of diabetic retinopathy: XVII. The 14-year incidence and progression of diabetic retinopathy and associated risk factors in type 1 diabetes. Ophthalmology 1998;105(10):1801–1815.
7. McCulloch DK. Pathogenesis and natural history of diabetic retinopathy. UpToDate.com Jul 2006, accessed Nov 15, 2006.
8. Frank RN. Diabetic retinopathy. N Engl J Med 2004;350(1):48–58.
9. Anonymous. The effect of intensive treatment of diabetes on the development and progression of long-term complications in insulin-dependent diabetes mellitus. The diabetes control and complications trial research group. N Engl J Med 1993;329(14):977–986.
10. McCulloch DK. Glycemic control and vascular complications in type I diabetes mellitus. UpToDate.com Jul 2006, accessed Nov 15, 2006.
11. Brownlee M. Lilly lecture 1993. Glycation and diabetic complications. Diabetes 1994;43(6): 836–841.
12. Brownlee M. The pathological implications of protein glycation. Clin Invest Med 1995;18(4): 275–281.
13. Greene DA, Lattimer SA, Sima AA. Sorbitol, phosphoinositides, and sodium-potassium-ATPase in the pathogenesis of diabetic complications. N Engl J Med 1987;316(10):599–606.
14. Suzen S, Buyukbingol E. Recent studies of aldose reductase enzyme inhibition for diabetic complications. Curr Med Chem 2003;10(15):1329–1352.
15. Kubo E, Urakami T, Fatma N, et al. Polyol pathway-dependent osmotic and oxidative stresses in aldose reductase-mediated apoptosis in human lens epithelial cells: Role of AOP2. Biochem Biophys Res Commun 2004;314(4):1050–1056.
16. Kohner EM, Patel V, Rassam SM. Role of blood flow and impaired autoregulation in the pathogenesis of diabetic retinopathy. Diabetes 1995;44(6):603–607.

17. Giusti C, Schiaffini R, Brufani C, et al. Coagulation pathways and diabetic retinopathy: Abnormal modulation in a selected group of insulin dependent diabetic patients. Br J Ophthalmol 2000;84(6):591–595.

18. Mizutani M, Kern TS, Lorenzi M. Accelerated death of retinal microvascular cells in human and experimental diabetic retinopathy. J Clin Invest 1996;97(12):2883–2890.

19. ETDRS. Classification of diabetic retinopathy from fluorescein angiograms. ETDRS report number 11. Early treatment diabetic retinopathy study research group. Ophthalmology 1991; 98(Suppl 5):807–822.

20. ETDRS. Fundus photographic risk factors for progression of diabetic retinopathy. ETDRS report number 12. Early treatment diabetic retinopathy study research group. Ophthalmology 1991;98(Suppl 5):823–833.

21. ETDRS. Early photocoagulation for diabetic retinopathy. ETDRS report number 9. Early treatment diabetic retinopathy study research group. Ophthalmology 1991;98(Suppl 5):766–785.

22. Davis MD. Vitreous contraction in proliferative diabetic retinopathy. Arch Ophthalmol 1965;74(6):741–751.

23. Ramsay RC, Goetz FC, Sutherland DE, et al. Progression of diabetic retinopathy after pancreas transplantation for insulin-dependent diabetes mellitus. N Engl J Med 1988;318(4):208–214.

24. Wang Q, Klein R Moss SE, et al. The influence of combined kidney-pancreas transplantation on the progression of diabetic retinopathy. A case series. Ophthalmology 1994;101(6):1071–1076.

25. McCulloch DK. Treatment of diabetic retinopathy. UpToDate.com Jun 2006, accessed Nov 11, 2006.

26. UKPDS. Tight blood pressure control and risk of macrovascular and microvascular complications in type 2 diabetes: UKPDS 38. UK Prospective Diabetes Study Group.[erratum appears in BMJ 1999 Jan 2;318(7175):29]. BMJ 1998;317(7160):703–713.

27. Chew EY, Klein ML, Murphy RP, et al. Effects of aspirin on vitreous/preretinal hemorrhage in patients with diabetes mellitus. Early treatment diabetic retinopathy study report no. 20. Arch Ophthalmol 1995;113(1):52–55.

28. ETDRS. Effects of aspirin treatment on diabetic retinopathy. ETDRS report number 8. Early tTreatment diabetic retinopathy study research group. Ophthalmology 1991;98(Suppl 5): 757–765.

29. Bergerhoff K, Clar C, Richter B. Aspirin in diabetic retinopathy. A systematic review. Endocrinol Metab Clin North Am 2002;31(3):779–793.

30. DRS. Photocoagulation treatment of proliferative diabetic retinopathy. Clinical application of Diabetic Retinopathy Study (DRS) findings, DRS Report Number 8. The Diabetic Retinopathy Study Research Group. Ophthalmology 1981;88(7):583–600.

31. Chieh JJ, Roth DB, Liu M, et al. Intravitreal triamcinolone acetonide for diabetic macular edema. Retina 2005;25(7):828–834.

32. Martidis A, Duker JS, Greenberg PB, et al. Intravitreal triamcinolone for refractory diabetic macular edema. Ophthalmology 2002;109(5):920–927.

33. Rhee DJ, Peck RE, Belmont J, et al. Intraocular pressure alterations following intravitreal triamcinolone acetonide. Br J Ophthalmol 2006;90(8):999–1003.

34. Nelson ML, Tennant MT, Sivalingam A, et al. Infectious and presumed noninfectious endophthalmitis after intravitreal triamcinolone acetonide injection. Retina 2003;23(5):686–691.

35. DRVS. Early vitrectomy for severe proliferative diabetic retinopathy in eyes with useful vision. Results of a randomized trial–Diabetic Retinopathy Vitrectomy Study Report 3. The Diabetic Retinopathy Vitrectomy Study Research Group. Ophthalmology 1988;95(10): 1307–1320.

36. Kuppermann BD, Thomas EL, de Smet MD, et al. Vitrase for vitreous hemorrhage studygroups. Pooled efficacy results from two multinational randomized controlled clinical trials of a single intravitreous injection of highly purified ovine hyaluronidase (Vitrase) for the management of vitreous hemorrhage. Am J Ophthalmol 2005;140(4):573–584.

37. Spaide RF, Fisher YL. Intravitreal bevacizumab (Avastin) treatment of proliferative diabetic retinopathy complicated by vitreous hemorrhage. Retina 2006;26(3):275–278.

38. Avery RL, Pearlman J, Pieramici DJ, et al. Intravitreal bevacizumab (Avastin) in the treatment of proliferative diabetic retinopathy. Ophthalmology 2006;113(10):1695.e1–15.

39. van Wijngaarden P, Coster DJ, Williams KA. Inhibitors of ocular neovascularization: Promises and potential problems. JAMA 2005;293(12):1509–1513.

40. Cunningham ET Jr, Adamis AP, Altaweel M, et al. A phase II randomized double-masked trial of pegaptanib, an anti-vascular endothelial growth factor aptamer, for diabetic macular edema. Ophthalmology 2005;112(10):1747–1757.

41. Adamis AP, Altaweel M, Bressler NM, et al. Changes in retinal neovascularization after pegaptanib (Macugen) therapy in diabetic individuals. Ophthalmology 2006;113(1):23–28.

42. Chun DW, Heier JS, Topping TM, et al. A pilot study of multiple intravitreal injections of ranibizumab in patients with center-involving clinically significant diabetic macular edema. Ophthalmology 2006;113(10):1706–1712.

43. Fong, Donald S. ADA position statement: Retinopathy in diabetes. Diabetes Care 2004;27(1):584–587.

44. Javitt JC, Canner JK, Frank RG, et al. Detecting and treating retinopathy in patients with type I diabetes mellitus. A health policy model. Ophthalmology 1990;97(4):483–494.

9
Diabetic Nephropathy

Y. Woredekal
SUNY Downstate Medical Center, Brooklyn, New York, U.S.A.

INTRODUCTION

Diabetes mellitus is associated with an increased risk of several comorbid conditions including coronary artery disease, hypertension, peripheral vascular disease, retinopathy, and nephropathy (1,2). The involvement of the kidney in diabetes, known as diabetic nephropathy, is a progressive disease and is often associated with hypertension. Diabetic nephropathy occurs as a result of both direct and indirect effect of hyperglycemia. Strict control of hyperglycemia, hypertension, and low protein diet has been shown to slow the progression of the renal disease.

In the United States and most western developed countries, diabetic nephropathy is the leading cause of end-stage renal disease (ESRD) in patients starting renal replacement therapy (3). The mortality rate of patients with diabetic nephropathy is high, and a marked increase in cardiovascular risk accounts for more than one-half of the mortality rate among these patients.

In this chapter we try to provide information on the pathogenesis, natural history, and management of diabetic nephropathy.

EPIDEMIOLOGY

A cumulative incidence of diabetic nephropathy has been documented after 20 to 25 years of diabetes in both type 1 and type 2 diabetic patients (4,5). The incidence of diabetic nephropathy is about 1% to 2% per year in patients with type 1 diabetes (6). Among the young of nonwhite origin with type 2 diabetes, such as Pima-Indians, Japanese, and African-Americans, the incidence of nephropathy is similar to that of type 1 diabetes (7,8). By contrast the incidence of diabetic nephropathy is much lower in elderly white type 2 diabetic patients than in nonwhite patients (9).

Recent studies have shown substantial reduction in incidence of diabetic nephropathy in type 1 diabetes (10,11); for example, a study from Sweden showed a substantial decline in proteinuria after 25 years of diabetes from 30% in patients in whom diabetes was diagnosed between 1961 and 1965 to 8.5% in those in whom the onset of diabetes was between 1966 and 1970 (10). Similar finding was also reported from Steno clinic in Denmark

(11). The decline in the incidence of diabetic nephropathy is attributed to the adoption in clinical practice of several measures that contribute to early diagnosis and prevention of the disease. In contrast to the decreasing incidence of diabetic nephropathy in type 1 diabetes, the incidence of diabetic nephropathy in type 2 diabetes has been increasing over the last 50 years. According to the 2006 United States Renal Data, diabetes is the cause of renal disease in 44.5% of incident ESRD cases, making the U.S. rate one of the highest worldwide (3).

There is a marked racial, ethnic, and international disparity in the epidemiology of diabetic nephropathy. Native Americans, Mexican-Americans, and African-Americans have a much higher risk of developing ESRD than non-Hispanic whites with type 2 diabetes (7–9).

NATURAL HISTORY

Diabetic nephropathy in type 1 diabetes follows a well outlined clinical course, starting with initial period of glomerular hyperfiltration associated with progressive proteinuria, followed by a gradual decline in glomerular filtration rate, eventually resulting in ESRD (12). Nephropathy usually becomes clinically evident after 15 to 25 years of diabetes and almost always progresses to ESRD. By contrast, because of the frequent insidious onset of type 2 diabetes and the common presence of coexisting vascular disease and hypertension, early renal involvement is frequently missed in this group of patients. However, in young patients with type 2 diabetes, recent studies have shown a course of nephropathy similar to that seen in type 1 diabetes (13,14). Renal involvement in type 1 diabetes has been divided into four stages.

Stage 1: Glomerular Hyperfiltration and Renomegaly

At the onset of type 1 diabetes mellitus, many patients have an increase in the glomerular filtration rate (GFR) and renal enlargement (15). Intensive insulin therapy normalizes hyperglycemia and corrects glomerular hyperfiltration (16,17). However, a substantial subset of individuals, after achieving acceptable level of glucose level continues to manifest a persistently elevated GFR (18,19). It is within this subgroup of patients with hyperfiltration that the initial reduction in GFR is noted, with progression to clinical nephropathy. Glomerular hyperfiltration has also been reported in patients with recent diagnosis of type 2 diabetes mellitus (20,21) and positively correlates with the development of nephropathy.

Stage 2: Microalbuminuria

Microalbuminuria is defined as an increased urinary albumin excretion (UAE) (30–299 mg/24 hr or 20–200 μg/min) not detected by standard bedside tests (dipstick) commonly used to detect proteinuria. The development of microaluminuria is the most important risk factor for the development of overt nephropathy. However, overt nephropathy is not its inevitable consequence. Although many patients, who manifest microalbuminuria, go on to develop overt nephropathy, a subset of patients' remains microalbuminuric or even regress to a normoalbuminuric state (22–24).

Earlier studies had shown that 80% of microalbuminuric type 1 diabetic patients progressed to proteinuria over a period of 5 to 15 years (25,26). In more recent studies, only 30% to 45% of microalbuminuric patients had progressed to proteinuria over 10 years (22). This change might be due to more intensive glycemic and blood pressure control.

Stage 3: Clinical Nephropathy—Proteinuria and Azotemia

Proteinuria, defined as UAE greater than 300 mg/day, is the universal hallmark of diabetic nephropathy. After 5 to 10 years of microalbuminuria, macroalbuminuria is detected by the urine dipstick in 30% to 40% of patients with type 1 diabetes. At this time blood pressure is usually elevated and renal function begins to decline. The rate of decline in function varies considerably among patients but averages 1 mL/min per month without therapeutic intervention. Nearly 100% of diabetic patients who have reached the azotemic phase of diabetic nephropathy have coincident retinopathy when examined by fluorecein angiography; the absence of diabetic retinopathy in advanced renal disease is a reason to doubt the diagnosis of diabetic nephropathy.

It should be kept in mind that because diabetic patients are at equal risk for unrelated renal disease, the quest for a renal diagnosis should be pursued, including renal biopsy, whenever the course does not fit the usual pattern of diabetic nephropathy. Renal biopsies from patients with type 1 diabetes and constant proteinuria show diffuse intercapillary glomerulosclerosis, mesangial expansion, and a thickened glomerular basement membrane (27,28).

Glomerular damage continues with increasing amount of protein in the urine. The kidneys' filtering capacity began to decline steadily and blood urea nitrogen and creatinine continue to rise in the blood.

Stage 4: ESRD

ESRD usually occurs 5 to 15 years after the onset of proteinuria. GFR has fallen approximately to 10 mL/min or lower and renal replacement therapy is needed. In diabetic patients with declining renal function, uremic signs and symptoms manifest at a higher creatinine clearance than nondiabetic patients.

PATHOGENESIS

The pathogenesis of diabetic nephropathy is likely due to genetic predisposition, and the interplay between hemodynamic and metabolic pathways in the renal microcirculation. Familial studies have demonstrated genetic susceptibility contribute to the development of diabetic nephropathy in both type 1 (29,30) and type 2 diabetes (31,32).

The diabetic offsprings of parents with diabetes and proteinuria have three to four times the prevalence of nephropathy compared to the siblings of diabetic parents without renal disease (29,30). The risk appears to be further increased if both parents have diabetic nephropathy, as opposed to only one parent with albuminuria (31). This has led to the suggestion that the predisposition to diabetic nephropathy may be inherited as a dominant trait.

The leading metabolic factor involved in the development of diabetic nephropathy is hyperglycemia. First, glucose in high concentration may be toxic to cells, altering cell growth and gene and protein expression, thus increasing extracellar matrix and growth factor production. Second, hyperglycemia may induce its adverse effect indirectly through the formation of metabolic end products such as oxidative and glycation products and also through activation of protein kinase and renin–angiotensin system.

Glomerular Hyperfiltration

Glomerular hyperfiltration has been proposed to play a role in the pathogenesis of diabetic nephropathy by directly promoting extracellular matrix (ECM) accumulation, by mechanism such as increased expression of transforming growth factor (TGF-β). In vitro, TGF-β modulates ECM production in glomerular mesangial and epithelial cells that are observed in persons with diabetic nephropathy (33,34).

Advanced Glycosylated End Products

Advanced glycosylated end products (AGEs) are formed from the nonenzymatic reaction of a sugar-derived carbonyl group with a reactive amino group resulting in the formation of an unstable Schiff base with subsequent Amadori rearrangement to form a more stable ketoamine. Over time, these intermediates undergo further modification to produce a range of poorly characterized compound products, termed AGE. Several binding sites and receptors for AGEs have been identified. Chronic hyperglycemia is responsible for the accumulation of high level of AGEs in patients with diabetes. In cultured glomerular endothelial and mesangial cells, in vitro, glycated albumin and AGE-rich proteins have been shown to enhance the expression of type IV collagen and TGF-β and increased PKC activity, which contribute to glomerular sclerosis and tubulointerstitial damage by means of an abnormal ECM production (35). Several therapeutic strategies have been tried either to block AGEs formation or to inhibit AGE action by inhibition of its interaction with its receptor. Forbes et al. demonstrated that the administration of ALT711, an AGE cross-link breaker, in diabetic rats readily reduced the glomerulosclerosis, tubulointerstitial fibrosis, and proteinuria (36).

Protein Kinase C

This is another pathway postulated to play a role in pathogenesis of diabetic nephropathy. Protein kinase C is a family of serin-threonine kinases, consisting of at least 10 structurally related isoforms that regulate a variety of cell functions including proliferation, gene expression, cell differentiation, cell migration, and apoptosis (37). Upregulation of PKC was observed in kidneys of rats with diabetic nephropathy (38). Activated PKC increases production of cytokines and extracellular matrix as well as vasoconstrictor endothelin-1 (39). These changes contribute to basement membrane thickening, vascular occlusion, and increased permeability. When experimental rodents were given a PKC inhibitor LY333531, reduction in glomerular hyperfiltration, UAE, and glomerular TGF-beta 1 and ECM production were noted, despite persistent hypertension and hyperglycemia (40).

Renin–Angiotensin System

Its role in the pathogenesis of diabetic nephropathy has been recognized for a while. This is best shown by the unique protective effects seen by inhibitors of the renin–angiotensin system (RAS) in diabetic renal disease (41). In experimental models, upregulation of the RAS in the presence of diabetes is associated with accelerated nephropathy. In humans, activity of the RAS can be modified by a number of genetic factors. For example, circulating angiotensin-converting enzyme (ACE) activity is strongly associated with polymorphisms in the ACE gene (42). The best characterized of these is the biallellic polymorphism defined by the presence of an extra 287-base pair sequence in intron 16 of the ACE gene called insertion or I, genotype or its absence so called deletion or D. Studies have shown that

D allele was associated with an increased prevalence of nephropathy and premature death in patients with both type 1 and type 2 diabetes (43,44). The GENEDIAB study of 449 patients with type 1 diabetes found that the D allele was associated with increased incidence and severity of diabetic nephropathy (with odds ratio of 1.9) independent of hypertension or glycemic control (43).

PATHOLOGY

Diabetic nephropathy causes unique changes in the kidney. It is characterized by increased glomerular basement membrane width, diffuse mesangial expansion, hyalinosis, microaneurysm, and hyaline arteriosclerosis (45). Areas of extreme mesangial expansion called Kimmelstiel–Wilson nodules or nodular mesangial expansion are observed in 40% to 50% of patients developing proteinuria (46). Tubular and interstitial changes are also common findings in diabetic nephropathy (47,48).

SCREENING AND DIAGNOSIS

Screening for diabetic nephropathy in patients with type 1 diabetes mellitus is recommended at 5 years after diagnosis of diabetes (49), while for those with type 2 diabetes screening should be started at the time of diagnosis, since at least 7% of newly diagnosed patients have microalbuminuria (50). Even in type 1 diabetic patients with poor glycemic control, high blood pressure, and poor lipid regulation, the prevalence of microalbuminuria before 5 years may be as high as 18% (51).

The first step in the screening and diagnosis of diabetic nephropathy is to measure albumin in a spot urine sample, collected either as the first urine in the morning or random. Results of albumin spot measurements may be expressed as a urinary albumin concentration (mg/L) or as a urinary albumin-to-creatinine ratio (mg/mmol) (52). The upper limit of 17 mg/L in a random urine specimen has a sensitivity of 100% and a specificity of 80% for diagnosis of microalbuminuria using a 24-hour–timed urine collection as the reference standard (53). All positive tests should be confirmed in two out of three samples collected over a 3- to 6-month period because of the known day-to-day variability in UAE. Furthermore, screening should be avoided in the conditions that may temporarily induce albuminuria, such as fever, urinary or systemic infection, marked hypertension, heart failure, pronounced hyperglycemia, or vigorous exercise.

Although the measurement of UAE is the cornerstone for the diagnosis of diabetic nephropathy, there are some patients with either type 1 or type 2 diabetes who have decreased GFR in the presence of normal UAE (54,55). Therefore, UAE and GFR should be estimated routinely for proper screening of diabetic nephropathy.

PREVENTION AND TREATMENT STRATEGIES

Significant progress has been made in recent years in understanding the pathophysiology, prevention, and treatment of diabetic nephropathy. Median survival after the onset of nephropathy has increased from 6 to 15 years (56). The basis for the prevention of diabetic nephropathy is the treatment of its known risk factors: hyperglycemia, hypertension, smoking, high protein diet, and dyslipidemia (Table 1).

Table 1   Measures Influencing
Progression of Diabetic Nephropathy

- Glycemic control
- Tight blood pressure control
- Low protein diet
- Lipid-lowering agent
- Cessation of cigarette smoking

Glycemic Control

Two major clinical trials, the diabetes control and complications trial (DCCT) (57), and the United Kingdom prospective diabetes study (UKPDS) (58), convincingly demonstrated that intensive glycemic control reduces the risk of developing microalbuminuria and nephropathy. It was also noted that the patients randomized to strict glycemic control had a long-lasting reduction of 40% in the risk for development of microalbuminuria and hypertension 7 to 8 years after the end of the DCCT (59).

Fioretto and her colleagues have shown regression of glomerular and tubular basement membrane thickening and reduction of mesangial matrix 10 years after solitary pancreas transplant in patients with type 1 diabetes and microalbuminuria (60). These changes were associated with a reduction in the UAE from 103 mg/day at baseline to 30 mg/day after 5 years and 20 mg/day after 10 years. The above structural changes were not seen at 5 years.

The effect of a strict glycemic control on the progression from micro- to macroalbuminuria and on the rate of renal function decline in macroalbuminuric patients is still controversial. Both the DCCT study and the Microalbuminuria Collaborative Study Group did not show reduction in the rate of progression to macroalbuminuria in patients with type 1 diabetes and microalbuminuria (57,61).

In general, the goal for glycemic control is to keep blood glucose level as close to normal as possible without causing significant hypoglycemia. The American Diabetes Association (ADA) recommended HbA1 c to be $< 7\%$ (62).

Intensive Blood Pressure Control

Multiple studies have shown the impact of good blood pressure control on prevention and progression of diabetic nephropathy. About 40% of type 1 and 70% of type 2 diabetic patients with normoalbuminuria have blood pressure level $> 140/90$ mm Hg (63). In the UKPDS, a reduction from 154 to 144 mm Hg of systolic blood pressure reduced the risk for the development of microalbuminuria by 29% (64).

As reviewed by Parving, in both type 1 and type 2 diabetic patients with overt diabetic nephropathy, blood pressure reduction, whether with ACE inhibitors or other antihypertensive medication, reduces albuminuria, delays progression of nephropathy, postpones renal insufficiency, and improves survival (65). Although slowing of the progression of renal function has been achieved by using other antihypertensive medications, the RAS has become the target of the most effective strategy for both hypertension control and, independently, for reduction of the pathophysiologic abnormalities that lead to renal protein leak in diabetic nephropathy (66).

In the landmark captopril study of type 1 diabetics, the ACE inhibitor significantly reduced the progression of diabetic nephropathy. Proteinuria decreased and the endpoints of doubling of the serum creatinine, ESRD, or death were reduced by 50% (67). Later on, the

EUCLID study, which was done in 18 European centers, randomized type 1 diabetic patients with normo- or microalbuminuria to treatment with an ACE inhibitor (lisinopril) or placebo (68). After 24 months, there was a significant difference favoring the lisinopril cohort both in terms of mean UAE and in the ratio of transition from normo- to microalbuminuria. Angiotensin receptor blockers (ARBs) were also effective in reducing the development of macroalbuminuria in microalbuminuric type 2 diabetic patients. Irbesartan (300 mg/day) reduced the risk of progression to overt diabetic nephropathy by 70% in a 2-year–follow-up study of 590 hypertensive microalbuminuric type 2 diabetic patients (69). Additionally, a 38% reduction in UAE was observed, with 34% of patients reversing to normoalbuminuria. Recent studies have indicated benefit from dual blockade of the RAS by ACE inhibitors plus ARBs as noted by greater reduction in proteinuria and blood pressure in both type 1 and type 2 diabetic patients (70–72). The combination of spironolactone, an aldosterone antagonist, with an ACE inhibitor was also more effective in reducing UAE and blood pressure in micro- and macroalbuminuric type 2 diabetic patients than the ACE inhibitor alone (73). Therefore, the use of either ACE inhibitors, ARBs, or combination of both is recommended as a first-line therapy for type 1 and type 2 diabetic patients with microalbuminuria, even if they are normotensive.

Current ADA recommendations are to lower blood pressure to 130/80 mm Hg in normoalbuminuric and to 126/70 mm Hg for proteinuric diabetic patients (74).

Low Protein Diet

It has long been known that protein restriction is effective in alleviating the symptoms of uremia and delaying the need for dialysis (75). Beyond symptomatic relief, a low protein diet is advocated to slow the decline of renal function (76,77). The proposed mechanism for slowing the progression of renal disease is reduction in hyperfilteration that occurs in the remaining nephrons after renal injury. In 5 year prospective study of patients with type 1 diabetes, ESRD or death occurred in 27% of patients on the usual protein diet as compared with 10% on a low protein diet (78) with a comparable glycemic and blood pressure control in both groups.

Although a clear benefit of dietary protein restriction has not been established in a large randomized prospective trial, current recommendation is dietary allowance of 0.8 g/kg/day of protein, accounting for 10% of total calories, with further restriction as GFR falls.

Lipid-Lowering Agents

Hyperlipidemia is commonly seen in patients with both type 1 and type 2 diabetes mellitus. A number of experimental studies have suggested a link between hyperlipidemia and the development of glomerulsclerosis (79,80). In both type 1 and type 2 diabetes, only a few prospective and controlled studies have shown a correlation between hyperlipidemia and worsening of renal function.

Thomas et al. prospectively followed 152 patients with type 1 diabetes for 8 years to examine the association of dyslipidemia to progression of nephropathy. In patients with microalbuminuria, progression was independently associated with triglycerides content of VLDL, and intermediate-density lipoprotein. In patients with macroalbuminuria, a significant decline in the renal function was independently associated with poor glycemic control, hypertension, and LDL size (81). Hadjadj et al. have also found similar findings when they prospectively followed 297 patients with type 1 diabetes without ESRD for 7 years. High triglycerides levels were an independent predictive factor of both renal and retinal complications. After adjusting for systolic blood pressure, glycemic control, stages of complications at baseline, and diabetes duration, the relative risk for progression was 2.01 (95%, CI: 1.07–3.77) for nephropathy and 2.3 (95%, CI: 1.03–5.12) for retinopathy for patients having serum triglyceride in the highest tertile, compared to the others (82).

Although large prospective trials of the effect of treatment of dyslipidemia on progression of diabetic nephropathy are not yet reported, some evidence indicates that lipid reduction by antilipidemic agents preserves GFR and decreases proteinuria in diabetic patients (83–84). A meta-analysis of lipid-lowering therapy on progression of renal disease assessed 13 prospective controlled trials, 7 of which were exclusively in diabetic patients (85). Lipid lowering was associated with a lower rate of decline in renal function compared to controls ($P = 0.008$) inducing beneficial effects equivalent to ACE inhibition in preservation of renal function. As for other component of renoprotection, longitudinal prospective trials are needed to validate the value of lipid-lowering agents. However, as cardiovascular disease is the number one cause of death in diabetic patients with nephropathy, optimizing lipid control is now a standard of care.

Cessation of Cigarette Smoking

Several studies have established the linkage between cigarette smoking and progression of diabetic nephropathy (86–89). Chase et al. assessed the effect of cigarette smoking on diabetic renal and retinal complication in 359 type 1 diabetic patients. The prevalence of increased albumin excretion rate was 2.8 times higher in smokers than in those who do not smoke. Even after correction for glycohemoglobin level and duration of diabetes, smoking was an independent risk factor for development and progression of diabetic nephropathy (86). Chuahirum et al. reported type 2 diabetic patients who smoked had a faster decline of renal function than nonsmokers (88,89). As is true for pulmonary and cardiovascular disease, quitting smoking should be the therapy of preventive measures for nephropathy in diabetic patients.

MANAGEMENT OF ADVANCED RENAL FAILURE

Although normalizing blood pressure, optimizing glycemic control, and adhering to low protein diet may slow the development and progression of diabetic nephropathy; many patients still progress to ESRD. Patients with diabetic nephropathy and declining renal function should be referred to nephrologists at an early stage and certainly by the time serum creatinine levels have raised to 2–3 mg/dL. This helps to optimize treatment and early consideration for renal replacement therapy. Reports from both Europe and the United States showed that a high proportion of patients with diabetic nephropathy were referred to nephrologists late in the course of their disease, and resulting in suboptimal care (90,91).

As the renal disease progresses, taking care of diabetic patients becomes more complicated and requires multidisciplinary medical team that consist of diabetologist, nephrologists, nutritionist, cardiologist, ophthalmologist, and podiatrist.

Pre-ESRD care (Table 2) of diabetic patients with advanced renal disease beyond glycemic and blood pressure control includes maintaining of hemoglobin above 11 gm/dL, by administering human recomobinant erythropoietin and supplemental iron, minimizing metabolic bone disease due to secondary hyperparathyroidism by using phosphate binders along with use of synthetic vitamin D and/or calcimimetics and maintaining of good nutritional status.

Table 2 Pre-ESRD Care for Diabetic Patients with
Advance Renal Disease

- Glycemic control
- Blood pressure control
- Maintenance of hemoglobin > 11 gm/dL
- Maintenance of calcium and phosphate balance
- Prevention of malnutrition
- Early preparation for renal replacement therapy

As renal function decreases, the doses of medications, especially those excreted by the kidney, have to be adjusted in order to prevent high blood levels and drug–drug interaction. Thus, diabetic patients with advanced renal disease should be closely followed and be referred to the treatment team responsible for preparing them for renal replacement therapy.

OPTIONS FOR RENAL REPLACEMENT THERAPY

Diabetic patients with ESRD have similar options for renal replacement therapy, as do nondiabetic patients. Choices in renal replacement therapy available for diabetic ESRD patients include hemodialysis, peritoneal dialysis, kidney transplantation, and a combined pancreas and kidney transplant (Table 3).

Before a patient is assigned a specific modality of renal replacement therapy, it is important that both patients and their families be properly informed about the advantages and disadvantages of each treatment option. Selecting a treatment for a particular patient is determined by considering the patient's age, level of education, severity of comorbid conditions, social and family support, and geographical location.

Regular scheduled meetings with both a nurse educator and nutritionist, coupled with participation in patient support groups, can play a vital role in guiding ESRD patients to make appropriate choices of treatment.

Once the decision for a preferred option is made, preparation for renal replacement therapy should be started. For instance, for those electing hemodialysis, it is important to establish vascular access in the nondominant arm when creatinine clearance is around 25 mL/min. For those who have live kidney donors, family members should be blood typed

Table 3 Options for Renal Replacement Therapy for
Diabetic Patients with ESRD

- Hemodialysis
  In-center hemodialysis
  Home hemodialysis
  Daily (nocturnal) hemodialysis
- Peritoneal dialysis
  CAPD
  CCPD
- Organ transplantation
  Kidney transplantation
  Simultaneous pancreas and kidney transplantation
  Pancreas after kidney transplantation

and tissue matched early so that preemptive transplantation can be done before initiating dialytic treatment. Long-term survival is greatly superior with a kidney transplant than in any dialytic regimen.

Although evidence from prospective, controlled, clinical trials is lacking, there is a widespread consensus among nephrologists that diabetic individuals develop uremic symptoms at a higher level of residual renal function, and that dialysis should be initiated earlier than in nondiabetics. As renal failure progresses, the diabetic kidney is progressively less able to compensate for hypoalbuminemia by regulation of volume and sodium balance, and as a result, hypertension and fluid overload may become refractory at a relatively high GFR. Concomitant gastroparesis and nephritic syndrome may exacerbate protein–calorie malnutrition. Many nephrologists believe that early initiation of dialysis protects against malnutrition during the pre-ESRD period and might prevent the increased morbidity and early mortality related to malnutrition among dialysis patients. The Canada-USA (CANUSA) study of peritoneal dialysis showed that nutritional status at initiation of dialytic therapy is correlated with residual renal function at its initiation (92). In general, it is advisable to start dialytic therapy for diabetic patients when the creatinine clearance is between 10 and 15 mL/min.

Maintenance Hemodialysis

As reported in the USRDS 2004 registry, 75% of all diabetic patients with ESRD are treated with hemodialysis (center or home), 7.4% with peritoneal dialysis (CAPD or CCPD), and 17.6% received kidney transplant (3). Hemodialysis treatment for diabetic patients is similar to that in nondiabetic patients. An ideal hemodialysis regime consists of dialyses thrice weekly, each lasting 3.5 to 4.5 hours, as determined by individual blood chemistry and clinical response, during which extracorporeal blood flow is maintained at 300 to 400 mL/min.

Survival and rehabilitation of diabetic patients on hemodialysis is inferior to that of nondiabetic patients, mainly because of preexisting severe vascular diseases. Although the preferred vascular access is an arteriovenous fistula, preexisting vascular disease limits its utility in diabetic patients, who have a primary fistula failure rate of 30% to 40%. A less desirable, but necessary alternative vascular access can be constructed using a polytetrafluoroethylene graft, which has a half-life of 1 to 2 years. Complication of vascular access is the leading cause of hospitalization in diabetic patients with ESRD undergoing hemodialysis treatment.

Glycemic control in diabetic patients on dialysis is difficult. Insulin dosage is more complex because of reduced renal insulin catabolism that result in prolonged exogenous insulin, as well as unrecognized gastroparesis that disconnects absorption of ingested food from timed insulin administration. This combination causes erratic glucose regulation complicated by frequent hypoglycemic episodes, potentially serious complications. Glycemic control should remain a priority in the dialyzed diabetic patient as it may retard further complications of microvascular disease. Survival during long-term management of ESRD in diabetic patients has been linked to the quality of glycemic control achieved (93).

Peritoneal Dialysis

Peritoneal dialysis is a satisfactory alternative mode of dialytic therapy available for diabetic ESRD patients. As is true for hemodialysis, preparation of the patient for continuous ambulatory peritoneal dialysis (CAPD) necessitates education, repetitive explanation, and facilitating surgery to insert an intraperitoneal permanent catheter. CAPD can be mastered as a home regimen in about 4 weeks. An alternative to manual cycling of dialysate is the use of a mechanical cycling device in a regimen termed continuous cyclic peritoneal dialysis (CCPD), which can be performed during sleep.

CAPD offers some advantages over hemodialysis such as freedom from machine, reduced cardiovascular stress, better preservation of renal function, avoidance of heparin, and less dietary restriction. On the other hand disadvantages of peritoneal dialysis include the risk of peritonitis, high rate of technical failure, and less adequate dialysis when residual renal function gets very low. Some nephrologists view peritoneal dialysis as the preferred choice of treatment for diabetic ESRD patients. Indeed, peritoneal dialysis may be life sustaining when vascular access sites for hemodialysis have been exhausted, or in those with sever congestive heart failure or angina. Peritoneal dialysis offers less vascular stress because of its relatively slow ultrafiltration rate coupled with less rapid solute removal.

During the course of both CAPD and CCPD, there is a constant risk of peritonitis as well as a gradual decrease in peritoneal surface area which may ultimately drove to be insufficient for adequate dialysis. Diabetic patients on CAPD experience twice as many hospitalization days as nondiabetic patients: peritonitis accounts for 30% to 50% of these hospital days (94). Of the two major options in dialytic therapy for diabetic patients, the USRDS consistently reports superior survival in those treated by hemodialysis, except in those younger than 45 years compared with peritoneal dialysis. However, there are few studies reporting equivalent patients survival between peritoneal dialysis and hemodialysis in the first 2 years of treatment (95,96).

Kidney Transplantation

In the 1970s and early 1980s many transplant programs excluded diabetic ESRD patients from consideration for renal transplantation. However, in centers that perform transplants in diabetic patients during this period, survival exceeded that of diabetic patients remaining on dialysis. Today, improved management of diabetic and uremic complications, established kidney transplantation is the preferred option of treatment for diabetic ESRD patients. Diabetic patients with ESRD should be referred to a transplant center to assess their candidacy. Absolute contraindications to transplantation include severe uncorrectable cardiac or pulmonary disease, unresolved chronic infections, metastatic/ untreatable cancer, and significant psychiatric disease (97). In many transplant centers there is no absolute age ceiling in considering someone for transplantation.

Type 1 diabetic patients with ESRD have several options for transplantation: they may be a candidate for kidney transplantation alone, simultaneous pancreas and kidney transplantation (SPK), or pancreas after kidney transplantation (usually a living donor kidney transplantation).

Although survival of diabetic ESRD patients after renal transplantation is continuously improving, it is 10% to 20% less over 5 years than of patients with other causes of renal disease. A further fall-off in survival of diabetic renal transplant recipients after 5 or more years is the consequence of advanced macrovascular disease. Annual death rate of transplant recipients is approximately one-third that of diabetic patients remaining on dialysis—a finding, which may reflect the selection of healthier patients for transplantation. But when diabetic patients who had been transplanted were compared with patients remaining on the transplant list, presumably with similar comorbidities, patient survival was significantly better in transplant recipients (98,99).

Over the past decade, highly successful results have been reported in type 1 diabetic patients for pancreatic transplants inserted concurrently with a renal allograft. Although combined pancreas and kidney transplant does not raise immediate perioperative mortality, perioperative morbidity is markedly increased over that of a kidney transplant alone.

Diabetic renal transplant recipients have been shown to have three times the risk of events related to ischemic heart disease than the general population (100). In addition to the traditional risk factors (hypertension, hyperlipidemia, cigarette smoking, etc.), factors associated with ESRD and dialytic therapy present before transplantation, such as left-ventricular hypertrophy due to chronic volume overload, oxidative stress, vascular calcification secondary to abnormality in calcium and phosphate metabolism, and hyper-homocysteinemia, can contribute to an increased cardiovascular risk.

Given the impact of cardiovascular disease in diabetics with kidney transplant, modifications of risk factors in order to decrease risk of progression and development of cardiovascular disease is important. In addition to the assessing the extent of cardiovascular disease present prior to transplantation, at least annual reassessment with noninvasive studies in asymptomatic high-risk patients should be performed.

REFERENCES

1. Parving HH, Hommel E, Mathiesen E, et al. Prevalence of microalbuminuria, arterial hypertension, retinopathy, and neuropathy in patients with insulin-dependent diabetes. Br Med J (Clin Res Ed) 1988;296:156–160.
2. Ismail N, Becker B, Strazelczyk P, et al. Renal disease and hypertension in non-insulin-dependent diabetes mellitus. Kidney Int 1999;55:1–28.
3. United States Renal Data System (USRDS). Annual Data Report. Bethesda, MD: National Institute of Health, National Institute of Diabetes, Digestive and Kidney Disease, 2006.
4. Anderson AR, Christiansen JS, Andersen JK, et al. Diabetic nephropathy in type 1 (insulin-dependent) diabetes. An epidemiological study: Diabetologia 1983;25:496–501.
5. Hasslacher C, Ritz E, Wahl B, et al. Similar risks of nephropathy in patients with type I or type II diabetes mellitus. Nephrol Dial Transplant 1989;4:859–863.
6. Breyer JA. Diabetic nephropathy in insulin-dependent diabetic patients. Am J Kidney Dis 1992;20:533–547.
7. Cowie CC, Port FK, Wolfe RA, et al. Disparities in incidence of diabetic end-stage renal disease according to race and type of diabetes. N Engl J Med 1989;321:1074–1079.
8. Nelson RG, Newman JM, Knowler WC, et al. Incidence of end stage renal disease in type 2 (non-insulin-dependent) diabetes mellitus in Pima Indians. Diabetologia 1988;31:730–736.
9. Ballard DJ, Humphrey LL, Melton IJ 3rd, et al. Epidemiology of persistent proteinuria in type I diabetes mellitus population based study in Rochester, Minnesota. Diabetes 1988;37:405–412.
10. Nordwall M, Bojestig M, Arnquist HJ, et al. Declining incidence of severe retinopathy and persisting decrease of nephropathy in an unselected population of type 1 diabetes-the Linkoping Diabetes Complications Study. Diabetologia 2004;47(7):1266–1272.
11. Hovind P, Tarnow L, Rossing K, et al. Decreasing incidence of severe diabetic microangiopaghy in type 1 diabetes. Diabetes Care 2003;26:1258–1264.
12. Mogensen CE, Schmitz O. The diabetic kidney: From hyperfiltration and microalbuminuria to end-stage renal failure. Med Clin North Am 1988;72:1465–1492.
13. Rossing K, Christensen PK, Hovind P, et al. Progression of nephropathy in type 2 diabetic patients. Kidney Int 2004;66:1596–1605.
14. Chiken RL, Eckert-Norton M, Bard M, et al. Hyperfiltration in African-American patients with type 2 diabetes. Cross-sectional and longitudinal data. Diabetes Care 1998;21:2129–2134.
15. Mogensen CE, Christensen CK. Predicting diabetic nephropathy in insulin-dependent diabetic patients. N Engl J Med 1984;311:89–94.

16. Tuttle KR, Bruton JL, Perusek MC, et al. Effect of strict glycemic control on renal hemodynamic response to amino acids and renal enlargement in insulin-dependent diabetes mellitus. N Engl J Med 1991;324(23):1626–1632.

17. Christensen CK, Christansen JS, Schmitz A, et al. Effect of continuous subcutaneous insulin infusion on kidney function and size in IDDM patients: A 2 year controlled study. J Diabet Complications 1987;1(3):91–95.

18. Rudberg S, Persson B, Dahlquist G. Increased glomerular filtration rate as a predictor of diabetic nephropathy: an 8- year prospective study. Kidney Int 1992;41:822–828.

19. Chiarelli F, Verrotti A, Morgese G. Glomerular hyperfiltration increases the risk of developing microalbuminuria in diabetic children. Pediatr Nephrol 1995;9:154–158.

20. Taniwaki H, Ishimura E, Emoto M, et al. Relationship between urinary albumin excretion and glomerular filtration rate in normotensive, nonproteinuric patients with type 2 diabetes mellitus. Nephron 2000;86:36–43.

21. Lee KU, Park JY, Hwang IR, et al. Glomerular hyperfiltration in Koreans with non-insulin-dependent diabetes mellitus. Am J Kidney Dis 1995;26(5):722–726.

22. Caramori ML, Fioretto P, Mauer M. The need for early predictors of diabetic nephropathy risk: Is albumin excretion rate sufficient? Diabetes 2000;49:1399–1408.

23. Gaede P, Tarnow L, Vedel P, et al. Remission to normoalbuminuria during multifactorial treatment preserves kidney function in Patients with type 2 diabetes and microalbuminuria. Nephrol Dial Transplant 2004;19(11):2784–2788.

24. Perkins BS, Ficociello LH, Silva KH, et al. Regression of microalbuminuria in type 1 diabetes. N Engl J Med 2003;348:2285–2293.

25. Parving HH, Oxenboll B, Svendsen PA, et al. Early detection of patients at risk of developing diabetic nephropathy: A longitudinal study of urinary albumin excretion. Acta Endocrinol (Copenh) 1982;100:550–555.

26. Viberti GC, Hill RD, Jarrett RJ, et al. Microalbuminuria as a predictor of clinical nephropathy in insulin-dependent diabetes mellitus. Lancet 1982;1:1430–1432.

27. Mauer SM, Steffes MW, Ellis EN, et al. Structural-functional relationships in diabetic nephropathy. J Clin Invest 1984;74:1143–1155.

28. Steffes MW, Osterby R, Chavers B, et al. Mesangial expansion as a central mechanism for loss of kidney function in diabetic patients. Diabetes 1989;38:1077–1081.

29. Seaquist ER, Goetz FC, Rich S, et al. Familial clustering of diabetic kidney disease: Evidence for genetic susceptibility to diabetic nephropathy. N Engl J Med 1989;320:1161–1165.

30. Quinn M, Angelico MC, Warram JH, et al. Familial factor determine the development of diabetic nephropathy in patients with IDDM. Diabetologia 1996;39:940–945.

31. Pettitt DJ, Saad MF, Bennett PH, et al. Familial predisposition to renal disease in two generatios of Pima Indians with type II (non-insulin dependent) diabetes mellitus. Diabetologia 1990;33:438–443.

32. Freedman BI, Tuttle AB, Spray BJ, Familial predisposition to nephropathy in African-Americans with non-insulin dependent diabetes mellitus. Am J Kidney Dis 1999;5:710–713.

33. Nakamura T, Miller D, Ruoslahti E, et al. Production of extracellular matrix by glomerular epithelial cells is regulated by transforming growth factor-beta. Kidney Int 1992;41:1213–1221.

34. Roberts AB, McCune BK, Sporn MB. TGF-beta: Regulation of extracellular matrix. Kidney Int 1992;41(3):577–579.

35. Chen S, Chohen MP, Lautenslager GT, et al. Gylcated albumin stimulates TGF-beta 1 production and protein kinase C activity in glomerular endothelial cells. Kidney Int 2001;59:671–681.

36. Forbes JM, Thallas V, Thomas MC, et al. The breakdown of preexisting advance glycation end products is associated with reduced renal fibrosis in experimental diabetes. FASEB J 2003;17:1762–1764.

37. Webb BIJ, Hirst SJ, Giembycz MA. Protein Kinase C isoenzymes: A review of their structure, regulation and role in regulating airway smooth muscle tone and mitogenesis. Br J Pharmacol 2000;130:1433–1452.

38. Koya, D, Jirousek MR, Lin Y-W, Ishii H, et al. Charcterzation of protein kinase C-beta isoform activation on the gene expression of transforming growth factor-beta, extracellular

matrix components, and prostandoids in the glomeruli of diabetic rats. J Clin Invest 1997;100: 115–126.

39. Igarashi M, Wakasaki H, Takahara N, et al. Glucose or diabetes activates p38 mitogen-activated protein kinase via different pathways. J Clin Invest 1999;103:185–195.

40. Kelly DJ, Zhang Y, Hepper C, et al. Protein kinase C-beta inhibition attenuates the progression of experimental diabetic nephropathy in the presence of continued hypertension. Diabetes 2003;52(2):512–518.

41. Cooper ME. Pathogenesis, prevention, and treatment of diabetic nephropathy. Lancet 1998; 352:213–219.

42. Rigat B, Hubert C, Alhenoc-Gelas F, et al. An insertion/deletion polymorphism in the angiotensin I-converting enzyme gene accounting for half the variance of serum enzyme levels. J Clin Invest 1990;86:1343–1346.

43. Marre M, Jeunemaitre X, Gallois Y, et al. Contribution of genetic polymorphism in the rennin-angiotensin system to the development of renal complications in insulin-dependent diabetes: Genetique de la Nephroapathie Diabetique (GENEDIAB) Study Group. J Clin Invest 1997;99:1585–1595.

44. Jeffers BW, Estacio RO, Raynolds MV, et al. Angiotensin-converting enzyme gene polymorphism in non-insulin-dependent diabetes mellitus and its relationship with diabetic nephropathy. Kindney Int 1997;52:473–477.

45. Mauer SM, Steffes MW, Brown DM. The kidney in diabetes. Am J Med 1981;70:603–612.

46. Kimmestiel P, Wilson C. Intercappilary lesion in the glomeruli of kidney. Am J Pathol 1936;12:83–97.

47. Brito PL, Fioretto P, Drummond K, et al. Proximal tubular basement membrane width in insulin-dependent diabetes mellitus. Kid Int 1998;53:754–761.

48. Katz A, Caramori ML, Sisson-Ross S, et al. An increase in the cell component of the cortical interstitium antedates interstitial fibrosis in type 1 diabetic patients. Kidney Int 2002;61: 2058–2066.

49. American Diabetes Association. Nephropathy in diabetes (position statement). Diabetes Care 2004;27(Suppl 2):S79–S83.

50. Adler AI, Stevens RJ, Manley SE, et al. Development and progression of nephropathy in type 2 diabetes: The United Kingdom Prospective Diabetes Study (UKPDS 64). Kidney Int 2003;63:225–232.

51. Stephenson JM, fuller JH. Microalbuminuria is not rare before 5 years of IDDM: EURODIAB IDDM Complications Study Group and the WHO Multinational Study of vascular Disease in Diabetes Study Group. Diabetes Complications 1994;8:166–173.

52. Gross JL, Zelmanovitx T, Oliveira J, et al. Screening for diabetic nephropathy: Is measurement of urinary albumin-to-creatinine ratio worthwhile? Diabetes Care 1999;22:1599–1600.

53. Zelmanovitz T, Gross JL, Oliveira J, et al. The receiver operating characteristics curve1 the evaluation of a random urine specimen as a screening test for diabetic nephropathy. Diabetes Care 1997;20:516–519.

54. Caramori ML, Fioretto P, Mauer M. Low glomerular filtration rate in normoalbuminuric type 1 diabetic patients is associated with more advanced diabetic lesions. Diabetes 2003;52: 1036–1040.

55. Maclsaac RJ, Tsalamandris C, Panagiotopoulos S, et al. Nonalbuminuric renal insufficiency in type 2 diabetes. Diabetes Care 2004;27:195–200.

56. Rossing P. Promotion, predition and prevention of progression of nephropathy in type 1 diabetes mellitus. Diabetic Med 1998;15:900–919.

57. The Diabetes Control and Complications Trial Research Group. The effect of intensive treatment of diabetes on the development and progression of long-term complications in insulin-dependent diabetes mellitus. N Engl J Med 1993;329:977–986.

58. UK Prospective Diabetes Study (UKPDS) Group. Intensive blood glucose control with sulphonylureas or insulin compared with conventional treatment and risk of complications in patients with type 2 diabetes (UKPDS 33). Lancet 1998;352:837–853.

59. Writing Team for the Diabetes Control and Complications Trial/Epidemiology of Diabetes Interventions and Complications Research Group. Sustained effect of intensive treatment

of type 1 diabetes mellitus on development and progression of diabetic nephropathy: The epidemiology of diabetes interventions and complications (EDIC) study. JAMA 2003;290: 2159–2167.

60. Fioretto P, Mauer SM, Bilous RW, et al. Reversal of lesions of diabetic nephropathy after pancreas transplantation. N Eng J Med 1998; 339:69–75.

61. Microalbuminuria Collaborative Study Group. Intensive therapy and progression to clinical albuminuria in patients with insulin dependent diabetes mellitus and microalbuminuria. BMJ 1995;311:973–977.

62. American Diabetes Association. Position statement: Standard of medical care for patients with diabetes mellitus. Diabetes Care 1999;22(Suppl 1):S32–S34.

63. Tarnow L, Rossing P, Gall MA, et al. Prevalence of arterial hypertension in diabetic patients before and after the JNC-V. Diabetes Care 1994;17:1247–1251.

64. UK Prospective Diabetes Study Group. Tight blood pressure control and risk f macrovascular and microvascular complications in type 2 diabetes: UKPDS 38. BMJ 1998;317: 703–713.

65. Parving HH. Is antihypertensive treatment the same for type 1 diabetes and type 2 diabetes patients? Diabetes Res Clin Pract 1998;39(Suppl 1):S43–S47.

66. Ritz E, Miltenberger-Miltenyi G, Wagner J, Rychlik I. Diabetes-renal function-what are the special problems? Basic Res Cardiol 1998;93(Suppl 2):125–130.

67. Lewis EJ, Huniscker LF, Bain BP, et al. The effect of angiotensin-converting enzyme inhibition on diabetic nephropathy. N Engl J Med 1993;329:1456–1462.

68. Chaturvedi N, Sjolie AK, Stephensen JM, et al. Effect of lisinopril on progression of retinopathy in normotesiv people with type 1 diabetes. The EUCLID Study Group. Lancet 1998;351: 836–838.

69. Heart Outcomes Prevention Evaluation (HOPE) Study Investigators. Effects of ramipril on cardiovascular and microvascular outcomes in people with diabetes mellitus results of the HOPE study and MICRO-HOPE substudy. Lancet 2000;355:253–259.

70. Jacobsen P, Andersen S, Jensen BR, et al. Additive effect of ACE inhibition and angiotensin II receptor blockade in type 1 diabetic patients with diabetic nephropathy. J Am Soc Nephrol 2003;14(4):992–999.

71. Mogensen CE, Neldam S, Tikkanen I, et al. Randomized controlled trial of dual blockade of renin-angiotensin system in patients with hypetension, microalbuminuria, and non-insulin dependent diabetes: The candesartan and lisinopril microalbuminuria (CALM) Study. BMJ 2000;321:1440–1444.

72. Rossing K, Jacobsen P, Pectraszek L, et al. Renoprotective effects of adding angiotensin II receptor blocker to maximal recommended doses of ACE inhibitors in diabetic nephropathy: A randomized double-blind crossover trial. Diabetes Care 2003;26:2268–2274.

73. Sato A, Hayashi K, Naruse M, et al. Effectiveness of aldosterone blockade in patients with diabetic nephropathy. Hypertension 2003;41:64–68.

74. American Diabetes Association. Position statement: Diabetic Nephropathy. Diabetes Care 1999;22(Suppl 1):S66–S69.

75. Walser M, Hill S. Can renal replacement therapy be deferred by a supplemental very low protein diet? J Am Soc Nephrol 1999;10:110–116.

76. Toeller M, Buyken A. Protein intake-new evidence for its role in diabetic nephropathy. Nephrol Dial Transplant 1998;13:1926–1927.

77. Barsotti G, Cupisti A, Barsotti M, et al. Dietary treatment of diabetic nephropathy with chronic renal failure. Nephrol Dial Transplant 1998;13(Suppl 8):49–52.

78. Hansen HP, Tauber-Lassen E, Jensen BR, et al. Effect of dietary protein restriction on prognosis in patients with diabetic nephropathy. Kidney Int 2002;62(2):220–228.

79. Kasiske BL, O'Donnell MP, Schmitz PG, et al. Renal injury of diet-induced hypercholesterolemia in rats. Kidney Int 1990;37:880–891.

80. Peric-Golia L, Peric-Golla M. Aortic and renal lesion in hypercholestrolemic adult male virgin Sprague-Dawley rats. Atherosclerosis 1983;46:57–65.

81. Thomas MC, Rosengard-Barlund M, Mills V, et al. Serum lipids and the progression of nephropathy in type 1 diabetes. Diabetes Care 2006;29(2):317–322.

82. Hadjadj S, Duly-Bouhanick B, Bekherraz A, et al. Serum triglycerides are a predictor factor for the developmet and the progression of renal and retinal complications in patients with type 1 diabetes. Diabetes Metab 2004;30(1):43–51.

83. Ansquer JC, Foucher C, Rattier S, et al. Fenofibrate reduces progression to microalbuminuria over 3 years in a placebo-controlled study in type 2 diabetes: Results from the Diabetes Atherosclerosis Intervention Study (DAIS). Am J Kidney Dis 2005;45(3):458–493.

84. Fried LF, forrest KY, Ellis D, et al. Lipid modulation in insulin-dependent diabetes mellitus: Effect on microvascular outcomes. Diabetes Complications 2001;15:113–119.

85. Fried LF, Orchard TJ, Kasiske BL. Effect of lipid reduction on the progression of renal disease: A meta analysis. Kidney Int 2001;59:260–269.

86. Chase P, Garg SK, Marshall G, et al. Cigarette smoking increases the risk of albuminuria among subjects with type 1 diabetes. JAMA 1991;265(5):614–617.

87. Sawicki PT, Didjurgeit U, Muhthauser I, et al. Smoking is associated with progression of diabetic nephropathy. Diabetes Care 1994;17(2):126–131.

88. Chuahirun T, Khanna A, Kimball K, et al. Cigarette smoking and increased urine albumin excretion are interrelated predictors of nephropathy progression in type 2 diabetes. Am J Kidney Dis 2003;41(1):13–21.

89. Chuahirun T, Simoni J, Hudson S, et al. Cigarette smoking exacerbates and its cessation ameliorates renal injury in type 2 diabetes. Am J Kidney Dis 2004;327(2):57–67.

90. Pommer w, Bressel F, Chen F, et al. There is room for improvement of pre-terminal care in diabetic patients with end-stage renal failure—the epidemiological evidence in Germany. Nephrol Dial Transplant 1997;12:1318–1320.

91. Crook ED, Harris J, Oliver B, et al. End-stage renal disease owing to diabetic nephropathy in Mississippi: An examination of factors influencing renal survival in a population prone in late referral. J Investig Med 2001;49:284–289.

92. Churchill DN, Taylor DW, Keshaviah PR, et al. Adequacy of dialysis and nutrition in continuous peritoneal dialysis; association with clinical outcome. J Am Soc Nephrol 1996;7:198–207.

93. Morioka T, Emoto M, Tabata T et al. Glycemic control is a predictor of survival for diabetic patient on hemodialysis. Diabetes Care 2001;24(5):909–913.

94. Joglar F, Saade M. Outcome of young and elderly diabetic patients on ambulatory peritoneal dialysis: The experience of a community hospital in Pueto Rico. P R Health Sci J 1996;15(2): 85–90.

95. Choi SR, Lee SC, Yoon SY et al. Comparative study of renal replacement therapy in Korean diabetic end stage renal disease patients. A single center study. Yonsei Med J 2003;44(3): 454–462.

96. Keshavian P, Collins AJ, Ma JZ, et al. Survival comparison between hemodialysis and peritoneal dialysis based on matched doses of delivered therapy. J Am Soc Nephrol 2002;Suppl 1:S48–S52.

97. Danovitch G. Handbook of Kidney Transplantation. Baltimore, MD: Lippincott Williams and Wilkins, 2001.

98. Wolfe R, Ashby V, Milford E, et al. Comparison of mortality in all patients on dialysis patients on dialysis awaiting transplantation, and recipients of a first cadaveric transplant. N Engl J Med 1999;341:1725–1730.

99. Meier-Kriesche H, Ojo A, Port F, et al. Survival improvement among patients with end-stage renal diseas: Trends over time for transplant recipients and wait-listed patients. J Am Soc Nephrol 2001;12:1293–1296.

100. Kasiske B, Chakkera H, Roel J. Explained and unexplained ischemicheart disease risk after renal transplantation. J Am Soc Nephrol 2000;11:1735–1743.

10
Neuropathy

J. L. Edwards, A. A. Little, and E. L. Feldman
Department of Neurology, University of Michigan, Ann Arbor, Michigan, U.S.A.

INTRODUCTION

Diabetic neuropathy (DN) is both a prevalent and a debilitating complication that exacts a profound physical, psychological, and financial toll on the type 1 diabetes mellitus (T1DM) patient. DN is widespread; it afflicts > 50% of the patients, 25 years after diagnosis with diabetes (1). DN is a causal factor in the development of foot ulcers, a frequent antecedent to nontraumatic limb amputations (2). DN is not limited to the peripheral nervous system; it also affects the autonomic nervous system, with a frequent loss of normal function in the urogenital, digestive, and cardiac systems (3). The estimated annual U.S. cost arising from diabetes is $132 billion and DN accounts for ~ $11 billion (www.diabetes.org) (4). This chapter will focus on the two most common forms of DN: diabetic polyneuropathy (DPN) and diabetic autonomic neuropathy (DAN). Classification, pathogenesis, epidemiology, clinical presentation, and treatment will be addressed particularly as it relates to T1DM.

CLASSIFICATIONS

DN is a collection of syndromes capable of affecting both the peripheral and the autonomic nervous systems. Figure 1 illustrates the general categories of DN. Each syndrome has a unique clinical manifestation, anatomical location, and prognosis.

DN is divided into two major categories: focal neuropathy and diffuse neuropathy. Focal neuropathy, the less prevalent form, is generally acute and self-limiting. Its onset is localized to single or multiple peripheral nerves, cranial nerves, brachial or lumbar plexuses, or nerve roots. Diffuse neuropathy, the more prevalent form, is further split into the more easily recognized DPN and the more indolent, yet serious, DAN.

DPN is a predominantly sensory neuropathy, with motor nerve fibers being affected only later in the course of the illness. Damage to the diabetic nerve is shown to be fiber-length dependent with DPN generally originating in the toes and moving upward until it reaches the calf. Upon reaching the calf, neuropathy is then detected in the fingers and progresses up both sets of limbs. This progression is commonly called the "stocking-glove" configuration. DAN is less understood despite its high degree of morbidity and mortality (5).

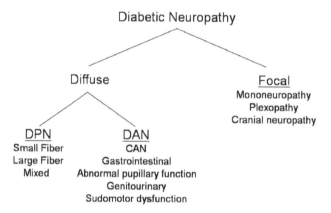

Figure 1 Hierarchy of diabetic neuropathy forms.

The high degree of innervation by the autonomic nervous system makes all organs susceptible to damage from DAN. The most prevalent forms of DAN are found as gastrointestinal
or urinary (parasympathetic nervous system) and cardiovascular (sympathetic nervous system) insult. DAN is more difficult to recognize than DPN, though often there is a high
degree of comorbidity between the two disorders.

PATHOGENESIS

Over the past decade, significant progress has been made in uncovering a unifying mechanism underlying the development of both DPN and DAN. Formation of reactive oxygen
species (ROS) as a consequence of continued hyperglycemia is a primary instigator in
complication-prone tissue damage (6). Complication-prone tissues with increased levels
of ROS are in a state now commonly referred to as "oxidative stress." Hyperglycemic oxidative stress originates in the energy-producing organelles, mitochondria (Mt), rendering
them especially prone to damage (7–10). Longer axons rich in Mt are among the first to be
damaged in DPN as is indicated by the nerve-length dependent stocking-glove pathology.
        Oxidative stress either disrupts or activates several pathways important in glucose
handling, including the (*i*) polyol, (*ii*) hexosamine, (*iii*) protein kinase C (PKC), and (*iv*)
advanced glycation end product (AGE) pathways. Figure 2 illustrates the proposed inter-
connection of these pathways (6). In the polyol pathway, conversion of glucose to sorbitol
induces osmotic stress. To bring osmotic equilibrium to the cell, other osmolytes, particularly myo-inositol and taurine, are effluxed from the cell. Taurine and myo-inositol have
antioxidant and signal-transduction activity, respectively (11–13). These deficiencies have
been implicated in Na^+/K^+ ATPase defects (14). The hexosamine pathway is accelerated
from increased conversion of glucose to fructose-6-phosphate and subsequently to UDP-
N-acetylglucosamine. UDP-*N*-acetylglucosamine modifies transcription factors causing an
increase in PAI-1 and TGF-β (15). Increased expression of these proteins is associated with
an aberrant circulation which is inherently tied to DN. PKC pathways are activated by hyperglycemia through diacylglycerol (16,17). Hyperactivity of PKC results in an increased
expression of vascular endothelial growth factor (VEGF), TGF-β, and NF-κB. Excess of
these proteins disturbs the neurovascular relationship such that inhibition of PKC partially
restores nerve conduction velocity (NCV) in rodents with DPN. The final pathway, the AGE
pathway, as the name suggests, is formed when glucose metabolites bond with proteins.
AGEs activate the AGE receptor and cause alterations of the extracellular matrix and induce

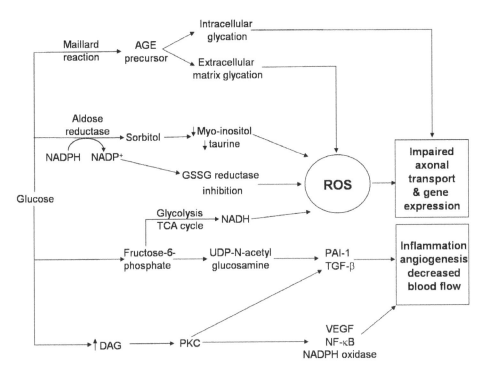

Figure 2 Biochemical pathogenesis of neuronal damage from hyperglycemia. *Source*: Adapted with permission from Ref. 6.

ischemia (18). All four pathways are induced through ROS formation and also produce ROS damage, thus deepening a deleterious cycle of aberrant cellular function.

Oxidative stress also disrupts lipid profiles by inducing lipid peroxidation. Oxidized lipids are known to cause ischemia and therefore reduce the delivery of proper nutrients to neurons. The combination of oxidative stress and ischemia are co-contributors to neuronal damage.

Although the culmination of hyperglycemia-induced oxidative stress and dyslipidemia are likely the major initiators in DPN and DAN, the manner in which neurons are damaged is still being investigated. Damage from oxidative stress is shown, in some cases, to initiate apoptosis or programmed cell death especially given that Mt are not only predisposed to oxidative damage but are also key components in the apoptosis signaling cascade (19). In certain diabetic models, apoptosis is not seen in the neuronal body, but rather neuroaxonal dystrophy is present. This discrepancy is most likely due to either an incomplete form of apoptosis or apoptosis localized to cell bodies of selected axons (20–22). Many investigators, including us, contend that the apoptotic process is incomplete but reoccurs over time with poor glucose control, resulting in cumulative injury to the cell body over time. This recurring cycle of injury results in impaired axonal transport, disrupted Mt distribution in the axon, and a subsequent dying back of axons toward the cell body yielding the stocking-glove presentation of signs and symptoms in DPN (9,23).

EPIDEMIOLOGY

Diffuse neuropathy is the most prevalent form found in diabetics. Prevalence and incidence is (*i*) higher in patients with diabetes than in the general public, (*ii*) dependent on the

Table 1 Reported Prevalence of Diabetic Peripheral Neuropathy

Study name	Diagnostic criteria	Initial prevalence (%)	Later assessment (%)	Reference
Rochester	Two or more abnormalities (symptoms, nerve conduction, QST, AFT)		54	(24)
DCCT	Confirmed clinical neuropathy	2.1	9.6	(25,26)
	Abnormal nerve conduction	21.8	40.2	
Pittsburgh	2 of 3 criteria:			
	symptoms, abnormal sensory signs, tendon reflex		58 (for age > 30 yr)	(25,26)
			18 (18–29 yr)	
EURODIAB	≥ 2 criteria		23.5	(27)
Danish	Loss of vibratory sensation		62	(28)

Abbreviations: QST, quantitative sensory testing; AFT, autonomic functional tests.

duration of diabetes, and (*iii*) generally correlated to glycemic control. Although studies vary on precise statistics due to mainly differing inclusion criteria regarding what does or does not constitute DN, all are consistent with these three points as major indicators of DN in T1DM.

Investigations into neuropathy confirm higher prevalence, though of varying magnitude in patients with T1DM than in the general population. Studies using multiple and various criteria for diagnosis indicate a range of DN in T1DM between 18% and 62% (Table 1). Onset of DN coordinates with patient age as the Pittsburgh Epidemiology of Diabetic Complications Study showed DPN in 18% of T1DM between 18 years to 29 years (25). The incidence rate rose to 58% for patients older than 30 years. Glycemic control and dyslipidemia are both linked to the onset and progression of DPN in adults (1). The Diabetes Control and Complications Trial (DCCT) demonstrated that patients in intensive therapy (HbA1C = 7) reduced their incidence of abnormal NCV by 44% over 5 years versus conventional treatment (HBA1C = 9). Moreover, intense glycemic control kept NCVs stable, whereas conventional treatment resulted in a significant decline over 5 years. For DPN, a 1% drop in HbA1C levels translates to a 27% reduction in DPN as determined by clinical examination (29). EURODIAB, a parallel study in T1DM, stands in good agreement with the DCCT. Variables such as duration of diabetes, age, HbA1C, etc., were analyzed for effect on the development of neuropathy. The highest correlation with neuropathy was found to be in metabolic control, duration of diabetes, and lipid profile (HDL and fasting triglyceride) (30–32).

To further explore the long-term effects of glycemic control, patients of both conventional and intense therapy were followed up 8 years after the DCCT in the Epidemiology of Diabetes Interventions and Complications (EDIC) study. After 8 years, the intense therapy group showed an increase in HbA1C that was equivalent to the conventional therapy group. EDIC indicates that even after glycemic control converges between conventional therapy and intensive therapy, frequency of DPN rose for both groups but still remains significantly lower in the intensive group than the conventional therapy (Fig. 3) (29). These long-term glycemic control studies clearly demonstrate the ability of intense therapy to prevent the onset and neutralize the progression of DPN, though restoration of nerve function remains rare.

Closely related to the pathophysiology of DPN is the occurrence of foot ulcers, which often leads to lower leg amputation. Although data are not available specific to T1DM, on

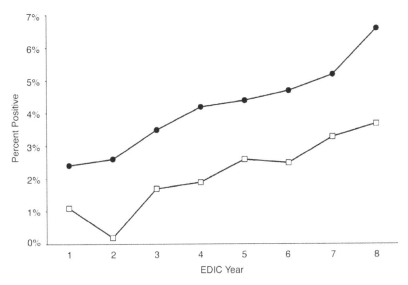

Figure 3 Frequency of neuropathy-positive MNSI questionnaires across 8 years of the EDIC study among former DCCT conventional therapy (●) and intensive therapy (□) subjects without confirmed clinical neuropathy at the end of the DCCT. $P < 0.0001$ on average for all EDIC years combined (29). *Source*: Adapted with permission from Ref. 29.

an average, all diabetic patients have a one in seven chance of developing a foot ulcer. Of these foot ulcers, 60% to 70% are attributable to DPN. The diabetic foot is closely related to comorbidity and mortality for the diabetic patient. In fact, the presence of a foot ulcer correlates to a 17% decrease in 3-year survival study after correcting for age and sex (33). Loss of vibration perception in the toe is the strongest corollary to increased mortality—trumping sex, race, BMI, duration of diabetes, and HbA1C (34).

The epidemiology of DAN shows the same general trends as DPN. However, because the condition is often more insidious, it could be that DAN is under-recognized by both patients and health-care providers. Most studies of DAN focus on cardiac autonomic neuropathy (CAN) due to a more defined clinical diagnosis than other types of DAN, such as those affecting the gastrointestinal and genitourinary tracts. Positive scores from six autonomic functional tests (AFT) described below are generally used to diagnose DAN. When heart rate variability is the sole criteria for DAN, occurrence in T1DM is generally high or overestimated (25.3%) (35). Use of three of the six criteria yielded DAN diagnosis of 16.8%.

Interestingly, data suggest that DPN is less prevalent in T1DM compared to T2DM (27% vs. 32%) (36), whereas symptomatic DAN is more prevalent in T1DM (11% for T1DM vs. 0.5% for T2DM). Denervation of the left ventricle of the heart, as determined by PET, is present in 40% of the patients with T1DM without other CAN symptoms (37,38). These data suggest that early autonomic dysfunction may contribute to silent myocardial ischemia. CAN accounts for an increased morbidity with a risk factor of myocardial ischemia ranging from 2 to > 4 in both T1DM and T2DM. In accordance with this, positive diagnosis of CAN increases the mortality risk ratio to between 2.1 and 9.2, with statistical significance in 12 of 14 studies (39). Increased risk factors for DAN include female gender, LDL/HDL, hypertension, and HbA1C. As mortality rates associated with DAN are staggeringly high for the T1DM patient, clinical screening using two or more indicators for the often nonsymptomatic CAN is advised.

CLINICAL PRESENTATION AND DIAGNOSIS

DPN is a collection of syndromes further categorized as either subclinical (class I) or clinical (class II). Subclinical DPN patients are asymptomatic but have slower NCVs and modest changes on quantitative sensory testing (QST). Patients with clinical DPN express symptoms and have abnormalities of either NCV or QST or most frequently both entities. Early diagnosis is imperative as glycemic control is the only proven way to prevent disease progression and the subsequent morbidity of DPN, including ulcer and amputation.

DPN symptoms manifest in two general forms commonly denoted as "positive" and "negative" symptoms. Positive symptoms include perceptions of prickling, pain, or numbness and are bothersome to the patient. Negative symptoms are frequently not noticed by the patient, who does not realize that he has a loss of sensory function with a decrease in thermal, tactile, or pain perception in response to the appropriate stimuli. Although normally progressing in the "stocking-glove" fashion described above, the form of clinical DPN is dependent on the type of fiber damaged. Large diameter–myelinated nerve fiber dysfunction results in decreased proprioception and vibratory sensation in the toes with reduced or absent Achilles reflexes. These patients experience "negative symptoms" and frequently their sensory loss is only discovered through clinical examination by a health professional. Aberrant small nerve fiber function response results in an impaired pain and thermal sensation. Patients with small fiber loss experience positive symptoms and on examination have a decreased perception of painful stimuli, such as pinprick, thermal sensation, and light touch.

Over time, patients with progressive DPN develop a condition frequently called the "diabetic foot." Loss of large and small myelinated fiber function leave the foot insensate. Loss of autonomic function results in anhydrosis and a dry, shiny skin. Arthropathy is common; poor ankle joint dorsiflexion or an equinus deformity leads to midfoot collapse. The progressive tightening of the Achilles tendon ultimately increases the load to the forefoot. The tarsometatarsal joint, the main junction between the forefoot and the hindfoot, will frequently collapse due to the extra load. The ensuing deformity is known as a rocker-bottom type deformity. These bone and joint changes comprise Charcot arthropathy, a frequent component of the diabetic foot. Loss of sensation with callus formation coupled with misplaced weight bearing secondary to arthropathy leads to ulcer formation (33). Charcot foot is generally underreported despite presentation in 15% of DPN patients (40). The diabetic foot is more susceptible to external trauma such as caused by tight shoes; a paradox is that patients with the diabetic foot are more apt to purchase ill-fitting shoes due to their lack of ability to feel shoeware, thereby inadvertently exacerbating their own condition. Foot ulcers are the leading cause of hospitalization in diabetic patients and generally the initiating event in the chain leading to lower limb amputation. Given the delayed healing of diabetic patients particularly in poor glycemic control, ulcers can turn gangrenous and lead to lower limb amputation. In fact, 80% of the lower extremity amputations are preceded by foot ulceration (41).

Focal neuropathy is common in patients with diabetes. This can take various forms but mononeuropathy is the most prevalent at either the wrist (median mononeuropathy— also known as carpal tunnel syndrome) or at the elbow (ulnar mononeuropathy) (42). These focal neuropathies are indistinguishable between patients with or without diabetes, suggesting that the diabetic state creates an environment more susceptible to compression injury rather than acting as a direct causal agent. Carpal tunnel syndrome is clinically present in nearly a quarter of patients with diabetes. When present as a cranial mononeuropathy, the third nerve is most often affected, resulting in pupillary-sparing diplopia, ptosis, and headaches.

Diagnosis of Diabetic Polyneuropathy

Diagnosis of DPN is based on history, examination, and, when possible, electrodiagnostic testing. The San Antonio Consensus Criteria remain the gold standard for diagnosis, although their use is limited to clinical trials and epidemiological studies (43); the criteria are too exhaustive for routine use in a clinical practitioner's office. The San Antonio Consensus Criteria are based on measurements in each of the following five categories: clinical symptoms, clinical examination, electrodiagnostic studies (EDX), QST, and AFT. EDX, also referred to as nerve conduction studies, are a quantitative and objective measure of peripheral nerve function. A major benefit of EDX is the ability to distinguish whether the origin of neuropathy is axonal or demyelinating. EDX most frequently show a mixed picture in DPN with primarily axonal damage and a low degree of dysmyelination (44). The most common criticism of EDX—that its restriction to large nerve fibers with small fibers is not questioned—is in most cases not valid.

QST assesses the loss of sensory functions which often go unnoticed by both patient and physician. The essence of the QST is the use of quantitative instruments to measure abnormal function with regards to sensing vibration and thermal changes. The simplest QST device is the quantitative 64 Hz tuning fork which measures the intensity of residual vibration on an eight-point scale rather than approximating dysfunction based on time elapsed from tuning fork strike (45). Most clinical trials and epidemiological studies employ the CASE IV system (WR Medical Electronics Co.). The CASE IV system measures both vibration detection threshold (great toe) and cool thermal detection threshold (dorsal foot) using a stepping algorithm; differences are expressed as just noticeable difference units that vary from 1 to 25. A discussion of AFT occurs later in this chapter.

Using the San Antonio Consensus Criteria, a patient has probable neuropathy if he has signs or symptoms and an abnormality of either EDX, QST, or AFT; he has definite neuropathy if he has signs or symptoms and two abnormalities among EDX, QST, or AFT. Because of the quantitative nature of the three groups of tests, patients can be followed longitudinally for a response to a therapeutic intervention or as part of a detailed epidemiological study of DN.

While the San Antonio Consensus Criteria are essential for clinical trials, in routine practice, a careful clinical examination of the feet with assessment of large fiber (vibration perception and proprioception) and small fiber (light touch, pain, and thermal perception) modalities and ankle reflexes is sufficient to make the diagnosis of DPN. Table 2 lists other possible etiologies underlying a distal symmetric polyneuropathy; depending on the patient presentation and history, the practitioner should consider other diagnostic possibilities. As DPN has no unique features from alternate forms of neuropathy, the most frequent unrelated forms of neuropathy that may be mistaken for DPN are B_{12} deficiency, uremia, hyperthyroidism, and alcoholic neuropathy. The three clinical pearls of DPN are (*i*) symmetry, (*ii*) slow progression, and (*iii*) sensory deficits more prominent than motor weakness. Deviations from these well-established attributes should be referred to the neurologist as the condition is less likely to be DPN.

In our own outpatient practice, we use the definition of DPN put forth by the American Diabetes Association i.e., "the presence of symptoms and/or signs of peripheral nerve dysfunction in people with diabetes after the exclusion of other causes" (1). To assess DPN we employ a simple standardized tool, the Michigan Neuropathy Screening Instrument (MNSI), with a questionnaire and clinical examination, allowing us to compare scores over time in the same patient. The MNSI has been independently tested and validated as a diagnostic tool (46,47) and is currently an important component of the DCCT/Epidemiology of Diabetes Interventions and Complications (DCCT/EDIC) Trial(29,48). The MNSI consists

Table 2 Differential Diagnosis of Diabetic Neuropathy

I. Distal symmetric polyneuropathy
   a. Metabolic
      i. *Diabetes mellitus*
      ii. Uremia
      iii. Folic acid/cyanocobalamin deficiency
      iv. Hypothyroidism
      v. Acute intermittent porphyria
   b. Toxic
      i. Alcohol
      ii. Heavy metal (Hg, Pb, etc.)
      iii. Industrial hydrocarbons
      iv. Various drugs
   c. Infectious or inflammatory
      i. Sarcoidosis
      ii. Leprosy
      iii. Periarteritis nodosa
      iv. Others: Systemic lupus erythematosus
   d. Others
      i. Dysproteinemias & paraproteinemias
      ii. Paraneoplastic syndrome
      iii. Leukemias and lymphomas
      iv. Amyloidosis
      v. Hereditary neuropathies
II. Pains and paresthesias without neurological deficit
   a. Early small fiber sensory neuropathy
   b. Psychophysiological disorder (depression, hysteria, etc.)
III. Autonomic neuropathy without somatic component
   a. Shy-Drager syndrome
   b. *Diabetic neuropathy with mild somatic involvement*
   c. Riley-Day Syndrome
   d. Idiopathic orthostatic hypotension
IV. Diffuse motor neuropathy without sensory deficit
   a. Guillain-Barre syndrome
   b. Primary myopathies
   c. Myasthenia gravis
   d. Heavy metal toxicity
V. Femoral neuropathy
   a. Degenerative spinal-disk disease (Paget's disease of the spine)
   b. Intrinsic spinal cord mass lesion
   c. Equina cauda lesions
   d. Coagulopathies
VI. Cranial neuropathy
   a. Carotid aneurysm
   b. Intracranial mass
   c. Elevated intracranial pressure
VII. Mononeuropathy multiplex
   a. Vasculidites
   b. Amyloidosis
   c. Hypothyroidism
   d. Acromegaly
   e. Coagulopathies

Source: Adapted with permission from Ref. 91.

Please take a few minutes to answer the questions below about the feeling in your legs and feet.
Check yes or no based on how you usually feel.

1.	Are your legs and/or feet numb?	1. yes ☐	2. no ☐
2.	Do you ever have burning pain in your legs and/or feet?	1. yes ☐	2. no ☐
3.	Are your feet too sensitive to touch?	1. yes ☐	2. no ☐
4.	Do you get muscle cramps in your legs and/or feet?	1. yes ☐	2. no ☐
5.	Do you ever have prickling feelings in your legs or feet?	1. yes ☐	2. no ☐
6.	Does it hurt when the bedcovers touch your skin?	1. yes ☐	2. no ☐
7.	When you get in the tub or shower, are you able to tell the hot water from the cold water?	1. yes ☐	2. no ☐
8.	Have you ever had an open sore on your foot?	1. yes ☐	2. no ☐
9.	Has your doctor ever told you that you have diabetic neuropathy?	1. yes ☐	2. no ☐
10.	Do you feel weak all over most of the time?	1. yes ☐	2. no ☐
11.	Are your symptoms worse at night?	1. yes ☐	2. no ☐
12.	Do your legs hurt when you walk?	1. yes ☐	2. no ☐
13.	Are you able to sense your feet when you walk?	1. yes ☐	2. no ☐
14.	Is the skin on your feet so dry that it cracks open?	1. yes ☐	2. no ☐
15.	Have you ever had an amputation?	1. yes ☐	2. no ☐

Figure 4 MNSI patient questionnaire. *Source*: Adapted with permission from Ref. 47.

of a 15-point patient questionnaire about sensation and peripheral vascular disease (Fig. 4). Scoring more than seven is the threshold to predict or diagnose DPN. Positive assessment on the MNSI should be followed by an eight-point MNSI clinical examination of the foot including foot inspection and vibration sensation (Fig. 5). Scoring more than two on the clinical examination properly diagnoses DPN with 95% confidence.

Many other tests besides the MNSI are available to diagnose and assess DPN. One frequently used tool developed by Peter Dyck and colleagues in the Rochester Diabetic Neuropathy Study is commonly referred to as the Neuropathy Impairment Score (NIS) plus 7. The simplest component of this scheme is the NIS of the lower limbs; this is an easily applied clinical exam evaluating both sensation and strength in the lower limbs. This can be added to seven quantitative tests to evaluate DPN severity (24), which include EDX and QST. The higher the number of abnormalities among the seven tests, the higher the severity of neuropathy. While the NIS plus 7 tests increase diagnostic accuracy, we prefer the MNSI because of its simplicity and availability to all practitioners.

Diagnosis of DAN

DAN is similar to DPN in that it can be divided into clinical and subclinical presentations. It can affect any organ receiving autonomic innervation. Common manifestations of DAN include: constipation, diarrhea, dysphagia, decreased urinary flow, and cardiac syndromes.

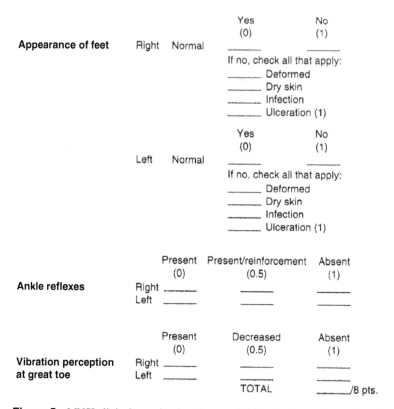

Figure 5 MNSI clinical examination. *Source*: Adapted with permission from Ref. 47.

Diagnosis is a manner of excluding other possible causes such as infection, inflammation, prostatic obstruction, or atherosclerotic disease.

The most frequently diagnosed syndrome among DAN is CAN. CAN is diagnosed through using a series of simple cardiovascular examinations or AFTs. The most popular include: the Valsalva maneuver, heart rate response to deep breathing, heart rate response to standing up, blood pressure response to standing up, and blood pressure response to sustained handgrip. Table 3 shows CAN diagnostic tests; the presence of CAN is frequently accompanied by other forms of DAN, particularly abnormal gastrointestinal and pupillomotor function. A more detailed discussion of CAN is presented at the end of this section.

Gastrointestinal autonomic neuropathy and genitourinary autonomic neuropathy are both parasympathetic forms of DAN whose injuries range from mild to, in rare cases, severe. Constipation is the most prevalent gastrointestinal presentation followed by diabetic diarrhea, heartburn, and dysphagia.

Diabetic diarrhea, while seemingly self-explanatory, may progress into more serious forms if left unaddressed. Severe symptoms include more than 20 bowel movements per day and stool volumes over 300 g per day. Such fluid losses result in dehydration if left untreated and can influence blood glucose control.

Gastroparesis or delayed gastric emptying is likely in T1DM patients, especially when unstable 2-hour postprandial blood glucose levels are present. After excluding dietary causes and implementing intense insulin therapy, the persistence of variable blood glucose may be attributed to aberrant gastric emptying. Diagnosis is generally not trivial, employing

Table 3 Diagnostic Tests for Cardiovascular Autonomic Neuropathy

Test	Diagnostic value
Resting heart rate	> 100 bpm
Beat-to-beat HR variation (HRV)	
Abstain from coffee overnight	
Do not test after hypoglycemic episode	
Supine position, 6 breaths per minute	Difference < 10 bpm or expiration: inspiration R-R ratio > 1.17
Heart rate response to standing	
R-R interval measured at 15 beats and 30 beats after standing (normally tachycardia is followed by reflex bradycardia)	30:15 ratio > 1.03
Heart rate response to Valsalva maneuver	
Patient forcibly exhales into manometer mouthpiece, exerting 40 mm Hg pressure for 15 seconds	Ratio of longest to shortest R-R interval < 1.2
Systolic BP response to standing	
Measure in supine position and 2 minutes after standing	Decrease > 30 mm Hg (10 to 29 is borderline)
Diastolic BP response to isometric exercise	
Establish patient's maximum handgrip pressure	
Exert 30% maximum for 5 minutes	Increase < 16 mm Hg in contralateral arm
Electrocardiography	QTc > 440 ms

Source: Adapted with permission from Ref. 5.

MRI scans or isotope labeling; the detection of [^{13}C]octanoic acid in breath analysis has proven to be an accurate indicator of gastric atony (49).

Genitourinary autonomic neuropathy encompasses such dysfunctions as retrograde ejaculation, erectile impotence, vaginal atrophy, dyspareunia, and cystopathy. Sexual dysfunction, affecting 50% of male diabetic patients and 30% of female diabetic patients is often an early sign of DAN (50,51). Sexual afflictions are common and have a high degree of comorbidity with other manifestations of diabetic complications. Retrograde ejaculation, the partial misdirection of sperm into the urinary tract, may be reported as cloudy urine, postcoitally. Diagnosis is made from low sperm count in ejaculate in conjunction with indications of sperm in urine. Erectile dysfunction is not uncommon in DAN patients but due diligence should be taken to exclude other causalities. Decreased vaginal lubrication and clitoral blood flow is the most common dysfunction for T1DM women (52). This may result in vaginal wall atrophy and dyspareunia.

Cystopathy is the term used to describe a collection of voiding problems whose progression is often symptomatic and presents as impaired bladder sensation, diminished urine flow, and increased postvoid residual volume (53). This incomplete emptying or infrequent urination typically results in dribbling, poor urinary stream, and frequent urinary infections. Bladder infections in men and postvoid residuals in both men and women with T1DM are strong indications of diabetic cystopathy (54).

CAN is an extremely insidious form of neuropathy due to the combination of its asymptomatic nature and high contribution to mortality (55). CAN can take a variety of forms with various degrees of morbidity and mortality rates (56). Blood pressure and heart rate variations are the most prominent defects resulting from CAN (57,58). Orthostatic hypotension, defined as a drop of 20 mm Hg 3 minutes after standing, is not common (3%)

and is generally present in elderly diabetic patients with preexisting CAN (59). Anemia, a result of erythropoietin deficiency from T1DM patients with renal denervation, is known to augment orthostatic hypotension. Frequently, the common symptoms of hypotension including dizziness and weakness are often difficult to distinguish from hypoglycemia; if blood glucose levels are not low, symptoms of dizziness should alert the clinician to the possibility of CAN.

Abnormal heart rate can appear in advanced CAN as abnormal cardiovascular exercise performance and/or what has been termed cardiac denervation syndrome (CDS). Failure to increase heart rate in response to exercise may be assessed by assessing heart rate variability or by a multigated angiopathy thallium scan. CDS is a combination of defects to the sympathetic and parasympathetic systems which is displayed as an elevated stable heart rate regardless of exercise, stress, or sleep (60). CDS first appears as an increase in resting heart rate ($\sim$ 110 bpm) from parasympathetic defect. This slowly progresses into a decrease in heart rate (90 bpm) due to sympathetic regression. CDS patients are more likely to encounter cardiac arrhythmias, myocardial ischemia, and sudden death. The increased risk of mortality found in T1DM patients is considered to be closely tied to syndromes such as CAN (61,62). Interestingly, the incidence of myocardial infarction for T1DM patients is higher in the evening than the morning. This suggests a decrease in morning sympathetic activity and an impaired evening parasympathetic activity (27,63). The ADA suggests testing for CAN 5-years postdiagnosis and every year thereafter for patients with T1DM.

TREATMENT

Treatment for reversing all types of DN is, at present time, generally limited, though avenues to significantly slow and even stop its progression are available to the patient. For those patients already displaying signs and symptoms of one or more syndromes of DN, treatments are available, in most cases, to mitigate the symptoms if not the root cause of the neuropathy. Prospective therapies currently being investigated will be mentioned.

Glycemic Control

As discussed above, the DCCT study has proven that intensive therapy ($\geq$ 3 insulin injections/day or insulin pump) decreases the incidence of DPN by 60% over a 10-year period when compared to conventional therapy ($\leq$ 2 insulin injections/day) (64–66). Besides reducing the onset of DPN, glycemic control was shown to maintain stable NCVs whereas NCVs for the conventional group declined over time. After completion of the DCCT, long-term observational follow-up of 1375 of the 1425 DCCT patients occurred in the EDIC study (67). DPN was followed in EDIC annually using the MNSI (47,68). While glycemic control merged in EDIC with an average HbA1 C of eight percent for both the intensive and conventional treatment arms, the beneficial effects of prior intensive treatment persisted for 8 years. Patients in the initial DCCT-intensive cohort have a 50% risk reduction for developing DPN when compared to patients in the initial DCCT-conventional cohort (29). This phenomenon is termed metabolic memory, and implies that the salutary effects of early glycemic control persist over many years. There are also selected reports of regression in mild forms of CAN in very small patient studies through tight glycemic control over a 3-year period, though this was not achieved in those patients with severe disease (56,69). The EDIC cohort is currently undergoing complete autonomic function testing, thus enabling the T1DM community to know in the future whether the phenomenon of metabolic memory also applies to the autonomic nervous system.

Pancreas and islet transplantation, while available to only a small set of T1DM patients, generally also receiving a kidney transplant, has given a unique insight into the role of reestablishing normalized metabolism after prolonged exposure to hyperglycemia as it relates to both DPN and CAN. T1DM patients who received a successful transplant and maintained insulin independence were compared to those patients who underwent kidney transplant only or an unsuccessful pancreas transplant (70). Normalization of metabolic function over a 10-year period maintained scores on the neurological examination and cardiorespiratory index and increased scores in sensory and motor nerve indices (71). Patients in the control group for this study demonstrated a decline in all four tests over time. These results further confirm the beneficial effects of euglycemia in the prevention of nerve function loss and raise the interesting possibility that return of function is possible over time.

Symptomatic Treatment of Peripheral Neuropathy

Pharmacologic Approaches: Symptomatic Treatment of Pain Associated with DPN

Pain is a common and potentially disabling symptom of DPN. In our practice, we use a stepwise treatment paradigm, titrating a drug to either efficacy within the recommended dose or to the onset of side effects. Table 4 lists the common therapies employed in our clinical practice; all have been tested in double-blind placebo-controlled trials [reviewed in (1,72,73)]. The two therapies in bold are now approved by the Food and Drug Administration (FDA) for the treatment of painful DPN.

Two new compounds are now FDA-approved and can be considered for initial treatment of painful DPN. There has not yet been a direct comparison of these two compounds with each other, or with other known therapies; because study designs vary prominently among the different trials (i.e., patient selection and the choice of primary end points), a direct comparison can not be made based on the published literature.

The two recently approved FDA drugs are duloxetine, a dual uptake inhibitor (serotonin and norepinephrine) (74), and pregabalin, an antiepileptic drug with a putative mode of action of decreasing glutamate levels in the spinal cord (75). While different scales were

Table 4 Treatment Options for Painful Neuropathy

Antidepressants
- *Duloxetine 60 mg, qid*
- Amitriptyline: 50–150 mg at night
- Nortriptyline: 50–150 mg at night
- Imipramine: 100 mg, qid
- Desipramine: 100 mg, qid

Antiepileptic drugs
- Pregabalin 150 mg, bid
- Gabapentin: 600–1200 mg, tid
- Topiramate: 200 mg, bid

Others
- Mexiletine: 150–450 mg, qid
- Tramadol, 50–100 mg, bid
- Transcutaneous electrical nerve stimulation
- Acupuncture

used in the individual phase III double-blind placebo-controlled trials for each therapy, the published data suggest the two medications are equally efficacious (74,75). Duloxetine is begun at a daily dose of 30 mg with a meal and slowly titrated to 60 mg a day. The major side effect, nausea, can be limiting; if this occurs, patients can begin on 20 mg a day, with a slow titration. This approach is sometimes better tolerated. Like all similar compounds, sedation and sleepiness are common side effects; duloxetine should not be taken with other serotonin or norepinephrine uptake inhibitors (74).

Pregabalin is a Schedule 5 drug and is begun at 50 to 100 mg per day. It can be increased to 150 mg two times per day after 1 week. Like its predecessor, gabapentin, effects include sedation, dizziness, and in some patients, lower extremity edema. Unlike gabapentin, however, pregabalin could be habit forming, and it is recommended that the drug be discontinued slowly (75).

Several other classes of drugs are commonly used in the symptomatic treatment of painful DPN (1,73). Only those drugs that have undergone a double-blind placebo-controlled trial will be briefly discussed. Of the commonly used classes of drugs, the tricyclic antidepressants (TCAs) are inexpensive and in Europe remain the first line in pharmacotherapy. In a meta-analysis of 21 clinical trials, the TCAs were most effective in relieving pain in patients with DPN (76). Amitriptyline, nortriptyline, and imipramine all possess more anticholinergic activity than desipramine. A TCA can be begun as first line therapy and titrated to either efficacy (within FDA-recommended dosing) or side effects, which include sedation, dry mouth, and nausea (76). The usual dosage schedule for TCAs is 10 to 25 mg at bedtime initially, slowly increasing the dose to a single bedtime dose of 100 or 150 mg. The TCAs should not be used in patients with known cardiac arrhythmias, congestive heart failure, orthostatic hypotension, or angle-closure glaucoma. Of note, the TCAs cannot be used in conjunction with monoamine oxidase inhibitors.

Anticonvulsants are useful in the treatment of painful DPN. Gabapentin, the predecessor of pregabalin, is begun at a dose of 300 mg tid and can be slowly titrated to a dose of up to 1200 mg tid. Many patients experience relief at doses ranging between 600 and 900 mg tid (77). For patients who prefer qid dosing, 600 to 900 mg may be effective. Dizziness, somnolence, headache, diarrhea, nausea, and confusion along with lower extremity edema are known side effects. Like gabapentin, the anticonvulsant topiramate is also effective in controlling painful DPN (78). Begun at 25 to 50 mg once a day, the dose can be very slowly titrated up to 200 mg bid. Patients experience the same side effects as with gabapentin, with the additional sensation of "fullness" to the extent that this drug is considered by some to be effective in weight loss.

If a patient continues to experience pain while taking therapeutic doses of two or three medications, use of the antiarrhythmic drug mexiletine can be considered (79). Mexiletine can be used only after stopping all anticonvulsants and under the consultation of a cardiologist. An initial dose of 150 mg daily can be slowly titrated to a final dose of 600 to 800 mg in three or four divided doses. This drug must be used with caution and in conjunction with careful cardiac monitoring. Another alternative therapy is tramadol, a drug with very low binding to μ-opioid receptors. It is most frequently used for breakthrough pain by patients at doses of 50 to 100 mg every 4 to 6 hours, up to 400 mg per day (80). Patients are routinely on other therapy for painful DPN and find that the intermittent use of tramadol adds symptomatic relief. The side effects of confusion, extreme fatigue, and/or somnolence can limit the use of this therapy.

There is a clear noticeable absence of high quality controlled clinical trials for the nondrug treatments, such as transcutaneous electrical nerve stimulation and acupuncture (81). However, these treatments are available, particularly in pain clinics, and have been reported to be effective in selected patients with DPN (73,81).

Foot Care

All patients with diabetes should receive at least an annual foot examination and patients with known DPN should undergo a careful foot examination at every office visit. Patient education on shoeware, daily foot inspection, and referral to a podiatrist for nail trimming are all essential components of a comprehensive prevention program. Patients with significant sensory loss should be encouraged to check their feet frequently during the day, at least three times, and ensure that there are no objects present in their shoes. Immediate attention is required at the first signs of local foot infection.

Symptomatic Treatment of Autonomic Neuropathy

As the pathology of DAN can present itself in virtually any organ, the treatment will vary according to the affected organ system and symptoms. While a majority of these symptoms may be addressed with one or more medications, many can be rectified using over-the-counter remedies or lifestyle changes.

Gastrointestinal disturbances in T1DM should be approached in a multifaceted approach consisting of glycemic control for prevention or progression of all symptoms, lifestyle changes to minimize occurrences, and, when necessary, medication. In gastroparesis, blood glucose levels play an additional role besides hindering further progression. In fact, euglycemia advances gastric motor function, further easing postprandial stability (82). Consumption of multiple smaller meals rather than a few large portion meals is recommended. As fat slows digestion or metabolism, low fat small meals are ideal for the T1DM patient. Administration of rapid-acting insulin to a T1DM patient with gastroparesis may induce hypoglycemic episodes. While pramlintide has proven effective in controlling postprandial blood glucose levels in T1DM patients, it should be avoided in gastroparetic patients as its mode of action is to delay gastric emptying, the delay of which may further exacerbate the patient's symptoms. Other drugs with possible utility are listed in Table 5. Diabetic diarrhea is also a common manifestation of DAN (83). Exclusion of alternate causes should be examined before attributing this to DAN. Table 5 describes other underlying causes as well as drugs suitable for use for diabetic diarrhea. Administration of these various drugs depends on symptomatic origin.

Genitourinary problems derived from DAN are also quite common. Loss of afferent innervation of the bladder leads to decreased voiding frequency. To account for this, the patient may use timed voiding in conjunction with the Crede maneuver to initiate voiding. As appearance of urinary tract infections is a possible pathology, self-catheterization is a possible remedy. Two drugs, bethanechol (10-mg qid) and doxazosin (1–2 mg, bid/tid) may be useful in alleviating symptoms.

Although T1DM has a high incidence rate of erectile dysfunction, it should not be taken as the causative factor without the exclusion of other possible agents. In this way, a therapy may be specifically targeted to the particular cause. The common alternative origin to erectile dysfunction is psychosomatic for which the patient should be directed to proper counseling (84). Low testosterone levels may also contribute to erectile dysfunction in which case testosterone supplementation is advised. Arteriosclerosis resulting in low genital blood flow should be directed to a vascular surgeon. The presentation of erectile dysfunction has comorbidity with other nonsymptomatic forms of DAN and atherosclerosis (85). Therefore, a thorough cardiac screening should be performed on all T1DM patients with erectile dysfunction.

To treat erectile dysfunction, glycemic control should be instituted along with cessation of alcohol or tobacco. Prescription drugs which are known to cause erectile

Table 5 Treatments of Gastroparesis and Diabetic Diarrhea

Treatment	Dose regimen	Possible side effects
Gastroparesis		
Behavioral advice		
Improve glycemic control		
Eat frequent small meals		
Reduce dietary fat (< 40 g/day)		
Reduce dietary fiber		
Metoclopramide	10 mg, 30–60 min ac	Galactorrhea, extrapyramidal symptoms
Erythromycin	250 mg, 30 min ac	Abdominal cramps, nausea, diarrhea, rash
Jejunostomy and liquid diet		
Diabetic Diarrhea		
Exclude other underlying causes:		
Bacterial overgrowth		
Drug-related (acarbose, metformin, lactose intolerance)		
Osmotic (resolves with fasting)		
Secretory (consider neuroendocrine tumors)		
Metronodiazole	250 mg, tid, ≥ 3 wk	Fungal overgrowth
Clonidine	0.1 mg, bid or tid	Orthostatic hypotension
Loperamide	2 mg, qid	Toxic megacolon
Cholestyramine	4 g, 1–6 times daily	
Octreotide	50 μg, tid	Aggravated nutrient malabsorption

dysfunction, particularly antidepressant agents, should, when possible, be reduced or replaced with drugs having less propensity toward sexual dysfunction. There are currently multiple medications available for the treatment of erectile dysfunction. Pharmaceutical agents such as sildenafil and tadalafil are effective in 50% to 60% of the patients (86,87). These must not be given with organic nitrates as hypotension and fatal cardiac events may occur. Other options include prostacyclin injections, yohimbine, suction devices, and prosthetic devices. Retrograde ejaculation has been successfully treated with antihistamines. Female sexual dysfunction, commonly decreased lubrication of the vaginal walls, is treated with vaginal lubricants and estrogen creams.

Treatment of CAN is difficult due to its often hidden symptoms. Besides the ubiquitous recommendation of glycemic control, treatment is generally specific to the presentation of symptoms. Use of glycemic control, aspirin and angiotensin converting enzyme inhibitors for patients with microalbuminuria was shown to dramatically reduce CAN by a risk factor of 0.32 (88). Although this intervention was specific to T2DM, it may be applicable to T1DM. Other experimental techniques for broad reduction of CAN include the use of antioxidants (α-lipoic acid) or aldose reductase inhibitors. While many aldose reductase inhibitor trials have been withdrawn due to adverse or only marginal effects, the clinical trial of epalrestat showed optimistic results. In this study, epalrestat was well-tolerated, delayed onset of CAN, and ameliorated some symptoms (89).

Orthostatic hypotension can be treated with environmental changes though success is limited. Elevating the head by 30° at night, standing in stages, and the use of waist-high body stockings are all possible therapies. High sodium diet or fluorohydrocortisone as a plasma volume enhancer and the discontinuation or switching of long-term hypotensive agents to more short-term agents (e.g., captopril) have been used. Volume enhancement does not offer relief until the onset of edema, which itself has an increased risk of heart failure. Erythropoietin has been shown to alleviate symptoms especially with anemic T1DM (90).

SUMMARY

At the current time, a patient with T1DM has a > 50% probability of developing DN, capable of affecting sensory input (DPN), heart function (CAN), and genitourinary and gastric function (DAN). Diagnosis for DPN can be accomplished by a simple patient questionnaire and focused clinical examination. Diagnosis of DAN can also be begun at the bedside, but more formal testing is usually mandated, as the presence of DAN portends a high comorbidity with cardiac ischemia and arrhythmias. The high rate of DN causes an extreme financial burden to the U.S. economy, driving the search for more palpable options to reverse DN.

The only known course proven to prevent the progression of DN is intense glycemic control. Present treatments are limited to alleviating symptoms rather than eliminating initiating causes. Clinical trials are currently underway for drug therapies that would dampen the influence of the deleterious biochemical pathways linked to hyperglycemia.

ACKNOWLEDGEMENTS

We thank Ms. Judith Boldt for her expert secretarial assistance. This work was supported by the National Institutes of Health (NS36778 and NS38849), the Juvenile Diabetes Research Foundation Center for the Study of Complications in Diabetes, and the Program for Understanding Neurological Diseases (PFUND).

REFERENCES

1. Boulton AJ, Vinik AI, Arezzo JC, et al. Diabetic neuropathies: A statement by the American Diabetes Association. Diabetes Care 2005;28:956–962.
2. Thomas PK. Diabetic peripheral neuropathies: Their cost to patient and society and the value of knowledge of risk factors for development of interventions. Eur Neurol 1999;41(Suppl 1):35–43.
3. Vinik AI, Erbas T. Recognizing and treating diabetic autonomic neuropathy. Cleve Clin J Med 2001;68:928–944.
4. American Diabetes Association. Economic consequences of diabetes mellitus in the U.S. in 1997. Diabetes Care 1998;21:296–309.
5. Freeman R. Autonomic peripheral neuropathy. Lancet 2005;365:1259–1270.
6. Feldman EL. Oxidative stress and diabetic neuropathy: A new understanding of an old problem. J Clin Invest 2003;111:431–433.
7. Vincent AM, Feldman EL. New insights into the mechanisms of diabetic neuropathy. Rev Endocr Metabol Dis 2004;5:227–236.
8. Vincent AM, McLean LL, Backus C, et al. Short-term hyperglycemia produces oxidative damage and apoptosis in neurons. FASEB J 2005;19:638–640.
9. Vincent AM, Russell JW, Low P, et al. Oxidative stress in the pathogenesis of diabetic neuropathy. Endocr Rev 2004;25:612–628.

10. Leinninger GM, Backus C, Sastry AM, et al. Mitochondria in DRG neurons undergo hyper-glycemic mediated injury through BIM, BAX, and the fission protein DRP1. Neurobiol Dis 2005;23:11–22.

11. Aruoma OI, Halliwell B, Hoey BM, et al. The antioxidant action of taurine, hypotaurine, and their metabolic precursors. Biochem J 1988;256:251–255.

12. Stevens MJ, Lattimer SA, Kamijo M, et al. Osmotically-induced nerve taurine depletion and the compatible osmolyte hypothesis in experimental diabetic neuropathy in the rat. Diabetologia 1993;36:608–614.

13. Thomas TP, Feldman EL, Nakamura J, et al. Ambient glucose and aldose reductase-induced *myo*-inositol depletion modulate basal and carbachol-stimulated inositol phospholipid metabolism and diacylglycerol accumulation in human retinal pigment epithelial cells in culture. Proc Natl Acad Sci USA 1993;90:9712–9716.

14. Yorek MA, Wiese TJ, Davidson EP, et al. Reduced motor nerve conduction velocity and NA^+-K^+–ATPase activity in rats maintained on L-fucose diet. Diabetes 1993;42:1401–1406.

15. Cameron NE, Eaton SE, Cotter MA, et al. Vascular factors and metabolic interactions in the pathogenesis of diabetic neuropathy. Diabetologia 2001;44:1973–1988.

16. Koya D, King GL. Protein kinase C activation and the development of diabetic complications. Diabetes 1998;47:859–866.

17. Lee TS, Saltsman KA, Ohashi H, et al. Activation of protein kinase C by elevation of glucose concentration: Proposal for a mechanism in the development of diabetic vascular complications. Proc Natl Acad Sci USA 1989;86:5141–5145.

18. Singh R, Barden A, Mori T, et al. Advanced glycation end-products: A review. Diabetologia 2001;44:129–146.

19. Russell JW, Sullivan KA, Windebank AJ, et al. Neurons undergo apoptosis in animal and cell culture models of diabetes. Neurobiol Dis 1999;6:347–363.

20. Cheng C, Zochodne DW. Sensory neurons with activated caspase-3 survive long-term experi-mental diabetes. Diabetes 2003;52:2363–2371.

21. Zochodne DW, Verge VM, Cheng C, et al. Does diabetes target ganglion neurones? Progressive sensory neurone involvement in long-term experimental diabetes. Brain 2001;124:2319–2334.

22. Raff MC, Whitmore AV, Finn JT. Axonal self-destruction and neurodegeneration. Science 2002;296:868–871.

23. Sullivan KA, Feldman EL. New developments in diabetic neuropathy. Curr Opin Neurol 2005;18:586–590.

24. Dyck PJ, Davies JL, Litchy WJ, et al. Longitudinal assessment of diabetic polyneuropathy using a composite score in the Rochester diabetic neuropathy study cohort. Neurology 1997;49: 229–239.

25. Maser RE, Steenkiste AR, Dorman JS, et al. Epidemiological correlates of diabetic neuropa-thy. Report from Pittsburgh Epidemiology of Diabetes Complications Study. Diabetes 1989;38: 1456–1461.

26. Maser RE, Becker DJ, Drash AL, et al. Pittsburgh Epidemiology of Diabetes Complications Study. Measuring diabetic neuropathy follow-up study results. Diabetes Care 1992;15:525–527.

27. Tesfaye S, Chaturvedi N, Eaton SE, et al. Vascular risk factors and diabetic neuropathy. N Engl J Med 2005;352:341–350.

28. Olsen BS, Johannesen J, Sjolie AK, et al. Metabolic control and prevalence of microvascular complications in young Danish patients with Type 1 diabetes mellitus. Danish Study Group of Diabetes in Childhood. Diabet Med 1999;16:79–85.

29. Martin CL, Albers J, Herman WH, et al. Neuropathy among the diabetes control and complica-tions trial cohort 8 years after trial completion. Diabetes Care 2006;29:340–344.

30. Tesfaye S, Stevens LK, Stephenson JM, et al. Prevalence of diabetic peripheral neuropathy and its relation to glycaemic control and potential risk factors: The EURODIAB IDDM Complications Study. Diabetologia 1996;39:1377–1384.

31. Kempler P, Tesfaye S, Chaturvedi N, et al. Autonomic neuropathy is associated with in-creased cardiovascular risk factors: The EURODIAB IDDM Complications Study. Diabet Med 2002;19:900–909.

32. Witte DR, Tesfaye S, Chaturvedi N, et al. Risk factors for cardiac autonomic neuropathy in type 1 diabetes mellitus. Diabetologia 2005;48:164–171.
33. Ramsey SD, Newton K, Blough D, et al. Incidence, outcomes, and cost of foot ulcers in patients with diabetes. Diabetes Care 1999;22:382–387.
34. Coppini DV, Young PJ, Weng C, et al. Outcome on diabetic foot complications in relation to clinical examination and quantitative sensory testing: A case-control study. Diabet Med 1998;15: 765–771.
35. Ziegler D, Gries FA, Spuler M, et al. The epidemiology of diabetic neuropathy. DiaCAN Multicenter Study Group. Diabet Med 1993;10(Suppl 2):82S–86S.
36. Young MJ, Boulton AJM, Macleod AF, et al. A multicentre study of the prevalence of diabetic peripheral neuropathy in the United Kingdom hospital clinic population. Diabetologia 1993;36150–154.
37. Allman KC, Stevens MJ, Wieland DM, et al. Noninvasive assessment of cardiac diabetic neuropathy by carbon-11 hydroxyephedrine and positron emission tomography. J Am Coll Cardiol 1993;22:1425–1432.
38. Stevens MJ, Raffel DM, Allman KC, et al. Cardiac sympathetic dysinnervation in diabetes: Implications for enhanced cardiovascular risk. Circulation 1998;98:961–968.
39. Jermendy G, Toth L, Voros P, et al. Cardiac autonomic neuropathy and QT interval length. A follow-up study in diabetic patients. Acta Cardiol 1991;46:189–200.
40. Shaw JE, Vileikyte L, Connor H, et al. The diabetic foot 1994. Diabet Med 1995;12:88–90.
41. Frykberg RG. Epidemiology of the diabetic foot: Ulcerations and amputations. Adv Wound Care 1999;12:139–141.
42. Wilbourn AJ. Diabetic entrapment and compression neuropathies. In: Dyck PJ, Thomas PK, eds. Diabetic Neuropathy. Philadelphia: W.B. Saunders, 1999, pp. 481–508.
43. Consensus Panel. Consensus Statement. Report and recommendations of the San Antonio Conference on Diabetic Neuropathy. Diabetes 1988;37:1000–1004.
44. Walker FO. Nerve conduction studies in diabetic neuropathy. Neurology 1995;45:849.
45. Valk GD, de Sonnaville JJ, van Houtum WH, et al. The assessment of diabetic polyneuropathy in daily clinical practice: Reproducibility and validity of Semmes Weinstein monofilaments examination and clinical neurological examination. Muscle Nerve 1997;20:116–118.
46. Bax G, Fagherazzi C, Piarulli F, et al. Reproducibility of Michigan Neuropathy Screening Instrument (MNSI). A comparison with tests using the vibratory and thermal perception thresholds. Diabetes Care 1996;19:904–905.
47. Feldman EL, Stevens MJ, Thomas PK, et al. A practical two-step quantitative clinical and electrophysiological assessment for the diagnosis and staging of diabetic neuropathy. Diabetes Care 1994;17:1281–1289.
48. Genuth S. Insights from the diabetes control and complications trial/epidemiology of diabetes interventions and complications study on the use of intensive glycemic treatment to reduce the risk of complications of type 1 diabetes. Endocr Pract 2006;12(Suppl 1):34–41.
49. Folwaczny C, Wawarta R, Otto B, et al. Gastric emptying of solid and liquid meals in healthy controls compared with long-term type-1 diabetes mellitus under optimal glucose control. Exp Clin Endocrinol Diabetes 2003;111:223–229.
50. McCulloch DK, Campbell IW, Wu FC, et al. The prevalence of diabetic impotence. Diabetologia 1980;18:279–283.
51. Ellenberg M. Sexual function in diabetic patients. Ann Intern Med 1980;92:331–333.
52. Enzlin P, Mathieu C, Vanderschueren D, et al. Diabetes mellitus and female sexuality: A review of 25 years' research. Diabet Med 1998;15:809–815.
53. Kaplan SA, Blaivas JG. Diabetic cystopathy. J Diabet Complications 1988;2:133–139.
54. Joshi N, Caputo GM, Weitekamp MR, et al. Infections in patients with diabetes mellitus. N Engl J Med 1999;341:1906–1912.
55. Jermendy G. Clinical consequences of cardiovascular autonomic neuropathy in diabetic patients. Acta Diabetol 2003;40(Suppl 2):S370–S374.
56. Stevens MJ, Raffel DM, Allman KC, et al. Regression and progression of cardiac sympathetic dysinnervation in diabetic patients with autonomic neuropathy. Metabolism 1999;48:92–101.

57. Pop-Busui R, Kirkwood I, Schmid H, et al. Sympathetic dysfunction in type 1 diabetes: Association with impaired myocardial blood flow reserve and diastolic dysfunction. J Am Coll Cardiol 2004;44:2368–2374.
58. Hilsted J. Pathophysiology in diabetic autonomic neuropathy: Cardiovascular, hormonal, and metabolic studies. Diabetes 1982;31:730–737.
59. Hornung RS, Mahler RF, Raftery EB. Ambulatory blood pressure and heart rate in diabetic patients: An assessment of autonomic function. Diabet Med 1989;6:579–585.
60. Watkins PJ, Mackay JD. Cardiac denervation in diabetic neuropathy. Ann Intern Med 1980;92:304–307.
61. Kennedy WR, Navarro X, Sakuta M, et al. Physiological and clinical correlates of cardiorespiratory reflexes in diabetes mellitus. Diabetes Care 1989;12:399–408.
62. Maser RE, Mitchell BD, Vinik AI, et al. The association between cardiovascular autonomic neuropathy and mortality in individuals with diabetes: A meta-analysis. Diabetes Care 2003;26:1895–1901.
63. Aronson D, Weinrauch LA, D'Elia JA, et al. Circadian patterns of heart rate variability, fibrinolytic activity, and hemostatic factors in type I diabetes mellitus with cardiac autonomic neuropathy. Am J Cardiol 1999;84:449–453.
64. Albers JW, Kenny DJ, Brown M, et al. Effect of intensive diabetes treatment on nerve conduction in the diabetes control and complications trial. Ann Neurol 1995;38:869–880.
65. The Diabetes Control and Complications Trial Research Group. The effect of intensive treatment of diabetes on the development and progression of long-term complications in insulin-dependent diabetes mellitus. N Engl J Med 1993;329:977–986.
66. Diabetes Control and Complications Trial (DCCT) Research Group. The effect of intensive diabetes therapy on the development and progression of neuropathy. Ann Intern Med 1995;122:561–568.
67. Epidemiology of Diabetes Interventions and Complications (EDIC). Design, implementation, and preliminary results of a long-term follow-up of the Diabetes Control and Complications Trial cohort. Diabetes Care 1999;22:99–111.
68. Writing Team for the Diabetes Control and Complications Trial/Epidemiology of Diabetes Interventions and Complications Research Group. Effect of intensive therapy on the microvascular complications of type 1 diabetes mellitus. JAMA 2002;287:2563–2569.
69. Burger AJ, Weinrauch LA, D'Elia JA, et al. Effect of glycemic control on heart rate variability in type I diabetic patients with cardiac autonomic neuropathy. Am J Cardiol 1999;84:687–691.
70. Kendall DM, Rooney DP, Smets YF, et al. Pancreas transplantation restores epinephrine response and symptom recognition during hypoglycemia in patients with long-standing type I diabetes and autonomic neuropathy. Diabetes 1997;46:249–257.
71. Navarro X, Sutherland DE, Kennedy WR. Long-term effects of pancreatic transplantation on diabetic neuropathy. Ann Neurol 1997;42:727–736.
72. Simmons Z, Feldman EL. Update on diabetic neuropathy. Curr Opin Neurol 2002;15:595–603.
73. Argoff CE, Backonja MM, Belgrade MJ, et al. Consensus guidelines: Treatment, planning, and options. Diabetic peripheral neuropathic pain. Mayo Clin Proc 2006;81:S12–S25.
74. Goldstein DJ, Lu Y, Detke MJ, et al. Duloxetine vs. placebo in patients with painful diabetic neuropathy. Pain 2005;116:109–118.
75. Freynhagen R, Strojek K, Griesing T, et al. Efficacy of pregabalin in neuropathic pain evaluated in a 12-week, randomised, double-blind, multicentre, placebo-controlled trial of flexible- and fixed-dose regimens. Pain 2005;115:254–263.
76. Max MB, Lynch SA, Muir J, et al. Effects of desipramine, amitriptyline, and fluoxetine on pain in diabetic neuropathy. N Engl J Med 1992;326:1250–1256.
77. Backonja M, Beydoun A, Edwards KR, et al. Gabapentin for the symptomatic treatment of painful neuropathy in patients with diabetes mellitus: A randomized controlled trial [see comments]. JAMA 1998;280:1831–1836.
78. Raskin P, Donofrio PD, Rosenthal NR, et al. Topiramate vs placebo in painful diabetic neuropathy: Analgesic and metabolic effects. Neurology 2004;63:865–873.

79. Oskarsson P, Ljunggren JG, Lins PE. Efficacy and safety of mexiletine in the treatment of painful diabetic neuropathy. The Mexiletine Study Group. Diabetes Care 1997;20:1594–1597.

80. Harati Y, Gooch C, Swenson M, et al. Double-blind randomized trial of tramadol for the treatment of the pain of diabetic neuropathy. Neurology 1998;50:1842–1846.

81. Abuaisha BB, Costanzi JB, Boulton AJ. Acupuncture for the treatment of chronic painful peripheral diabetic neuropathy: A long-term study. Diabetes Res Clin Pract 1998;39:115–121.

82. Rayner CK, Samsom M, Jones KL, et al. Relationships of upper gastrointestinal motor and sensory function with glycemic control. Diabetes Care 2001;24:371–381.

83. Lysy J, Israeli E, Goldin E. The prevalence of chronic diarrhea among diabetic patients. Am J Gastroenterol 1999;94:2165–2170.

84. Schiavi RC. Psychological treatment of erectile disorders in diabetic patients. Ann Intern Med 1980;92:337–339.

85. Vinik A, Erbas T, Stansberry K. Gastrointestinal, genitourinary, and neurovascular disturbances in diabetes. Diabetes Rev 1999;7:358–378.

86. Sildenafil Study Group. Oral sildenafil in the treatment of erectile dysfunction. N Engl J Med 1998;338:1397–1404.

87. Rendell MS, Rajfer J, Wicker PA, et al. Sildenafil for treatment of erectile dysfunction in men with diabetes: A randomized controlled trial. Sildenafil Diabetes Study Group. JAMA 1999;281: 421–426.

88. Gaede P, Vedel P, Parving HH, et al. Intensified multifactorial intervention in patients with type 2 diabetes mellitus and microalbuminuria: The Steno type 2 randomised study. Lancet 1999;353:617–622.

89. Bril V, Buchanan RA. Aldose reductase inhibition by AS-3201 in sural nerve from patients with diabetic sensorimotor polyneuropathy. Diabetes Care 2004;27:2369–2375.

90. Hoeldtke RD, Streeten DH. Treatment of orthostatic hypotension with erythropoietin. N Engl J Med 1993;329:611–615.

91. Feldman EL, Stevens MJ, Russell JW, Greene DA. Somatosensory neuropathy. In: Porte D Jr, Sherwin RS, Baron A, eds. Ellenberg & Rifkin's Diabetes Mellitus, 6th edn. United States of America: McGraw-Hill, 2003, pp. 777.

11

Hypoglycemia in Type 1 Diabetes

V. J. Briscoe and S. N. Davis
*Vanderbilt School of Medicine, Division of Diabetes, Endocrinology and Metabolism,
Vanderbilt University, Nashville, Tennessee, U.S.A.*

INTRODUCTION

Hypoglycemia occurs when blood glucose levels are lower than the lowest limit of normal physiologic fluctuations. This level is approximately 70 mg/dL and is rarely encountered in healthy individuals. Iatrogenic hypoglycemia, however, is a common problem in the management of diabetes. It is also of special concern for adults with type 1 diabetes mellitus (T1DM) because complications associated with recurring hypoglycemia such as impaired physiologic defenses against hypoglycemia and an inability to recognize low-glucose levels [hypoglycemia unawareness (HU)] commonly occur. Hypoglycemia is one of the most feared complications of diabetes treatment and is often the cause for emergency care visits.

Plasma glucose concentration is normally rigidly regulated between 70 and 150 mg/dL, despite wide variations in glucose flux (e.g., fasting, postprandial, and exercising). Conversely, once plasma glucose concentrations fall below the euglycemic threshold, physiologic adaptive reactions to hypoglycemia elicit an array of neuroendocrine, autonomic nervous system (ANS), and metabolic responses to raise blood glucose levels back to normal.

Glucose (a major metabolic fuel) enters the brain from the circulation where it is metabolized for energy and stored (in negligible amounts) as glycogen. Hypoglycemic symptoms occur because of the brain's dependency on an adequate supply of glucose for normal function. The Whipple's triad has historically been used as a guide to define acute hypoglycemia. The triad consists of (*i*) symptoms attributable to a low plasma glucose concentration, (*ii*) a measurably low plasma glucose concentration (less than 70 mg/dL), and (*iii*) the rapid resolution of the symptoms after correction of the biochemical abnormality (1–5).

The landmark Diabetes Control and Complications Trial (DCCT) demonstrated that intensive glucose control in T1DM could reduce complications associated with diabetes (i.e., microvascular and subsequently macrovascular complications) (4). Unfortunately, intensive glycemic control was also associated with a threefold increased risk of severe hypoglycemia (6). Intensively treated individuals can experience up to 10 episodes of symptomatic hypoglycemia per week and severe temporarily disabling hypoglycemia at least once a year (6–9). An estimated 2% to 4% of deaths of people with T1DM have been attributed to hypoglycemia (8). The increased frequency of iatrogenic hypoglycemia is a limiting factor in the implementation of intensive glycemic control.

Hypoglycemia is a common problem in clinical practice, affecting 90% of all patients who receive insulin (3). Understanding the physiologic counterregulatory responses induced by hypoglycemia coupled with frequent monitoring of blood glucose and physiologic insulin replacement therapy can help reduce the prevalence of iatrogenic hypoglycemia in T1DM (3–11). Also key to reducing hypoglycemia will be patient education regarding all aspects of diabetes self-care.

MAINTENANCE OF BLOOD GLUCOSE

Effective blood glucose regulation is fundamentally important for the maintenance of life. The ANS and neuroendocrine systems preserve this homeostasis through the interplay of glucose absorption from the intestine, glucose production by the liver, and glucose uptake in tissues (i.e., muscle, liver, and brain) (1–3).

After a carbohydrate load, blood glucose is increased as it is absorbed by the intestines. Insulin is released in response to this acute glucose elevation and stimulates skeletal muscle, hepatic, and adipose tissue glucose uptake from the circulation. Insulin lowers plasma glucose by (i) suppressing endogenous glucose production (EGP), both by direct action on the liver and indirect actions, to reduce substrate flux such as lactate, pyruvate, glycerol, and free fatty acids to the liver and (ii) increasing glucose uptake into peripheral tissues, predominantly into muscles (1–3).

In the postprandial state, the liver releases glucose into the circulation via glycogenolysis. However, after an overnight fast, gluconeogenesis becomes the primary source of EGP (1–3). About one-third of glucose uptake in the fasting state is by the central nervous system with the brain being the chief consumer, since glucose is the brain's primary fuel. The brain has limited glucose stores and thus, is dependent on endogenous (primarily hepatic) glucose output for its glucose supply. The transport of glucose into the tissues is facilitated by a specific family of proteins called glucose transporters.

PHYSIOLOGICAL RESPONSE TO HYPOGLYCEMIA

The physiologic counterregulatory response to hypoglycemia involves neuroendocrine, ANS, and metabolic processes. This includes the suppression of insulin release as well as secretion of glucagon and pancreatic polypeptide from the pancreas, epinephrine from the adrenal medullae, norepinephrine from sympathetic postganglionic nerve terminals and adrenal medulla, cortisol from the adrenal cortex, and growth hormone from the anterior pituitary gland (11–13). In humans, inhibition of insulin secretion is the initial defense against a falling glucose and occurs at a plasma glucose concentration of about 80 mg/dL. The brain is one of the first organs affected and is most vulnerable to any glucose deprivation.

In adults with T1DM, insulin levels do not decrease as glucose levels fall, because of persistent absorption of exogenous insulin. The lack of decline in plasma insulin concentrations as glucose levels fall constitutes the first deficit in the defense against hypoglycemia in T1DM.

Next to respond in the acute defense against hypoglycemia are glucagon and epinephrine. These hormones begin to rise at glucose levels just below 70 mg/dL. Glucagon (secreted from pancreatic alpha cells) is a rapid-acting stimulus that facilitates hepatic glucose production. Glucagon acts directly on the liver to (*i*) convert glycogen to glucose (increasing hepatic glycogenolysis) and (*ii*) by promoting gluconeogenesis, (providing available 3-carbon glucose substrates such as lactate, pyruvate, alanine, and glycerol). This glucagon-stimulated increase in glucose production and thus the increased plasma glucose concentration lasts only for 2 to 3 hours (14).

The glucagon secretory response to hypoglycemia is irreversibly lost in patients with T1DM greater than 5-years duration (3–9). Hence, epinephrine (not glucagon) constitutes the main defense against hypoglycemia in these patients (3–9). As long as this mechanism is intact, epinephrine can adequately compensate for the glucagon deficiency.

Epinephrine sharply increases EGP during hypoglycemia. Secreted by the adrenal medullae, epinephrine binds to multiple receptors and causes an array of hemodynamic and metabolic effects. Through its actions (direct and indirect) on diverse target tissues, the hormone stimulates both glucose production and the limitation of glucose utilization by mainly beta adrenergic receptors in humans (1–3,7–9).

Epinephrine increases hepatic glucose production by direct stimulation of hepatic glycogenolysis. It also increases plasma glucose via hepatic gluconeogenesis; this process occurs mostly through an indirect mechanism, which consists of mobilization of lactate, alanine, glycerol (as gluconeogenic substrates), and nonesterified fatty acids (which provide energy for the process) (15–18). Another important physiologic function of epinephrine is its ability to limit glucose utilization in insulin-sensitive tissues (i.e., skeletal muscle). The epinephrine-stimulated increase in glucose production and glycogenolysis is relatively transient. However, because epinephrine also reduces glucose clearance, the hyperglycemic effect of the hormone is more persistent (8).

During hypoglycemia, norepinephrine is released from the adrenal medullae and through spillover from the sympathetic nervous system. Norepinephrine results in net vasoconstriction with increases in diastolic as well as systolic blood pressure. This effect differs from epinephrine, where there is net vasodilatation with increases in systolic blood pressure but decreases in diastolic blood pressure. Otherwise, norepinephrine, produces metabolic hyperglycemic effects through mechanisms analogous to those of epinephrine (3,7–9), as discussed above.

The increased sympathetic nervous system response is primarily responsible for the activation of lipolyis that results in release of free fatty acids (FFA) and glycerol. The elevated FFA levels result in significant glucose sparing as tissues can oxidize FFA instead of glucose. The inverse relationship that exists between fatty acid oxidation and glucose oxidation in insulin-sensitive tissues (including muscle) occurs by the inhibition of pyruvate dehydrogenase activity. Glycerol also becomes an important substrate for gluconeogenesis during prolonged hypoglycemia. Thus, it has been estimated that the increased lipolysis contributes up to 25% of the total defense against hypoglycemia (3,7–9).

Cortisol and growth hormone increase glucose production and restrain glucose disposal during hypoglycemia. However, these hormones have little or no role in the defense against acute hypoglycemia but become more important during prolonged hypoglycemia (9). Their effects do not become evident until 3 to 4 hours of prolonged hypoglycemia. The metabolic counterregulatory actions of cortisol and growth hormone are similar and include stimulation of gluconeogenesis and inhibition of glucose uptake. However, their effects are limited, having only approximately 20% compared to that of epinephrine (9).

Cortisol limits glucose utilization in muscle and other tissues through both direct and indirect actions. The latter occurs as a result of cortisol-stimulated lipolysis. Cortisol inhibits protein synthesis and promotes protein breakdown with increases of gluconeogenic precursors including lactate, alanine, and other amino acids from muscle and glycerol from fat. In addition to stimulating hepatic gluconeogenesis, cortisol also promotes glycogen

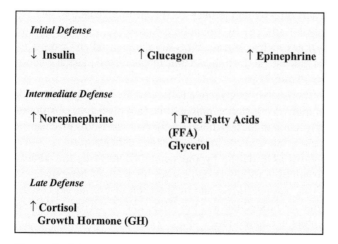

Initial Defense

↓ Insulin   ↑ Glucagon   ↑ Epinephrine

Intermediate Defense

↑ Norepinephrine   ↑ Free Fatty Acids
                              (FFA)
                              Glycerol

Late Defense

↑ Cortisol
  Growth Hormone (GH)

Figure 1   Diagrammatic outline of normal counterregulatory responses to hypoglycemia.

synthesis and exerts permissive effects on the gluconeogenic and glycogenolytic actions of glucagon and epinephrine. The net result is that cortisol produces an acute insulin-resistant state that serves to raise plasma glucose concentrations (Fig. 1) (1–3).

Growth hormone, after its initial insulin-like action, reduces glycemic sensitivity to insulin through mechanisms that are not well-understood but may include the effect of the hormone on stimulating lipolysis. The hormone's counterregulatory effects involve antagonizing insulin's actions to (*i*) effect to increase glucose utilization and (*ii*) reduce glucose production.

SYMPTOMS OF HYPOGLYCEMIA

For most adults with T1DM, hypoglycemia is an unfortunate fact of life (1–6). Those attempting to achieve better glycemic control suffer many episodes of mild-to-moderate hypoglycemia. Early detection and recognition of hypoglycemic symptoms is critical for the individual to self-treat the hypoglycemic episode before becoming disabled.

The two categories of hypoglycemic symptoms are neurogenic and neuroglycopenic. The neurogenic symptoms are activated by the ANS (usually occur at ∼ 60 mg/dL in nondiabetic individuals) and are mediated in part by sympathoadrenal release of cate-cholamines (norepinephrine and epinephrine) from the adrenal medullae and acetylcholine from postsynaptic sympathetic nerve endings (7–9). These symptoms are triggered by a falling glucose. This defense is critical for the recognition of symptoms that will alert the individual to treat the hypoglycemic episode. Neurogenic signs and symptoms include shakiness, anxiety, nervousness, palpitations, sweating, dry mouth and pallor, and pupil di-lation (7,10,20). Cholinergic-medicated neurogenic symptoms include diaphoresis, hunger, and paresthesias (Table 1) (3,7,20). Recent work by Aftab-Guy et al. (12) has demonstrated that simulating epinephrine levels found during moderate hypoglycemia on a background of hyperinsulinemic euglycemia only produces about 20% of the neurogenic symptom scores usually observed during moderate hypoglycemia. This indicates that the genesis of hypoglycemic symptoms is multifocal and probably arises mainly from CNS efferent pathways (12).

The second category of hypoglycemic symptoms includes neuroglycopenic symp-toms, which usually occur at approximately 50 mg/dL in nondiabetic individuals. These

Table 1 Neurogenic Symptoms
of Hypoglycemia

Sweating
Shakiness
Tremulousness
Paresthesias
Anxiety
Nervousness
Palpitations
Hunger

are generated as a result of brain neuronal glucose deprivation (3–7,10–12). The brain is vulnerable to any glucose deprivation and neuroglycopenia causes a rapid impairment of cerebral function. These symptoms include abnormal mentation, irritability, confusion, difficulty speaking, ataxia, paresthesias, headaches, stupor, and eventually (if untreated) seizures, coma, and even death (3,7–10,20–23). Neuroglycopenic symptoms can also include a wide array of transient and at times idiosyncratic focal neurological deficits (e.g., diplopia, hemiparesis) (3,7,20) (Table 2).

HYPOGLYCEMIA AND GLYCEMIC THRESHOLDS

The glycemic thresholds responsible for the activation of the physiologic defenses against hypoglycemia are dynamic (9). Patients with a higher HbA1c may perceive symptoms of hypoglycemia at a higher plasma glucose level than those with more intensive control (23). Some of these patients (with the higher HbA1c) may even generate hypoglycemic symptoms when their plasma glucose is above the normal range. This phenomenon is called "relative hypoglycemia" and is associated with release of counterregulatory hormones. It commonly occurs when patients are attempting to intensify their metabolic control to achieve near normoglycemia. "Relative hypoglycemia" is self-limiting and usually takes 2 to 4 weeks for the brain to readjust to the improved but relatively reduced circulating glucose levels (9,11,23,24). The opposite situation holds true in intensively controlled individuals with diabetes. These individuals may not recognize hypoglycemia until their plasma glucose is considerably lower to the normal physiologic glycemic thresholds (7,11). These changes

Table 2 Neuroglycopenic Symptoms
of Hypoglycemia

Irritability
Confusion
Dizziness
Weakness
Difficulty thinking
Slurred speech
Headaches
Sleepiness
Seizures
Coma

in glycemic thresholds can be caused acutely by antecedent hypoglycemia or chronically by persistent hyperglycemia (1–7).

HYPOGLYCEMIA UNAWARENESS

HU is a major limiting factor in the management of adults with T1DM. Recommendation of strict glycemic goals may not be appropriate for patients experiencing HU because it may contribute to an increased prevalence of severe hypoglycemia. HU is characterized by the loss of autonomic warning symptoms that defend against the development of neuroglycopenia. This failure to perceive autonomic warning signals like sweating, anxiety, or tremor, has been proposed to contribute to the increased frequency and severity of hypoglycemia in patients with T1DM. Duration of diabetes, antecedent hypoglycemia, and tight glycemic control are known risk factors for HU. The mechanism responsible for HU remains controversial. Work from Boyle et al. (21) has demonstrated that somewhat paradoxically, brain glucose uptake during hypoglycemia is increased in intensively treated patients with T1DM as compared with patients with poor metabolic control or healthy subjects. The explanation for this finding is that in T1DM patients with good glycemic control, there is acceleration of cerebral glucose transport during hypoglycemia. This perfusion of glucose preserves cerebral function, making available an adequate glucose supply to the brain. Hence, it (the brain) does not signal for a counterregulatory response and the patient is asymptomatic thereby creating HU (21). Segel et al. (22), using a different experimental methodology (PET as opposed to Kety Schmidt technique), however, reported no difference in net brain glucose uptake with hypoglycemia in patients with T1DM. Thus, it may be that regional differences in brain glucose uptake rather than global changes in brain glucose uptake are responsible for causing HU (9).

MECHANISMS OF COUNTERREGULATORY RESPONSES TO HYPOGLYCEMIA IN T1DM

Glucose counterregulation is fundamentally altered in T1DM as individuals become absolutely insulin deficient and insulin levels no longer fall as glucose levels decrease (Fig. 2).

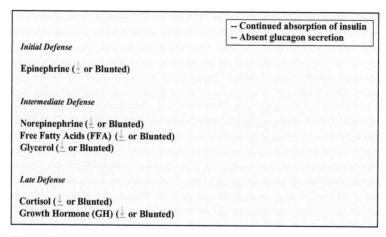

Figure 2 Diagrammatic outline of defective counterregulatory responses to hypoglycemia in T1DM.

Hence, the first defense against hypoglycemia is lost. Within a similar time frame (about 5 years), the glucagon response to falling glucose levels is also lost. Thus, an important second defense against hypoglycemia also fails. It should be noted that pancreatic alpha cells are present in equal numbers and size as compared to age and weight matched non-diabetic individuals. Glucagon responses to other physiologic stress such as exercise and amino acid infusion are preserved in T1DM. The mechanism of this selective and therefore functional (rather than anatomic) defect in glucagon secretion is controversial. Hypotheses, with supporting data, have included autonomic neuropathy and a failure of insulin "shut off" as the mechanism responsible for the lack of glucoagon release during hypoglycemia in T1DM (3,7–11,20).

Epinephrine (not glucagon), therefore, constitutes the main defense against hypoglycemia in patients with T1DM for greater than 5-years duration. Unfortunately, epinephrine responses to hypoglycemia also become impaired in T1DM patients undergoing intensive insulin treatment. This places intensively treated T1DM patients at a significant risk for recurrent hypoglycemia (16,17). These frequent bouts of hypoglycemia further reduces the counterregulatory responses to subsequent hypoglycemia by $\geq 50\%$. Thus, a vicious cycle is created whereby hypoglycemia induces further hypoglycemia (3,7,16,20). Reductions in ANS counterregulatory responses have significant clinical consequences. T1DM patients with deficient glucagon and epinephrine response to hypoglycemia have a 25-fold or greater risk of severe hypoglycemia (i.e., an individual is incapacitated and needs external assistance to raise their plasma glucose levels) during intensive insulin therapy (4).

ANTECEDENT HYPOGLYCEMIA AND HYPOGLYCEMIA-ASSOCIATED AUTONOMIC FAILURE

Cryer earlier coined the term "hypoglycemia-associated autonomic failure (HAAF)" to describe the syndrome of acquired counterregulatory deficits associated with prior hypoglycemia. This syndrome is experienced by individuals with T1DM and involves blunted neuroendocrine counterregulatory responses to hypoglycemia, lowered glycemic thresholds for activation of counterregulatory defenses, and HU. To test the hypothesis that hypoglycemia itself causes reduced neuroendocrine and symptomatic responses to subsequent hypoglycemia, Heller and Cryer measured counterregulatory responses during repeated hypoglycemic clamp studies (13). These experiments determined that two episodes of antecedent moderate hypoglycemia (50 mg/dL) resulted in significant reductions of plasma epinephrine, glucagon, pancreatic polypeptide, and cortisol responses to next day hypoglycemia. Neurogenic and neuroglycopenic symptom responses were also reduced after antecedent hypoglycemia (13). Importantly, Dagogo-Jack et al. also demonstrated that antecedent hypoglycemia can reduce ANS, neuroendocrine, and symptomatic counterregulatory responses to subsequent hypoglycemia in T1DM (25). These seminal observations have been conceptually supported by numerous subsequent studies from many different laboratories (10–16).

Davis et al. (17) demonstrated that the magnitude of antecedent hypoglycemia produced proportional blunting of counterregulatory responses to subsequent hypoglycemia; hence, the greater the depth of antecedent hypoglycemia, the greater the magnitude of subsequent counterregulatory failure. The ANS is extremely sensitive to the effects of antecedent hypoglycemia as minimal episodes of hypoglycemia of only 70 mg/dL can blunt subsequent counterregulatory response by 30% in men. Likewise, two episodes of short duration (20 minutes) of antecedent hypoglycemia of approximately 50 mg/dL can also produce significant blunting of subsequent ANS, neuroendocrine, and metabolic but not

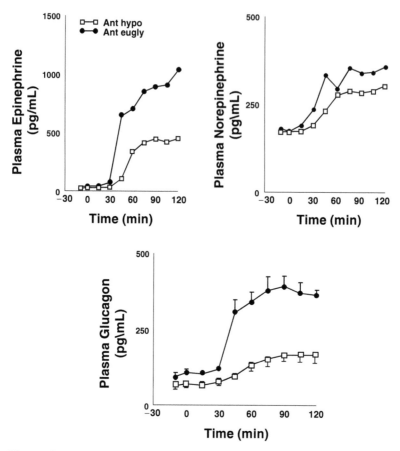

Figure 3 Effects of peripherally infused insulin (1.5 mU/kg/min) on arterialized plasma epinephrine, norepinephrine, and glucagon levels in overnight-fasted man following previous day antecedent euglycemia (ant eugly) or antecedent hypoglycemia (ant hypo). Plasma epinephrine was significantly increased ($P < 0.01$) following ant eugly. Plasma norepinephrine was significantly increased ($P < 0.05$) following ant eugly. Plasma glucagon significantly increased ($P < 0.05$) following ant eugly.

symptomatic counterregulatory responses (17). Thus, there appears to be a hierarchical effect of duration of antecedent hypoglycemia on blunting counterregulatory responses to subsequent hypoglycemia (18) (Fig. 3). ANS and neuroendocrine responses are more susceptible to the blunting effects of prior short-term hypoglycemia, whereas, more prolonged antecedent hypoglycemia is needed to blunt subsequent symptom responses. The resulting clinical consequence of the diminished ANS responses to hypoglycemia for T1DM patients (with already deficient glucagon response to hypoglycemia) is greater risk of severe hypoglycemia.

The timing and number of prior hypoglycemic episodes required to cause a blunting effect has also been investigated. Davis and Tate (19) studied whether one episode of hypoglycemia could modify counterregulatory responses to hypoglycemia induced that same day. Subjects were randomized to identical morning and afternoon hyperinsulinemic hypoglycemia separated by 2 hours or, morning and afternoon hyperinsulinemic euglycemia, or morning hyperinsulinemic euglycemia and afternoon hyperinsulinemic hypoglycemia. Morning hypoglycemia significantly reduced ANS and neuroendocrine responses (epinephrine, norepinephrine, glucagon, GH, cortisol, and pancreatic polypeptide) during afternoon hypoglycemia. Neuroglycopenic symptoms were also significantly reduced during afternoon hypoglycemia. Hence, one episode of prolonged, moderate, morning hypoglycemia produced substantial blunting of neuroendocrine and symptomatic responses to subsequent same day hypoglycemia (19).

The syndrome of HAAF is traditionally associated with reduced neuroendocrine counterregulatory responses. Recently, work has been focused on whether the actions as well as the levels of the key counterregulatory hormone, epinephrine, are also reduced. Korytkowski et al. (26) demonstrated that T1DM subjects with blunted counterregulatory responses to hypoglycemia had reduced β-adrenergic sensitivity compared to patients with normal counterregulatory responses. Also, Aftab-Guy et al. (12,27) have demonstrated that epinephrine has reduced effects in T1DM patients as compared to nondiabetic controls in stimulating glucagon release, activating lipolysis, increasing glucose production, reducing glucose uptake, and elevating blood pressure. Thus, it appears that T1DM patients have a widespread, pleotropic down regulation of epinephrine's key counterregulatory effects. In a subsequent study, Aftab-Guy et al. determined that these reduced epinephrine effects in T1DM were worsened by intensive glycemic control (28). It appears that reduced epinephrine action may be considered as an additional component to the HAAF syndrome. Several studies have investigated whether avoidance of hypoglycemia can reverse some or all of the elements of HAAF.

Fritsche et al. demonstrated that if hypoglycemic episodes are avoided for 4 months, β-adrenergic sensitivity and hypoglycemic symptom responses could increase despite a persistently blunted epinephrine response to hypoglycemia (29). Perhaps, indicating that increases in β-adrenergic sensitivity are a prelude to restoration of endocrine and autonomic function if hypoglycemic episodes are avoided (9). Other studies have also reported that some or all of the features of hypoglycemia-associated autonomic failure (i.e., blunted neuroendocrine counterregulatory responses) can be reversed with 3- to 6-months strict avoidance of antecedent hypoglycemia (3,7–9,20,30–32).

EXERCISE-RELATED HYPOGLYCEMIA

Exercise has numerous therapeutic benefits. Physical activity improves insulin sensitivity; helps maintain body weight, and can reduce postprandial hyperglycemia. However, despite these and numerous other benefits, exercise often results in hypoglycemia in adults with T1DM. Counterregulatory hormones are activated during exercise in a similar fashion to hypoglycemia. However, norepinephrine levels are higher and epinephrine levels are lower during exercise as compared to hypoglycemia. Nevertheless, the metabolic role of counterregulatory hormones during exercise is to allow the individual to match glucose production to the needs of the working muscles. Therefore, neuroendocrine mechanisms are invoked to stimulate EGP, while simultaneously limiting glucose uptake in muscles. If glucose production cannot match glucose uptake then hypoglycemia will develop.

Until recently, the mechanisms responsible for exercise-associated hypoglycemia in T1DM were thought to be due to a relative or absolute excess of insulin and inadequate glycogen repletion. Neuroendocrine counterregulatory responses are amplified during exercise in the presence of hypoglycemia (5). However, reports by Bottini et al. (33) and Schneider et al. (34) demonstrated that T1DM patients had reduced counterregulatory responses during exercise. Furthermore, the responses appeared to be attenuated by intensive metabolic control. These studies provided the first indication that deficient neuroendocrine

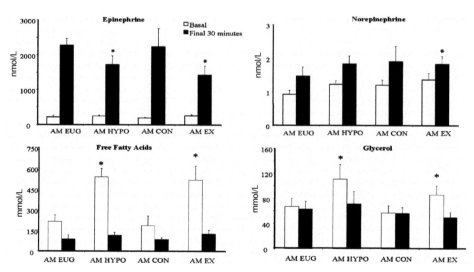

Figure 4 Effects of morning hyperinsulinemic euglycemia (AM EUG), hypoglycemia (AM HYPO), control (AM CON), or moderate intensity exercise (AM EX) on responses of epinephrine, norepinephrine, free fatty acid, and glycerol, during afternoon hyperinsulinemic hypoglycemia (50 mg/dL) in T1DM individuals. *$P < 0.05$, AM EX and AM HYPO are significantly reduced compared to AM CON and AM EUG groups. Values are means ± SE.

and ANS counterregulatory responses could be a contributing mechanism to exercise-associated hypoglycemia in T1DM.

Davis et al. and Galassetti et al. determined that neuroendocrine and metabolic responses during prolonged exercise (90 minutes at 50% Vo_{2max}) are reduced by about 50% after prior hyperinsulinemic hypoglycemia in nondiabetic (35) and T1DM (36) individuals. Conversely, two bouts of prior exercise for 90 minutes at 50% Vo_{2max} (31) or 60 minutes at 70% Vo_{2max} (37) have been shown to blunt counterregulatory responses to subsequent next-day hypoglycemia in both T1DM and nondiabetic subjects. Thus, the above studies confirmed that blunted counterregulation induced by prior moderate-intensity exercise is a mechanism responsible for subsequent hypoglycemia in T1DM (Fig. 4). And in fact, Sandoval et al. demonstrated that repeated episodes of prolonged exercise of both low (30% Vo_{2max}) and moderate (50% Vo_{2max}) intensities blunted key autonomic and metabolic (EGP and peripheral glucose uptake) counterregulatory responses to next-day hypoglycemia in T1DM (38). Thus, there appears to be a reciprocal feed-forward vicious cycle of counterregulatory failure that is generated following antecedent episodes of exercise and hypoglycemia (9).

Hypoglycemia can occur during exercise, and up to 24 hours after exercise (13). Hence, patients with T1DM who exercise late in the day may be at-risk for nocturnal or even next-day hypoglycemia. Following exercise, counterregulatory responses are diminished with the result that glucose rate of appearance during subsequent hypoglycemia is dramatically blunted (35). Similarly following antecedent hypoglycemia, counterregulatory defenses to preserve glucose production during exercise are diminished. Additionally, it should be noted that aerobic exercise will increase both insulin and noninsulin-mediated glucose uptake. In order to prevent hypoglycemia during exercise, reductions in replacement insulin doses during exercise are recommended (either basal insulin and/or preprandial subcutaneous injections). This can be supplemented with additional oral intake of carbohydrate of 10 to 20 g every 30 to 60 minutes depending upon the intensity of exercise. Insulin sensitivity increases about 2 hours after moderate-intensity exercise and thus consideration should be given to reducing basal and/or prandial insulin doses following exercise for the next 24 hours. Individuals who have had a previous episode of hypoglycemia are at greater risk of hypoglycemia during exercise. This may be countered by temporarily increasing glycemic targets, carefully monitoring glucose levels and adjusting insulin dosing by reducing preexercise insulin and consuming appropriate amounts of carbohydrate to replenish glycogen during and up to 24 hours following prolonged exercise.

COUNTERREGULATORY HORMONE RESPONSES TO HYPOGLYCEMIA IN WOMEN

There is a large sexual dimorphism in counterregulatory responses to hypoglycemia. It has been clearly demonstrated that both healthy young men and women with T1DM have reduced neuroendocrine, ANS, and EGP as compared to age and body mass indexed matched men (39–43). Davis et al. (2000) (43) illustrated that healthy and T1DM women have lower catecholamine, glucagon, cortisol, growth hormone, EGP, and lactate responses compared to age and BMI matched men. On the other hand, women have increased lipolytic responses to hypoglycemia. This sexual dimorphism also occurs during exercise and is not due to differences in glycemic thresholds for activation of counterregulatory responses (43) (Fig. 5).

In a series of separate glucose clamp studies at glycemic targets of 90, 70, and 50 mg/dL, Davis et al. (2000) (41) demonstrated that reduced central nervous system drive is responsible for the sexual dimorphic responses to hypoglycemia occurring in women. In a subsequent study, Sandoval et al. (2003) (42) determined that estrogen is the mechanism responsible for this sexual dimorphism in counterregulatory responses to hypoglycemia. Despite this, the prevalence of hypoglycemic episodes in T1DM for men and women are similar (4). This apparent paradox may be explained by the fact that women are more resistant to the blunting effects of antecedent hypoglycemia on the ANS as compared to men (43). Thus, two episodes of antecedent hypoglycemia in men will cause a twofold greater blunting of counterregulatory responses to subsequent hypoglycemia as compared to women. The result was that the usual sexual dimorphic response to hypoglycemia is abolished.

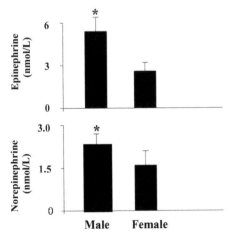

Figure 5 Effects of peripherally infused insulin and hypoglycemia on plasma epinephrine ($P < 0.01$) and norepinephrine ($P < 0.05$) responses in overnight-fasted T1DM individuals.

COUNTERREGULATORY HORMONE RESPONSES
TO HYPOGLYCEMIA IN OLDER ADULTS

Insulin therapy is often problematic for older adults with T1DM and the risk of severe or fatal hypoglycemia associated with the use of insulin increases exponentially with age (44,45). Older adults using multiple medications are likely to have comorbidities and those who are frequently hospitalized are at greater risk for iatrogenic hypoglycemia (46).

Meneilly et al. (44) investigated the effects of age on counterregulatory responses during hyperinsulinemic hypoglycemic clamp studies. They reported that older adults with diabetes had reduced glucagon and growth hormone responses during hypoglycemia, but reported increased epinephrine and cortisol responses when compared to age matched nondiabetic controls. Even with this mixed review, hypoglycemic symptom scores were similar in both the groups at all levels of glycemia (44).

Matyka et al. (46), on the other hand, found differences in hypoglycemic symptom responses when comparing healthy older men, aged 60 to 70, with younger men, aged 22 to 26. During clamp studies, neuroendocrine responses for the two groups were similar. However, symptoms began earlier in the younger men and were more intense (46). Measures of psychomotor coordination deteriorated earlier in the older subjects and to a greater degree (46). The usual 10 to 20 mg/dL plasma glucose difference between the subjective awareness of hypoglycemia and the onset of cognitive dysfunction was lost in the older men (46). This altered counterregulatory effect may contribute to the altered cognitive response to reductions in blood glucose. A lower glycemic threshold to hypoglycemia would be problematic in older persons. This would further limit the time available to self-treat and thereby increasing the risk of developing severe hypoglycemia (44,46). Additionally, in the older patient these neurological symptoms of hypoglycemia may be misinterpreted because of coexisting illnesses such as cerebrovascular diseases or dementia (44,46). In older individuals with diabetes who have comorbidities such as dementia, cerebral vascular accident, or depression, consideration should be given to these confounding factors when considering glycemic treatment goals (46). Polypharmacy or medication nonadherence, impaired renal and/or hepatic metabolism, and poor or erratic nutrition may increase hypoglycemic risks (44,45,47,48). The American Geriatrics Society (AGS) recommends an A1 C of ≤ 7% for older adults in good health and an A1 C of ≤ 8% for older adults with comorbidities and in frail health (47).

CLINICAL ASPECTS OF HYPOGLYCEMIA

Hypoglycemia constitutes a medical emergency and quick correction is important for survival of the individual. Recovery requires the appropriate glucoregulatory signaling from the brain, an enzmatically and structurally intact liver, and an adequate activation of the ANS and neuroendocrine systems. Normally, this acute physiologic counterregulatory response to hypoglycemia consists of suppression of insulin release and secretion of glucagon, epinephrine, and a host of other glucoregulatory substrates. However as discussed in detail, the response to hypoglycemia in adults with T1DM is altered. Treatment is often complicated by the dynamics of HU and HAAF and more fundamentally, by excessive action of exogenous insulin. This exogenous insulin that is delivered peripherally and not portally (as with endogenous insulin) is not responsive to change in blood glucose concentrations and has variable and nonphysiologic pharmacodynamics.

There are several different challenges to preventing hypoglycemia (47–52). One is related to the onset of short-acting insulin that is given preprandially. Short-acting (i.e., regular) insulin is designed for prandial use; however, its slow peak and long duration of action poorly mimic the short, sharp prandial burst of endogenous insulin produced by the healthy pancreas in response to eating. Thus, if enough insulin is taken to prevent an excessive increase in glucose level with a meal, too much insulin may remain in the circulation 2 to 4 hours later. Hence, the patient seeking to achieve control of immediate postprandial glycemia almost invariably realizes midmorning and midafternoon hypoglycemia before the next meal. Substitution of preprandial regular insulin with rapid-acting insulin (e.g., glulisine, lispro, or aspart) reduces the frequency of daytime hypoglycemia (49,50).

Another problem is basal insulin replacement and nocturnal hypoglycemia. Indeed, nighttime hypoglycemia can be a common occurrence in people with T1DM (4,51). Sleep can preclude detection of symptoms warning of impending hypoglycemia (47,48). Nocturnal hypoglycemia is a feared complication of T1DM for both patient and loved ones. Nocturnal hypoglycemia is frightening and can result in severe episodes such as seizures due to lack of perceived warning cues.

Nocturnal hypoglycemia may result from the use of conventional intermediate-acting insulins (such as NPH, Lente, or premix 70/30 or 50/50) for overnight insulin replacement in patients with T1DM. All have a marked peak and trough effect that do not match the physiologic pattern of nonprandial insulin secretion from the healthy pancreas. The predicted peak action is 4 to 8 hours after injection, with the subsequent decreased levels likely to leave the patient with relative insulin deficiency and hyperglycemia the next morning. The recent introduction of long-acting insulin analogs (e.g., glargine and detemir) has reduced the risk of nocturnal and some daytime hypoglycemia. To date, there is still debate as to whether continuous subcutaneous insulin infusion via a pump reduces the prevalence of hypoglycemia in T1DM adults. A study addressing this question is planned and should provide data in 2008. Recent advances in continuous glucose monitoring when linked to subcutaneous insulin delivery via a pump offer an exciting opportunity to reduce hypoglycemia in T1DM. The devices, Dexcom and Medtronic, allow frequent monitoring of plasma glucose trends (i.e., hyperglycemia and hypoglycemia) and alarm systems warning of impending hypoglycemia (53).

TREATMENT OF HYPOGLYCEMIA

Fear of hypoglycemia is a real concern of patients receiving insulin therapy. Intensive glycemic goals may make this concern "a reality" because there is a threefold greater incidence of severe disabling hypoglycemia for patients striving to achieve near normal glycemic targets as compared to conventional insulin replacement therapy (4,6). Education regarding all aspects of diabetes care will be paramount in equipping the patient to prevent and treat hypoglycemia. Carbohydrate counting, insulin dosing, concomitant medications, alcohol intake, exercise, and even driving should be included in the discussion. Reducing iatrogenic hypoglycemia will involve the patient, their support system, and health-care provider. The health-care providers will take on the role of facilitator as they educate and empower the patient to achieve diabetes self-care practices that will reduce diabetes-related complications (acute and long-term). Education will help alleviate fear of hypoglycemia that may impede ideal glycemic control (47).

Habitual review of signs, symptoms (often idiosyncratic to a particular individual), treatment, and troubleshooting regarding hypoglycemia is mandatory. Understanding the effects of insulin administration on daily routines, understanding that "diabetes" is now a part of who they are, will help empower the patient. It's not that perfection is expected; however, there is a need to understand consequences associated with certain behaviors. Lack of understanding of the diabetes-related therapeutic regimen will contribute to repeated incidents of hypoglycemia (47–51). The patients have to comprehend time-action profiles of their insulin(s) and realize that excessive treatment can be harmful. Also, while on the topic of hypoglycemia, it would be an oversight not to explain the importance of wearing diabetes alert identification, as it may be lifesaving.

Blood glucose monitoring is fundamentally important to all diabetes treatment regimens. However, for people who experience HU and those performing critical tasks such as driving or operating other heavy machinery, it is especially so (46,47). If a history of hypoglycemia is given, details regarding the timing of episodes need to be identified and treatment regimen adjusted accordingly. Sometimes, the hypoglycemic episodes—a missed or delayed meal, eating less food at the meal than planned, unplanned exercise, taking too much diabetes-related medication, or alcohol intake—have obvious remediable solutions. Appropriate regimen changes must be made. If these events are not addressed and intervention is not taken, then the risk of repeated episodes of hypoglycemia and the subsequent development of HU is high (50).

A review of the patient's self-monitoring blood glucose log will help interpret blood glucose patterns. Patients should always have a rapidly available source of glucose with them to treat hypoglycemia at the first sign of low glucose. Treatment of hypoglycemia (plasma glucose < 70 mg/dL), asymptomatic hypoglycemia and most episodes of mild-to-moderate symptomatic hypoglycemia are effectively self-treated by ingestion of some form of glucose. If blood glucose is < 70 mg/dL, give 15 to 20 g of quick-acting carbohydrates. Pure glucose is preferred; however, any form of carbohydrate that contains glucose will raise plasma glucose. Test the blood glucose in 15 minutes following treatment, if still below 70 mg/dL, retreat with 15 g of additional carbohydrate. The glycemic response to oral glucose is transient and therefore, ingestion of a small, complex carbohydrate snack shortly after the plasma glucose concentration is raised, is generally advisable, especially if the next meal is longer than an hour away. The "rule of 15" is a helpful treatment regimen when a patient is able to self-treat.

If a patient is unconscious or unable to take in oral carbohydrates, parental glucagon injection may be used. Glucagon kits require a prescription. Glucagon acts via mobilizing glucose stores from the liver via glycogenolysis. Thus, it is less effective in a glycogen-depleted states (e.g., prolonged starvation, immediately after exercise or alcohol ingestion). Glucagon kits need to be available for family members or caregivers, and they need to be knowledgeable in their use. Following administration of glucagon, oral carbohydrate should be administered to replenish hepatic glycogen. Furthermore, it should be remembered that the insulin responsible for the hypoglycemia is still active in the individual. Thus, steps should be taken to prevent any rebound hypoglycemia.

CONCLUSIONS

The ADA has glycemic target recommendations for individuals with T1DM. However, clinical judgment is required to determine what is reasonable and safe for the individual to achieve. The threat and incidence of iatrogenic hypoglycemia is a major limiting factor in implementing intensive glycemic management of diabetes. Aggressive glycemic therapy can create a vicious cycle of increased hypoglycemia, hence, reducing defenses against subsequent hypoglycemia. Many studies have demonstrated that antecedent hypoglycemia can result in transient autonomic failure. The compromised glucose counterregulatory systems in turn lead to HU. Nonetheless, it is possible to both improve glycemic control and minimize hypoglycemic risks by understanding the physiologic counterregulatory responses and aggressively monitoring glycemic therapy. Patient education is fundamental in the prevention and treatment of hypoglycemia when striving to achieve intensive glycemic control in adults with T1DM.

REFERENCES

1. Williams RH. Williams Textbook of Endocrinology. Philadelphia, PA: Saunders, 2003.
2. American Diabetes Association. Standards of medical care in diabetes. Diabetes Care 2006;29:S4–S42.
3. Cryer PE. Hypoglycemia risk reduction in type 1 diabetes. Exp Clin Endocrinol Diabetes 2001;109:S412–S423.
4. The Diabetes Control and Complication Trial Research Group. The effect of intensive treatment of diabetes on the development and progression of long term complication in insulin-dependent diabetes mellitus. N Engl J Med 1993;329:977–986.
5. Sotsky MJ, Shilo S, Shamoon H. Regulation of counterregulatory hormone secretion in man during exercise and hypoglycemia. J Clin Endocrinol Metab 1989;68:9–16.
6. Diabetes Control and Complications Trial (DCCT) Research Group. Hypoglycemia in the diabetes control and complications trial. Diabetes 1997;46:271–286.
7. Cryer PE, Davis SN, Shamoon H. Hypoglycemia in diabetes. Diabetes Care 2003;26(6),: 1902–1912.
8. Cryer PE. Hypoglycemia Pathophysiology, Diagnosis and Treatment. New York: Oxford University Press, 1997.
9. Diedrich L, Sandoval D, Davis SN. Hypoglycemia associated autonomic failure. Clin Auton Res 2002;12:358–365.
10. McAuley V, Deary IJ, Freier BM. Symptoms of hypoglycemia in people with diabetes. Diabet Med 2001;18:690–705.
11. Amiel SA, Sherwin RS, Simonson DC, et al. Effect of intensive insulin therapy on glycemic thresholds for counterregulatory hormone release. Diabetes 1988;37:901–907.
12. Aftab-Guy D, Sandoval D, Richardson MA, et al. Effects of glycemic control on target organ responses to epinephrine in type 1 diabetes. Am J Physiol Endocrinol Metab 2005;289: E258–E265.
13. Heller SR, Cryer PE. Reduced neuroendocrine and symptomatic responses to subsequent hypoglycemia after 1 episode of hypoglycemia in nondiabetic humans. Diabetes 1991;4: 223–226.
14. Davis SN, Shavers C, Collins L, et al. The effects of insulin on counterrgulatory response to equivalent hypoglycemia in patients with insulin-dependent diabetes mellitus. Am J Physiol Endocrinol Metab 1994;267:E402–E410.
15. Davis SN, Goldstein RE, Price L, et al. The effects of insulin on the counterregulatory response to equivalent hypoglycemia in patients with insulin-dependent diabetes mellitus. J Clin Endocrinol Metab 1993;77(5):1300–1307.
16. Cryer PE. Mechanisms of hypoglycemia-associated autonomic failure and its component syndromes in diabetes. Diabetes 2005;54:3592–3598.
17. Davis SN, Shavers C, Mosqueda-Garcia R, et al. Effects of differing antecedent hypoglycemia on subsequent counterregulation in normal humans. Diabetes 1997;46(8):1328–1335.
18. Davis SN, Mann S, Galassetti P, et al. Effects of differing durations of antecedent hypoglycemia on counterregulatory responses to subsequent hypoglycemia in normal humans. Diabetes 2000;49:1897–1903.
19. Davis SN, Tate D. Effects of morning hypoglycemia on neuroendocrine and metabolic responses to subsequent afternoon hypoglycemia in normal man. J Clin Endocrinol Metab 2001;86(5): 2043–2050.

20. Cryer PE. Current concepts: Diverse causes of hypoglycemia-associated autonomic failure in diabetes. N Engl J Med 2004;350(22):2272–2279.
21. Boyle PJ, Kepers SF, O'Connor AM, et al. Brain glucose uptake and unawareness of hypoglycemia in patients with insulin-dependent diabetes mellitus. N Engl J Med 1995;333: 1726–1732.
22. Segel SA, Fanelli CG, Dence CS, et al. Blood-to-brain glucose transport, cerebral glucose metabolism, and cerebral blood flow are not increased after hypoglycemia. Diabetes 2001;50:1911–1917.
23. Zammitt NN, Frier BM. Hypoglycemia in type 2 diabetes. Diabetes Care 2005;28(12): 2948–2961.
24. Korzon-Burakowska A, Hopkins D, Matyka K, et al. Effects of glycemic control on protective responses against hypoglycemia in type 2 diabetes. Diabetes Care 1998;21(2):283–290.
25. Dagogo-Jack SE, Craft S, Cryer PE. Hypoglycemia-associated autonomic failure in insulin-dependent diabetes mellitus. J Clin Invest 1993;91(3):819–828.
26. Korytkowski MT, Mokan M, Veneman TE, et al. Reduced beta-adrenergic sensitivity in patient with type 1 diabetes and hypoglycemia unawareness. Diabetes Care 1998;21(11):1939–1943.
27. Aftab-Guy DL, Galassetti PR, Sandoval DA, et al. Differing physiological effects of epinephrine in type 1 diabetes and healthy subjects. Diabetes 2002;51(2):A74.
28. Aftab-Guy DL, Sandoval D, Richardson MA, et al. Differing physiologic effects of epinephrine in type 1 diabetes and nondiabetic humans. Am J Physiol Endocrinol Metab 2005;288:E178–E186.
29. Fritsche A, Stefan N, Haring H, et al. Avoidance of hypoglycemia restores hypoglycemia awareness by increasing beta-adrenergic sensitivity in type 1 diabetes. Ann Intern Med 2001;134(9):729–736.
30. Cranston I, Lomas J, Maran A, et al. Restoration of hypoglycemia awareness in patients with long-duration insulin-dependent diabetes. Lancet 1994;344(8918):283–287.
31. Fanelli C, Pampanelli S, Epifano L, et al. Relative roles of insulin and hypoglycemia on induction of neuroendocrine responses to, symptoms of, and deterioration of cognitive function in hypoglycemia in male and female humans. Diabetologia 1994;37:797–807.
32. Dagogo-Jack S, Rattarasarn C, Cryer PE. Reversal of hypoglycemia unawareness, but not defective glucose counterregulation, in IDDM. Diabetes 1994;43(12):1426–1434.
33. Bottini P, Boschetti E, Pampanelli S, et al. Contribution of autonomic neuropathy to reduce plasma adrenaline responses to hypoglycemia in IDDM. Diabetes 1997;46:814–823.
34. Schneider S, Vitug A, Ananthakrishnan R, et al. Impaired adrenergic response to prolonged exercise in type I diabetes. Metabolism 1991;40:1219–1225.
35. Davis SN, Galassetti P, Wasserman DH, et al. Effects of antecedent hypoglycemia on subsequent counterregulatory responses to exercise. Diabetes 2000;49:73–81.
36. Galassetti P, Tate D, Neill RA, et al. Effect of antecedent hypoglycemia on neuroendocrine responses to subsequent exercise in type 1 diabetes. Diabetes 2001;50(Suppl 2):A54.
37. McGregor VP, Greiwe JS, Banarer S, et al. Limited impact of vigorous exercise on defenses against hypoglycemia: Relevance to hypoglycemia-associated autonomic failure. Diabetes 2002;51:1485–1492.
38. Sandoval DA, Aftab Guy DL, Richardson MA, et al. Effects of low and moderate antecedent exercise on counterregulatory responses to subsequent hypoglycemia in type 1 diabetes. Diabetes 2004;53:1798–1806.
39. Galassetti P, Neill RA, Tate D, et al. Sexual dimorphism in counterregulatory responses to hypoglycemia after antecedent exercise. J Clin endocrinol Metab 2001;86:3516–3525.
40. Amiel SA, Maran A, Powrie JK, et al. Gender differences in counterregulation to hypoglycemia. Diabetologia 1993;36:460–464.
41. Davis SN, Shavers C, Costa F. Gender-related differences in counterregulatory responses to antecedent hypoglycemia in normal humans. J Clin endocrinol Metab 2000;85(6):2148–2157.
42. Sandoval DA, Ertl AC, Richardson MA, et al. Estrogen blunts neuroendocrine and metabolic responses to hypoglycemia. Diabetes 2003;52(7):1749–1755.
43. Davis SN, Fowler S, Costa F. Hypoglycemic counterregulatory responses differ between men and women with type 1 diabetes. Diabetes 2000;49:65–72.

44. Meneilly GS, Cheung E, Tuokko H. Altered responses to hypoglycemia of healthy elderly people. Diabetes 1994;43:403–410.

45. Shorr RI, Ray WA, Daugherty JR, et al. Incidence and risk factors for serious hypoglycemia in older persons using insulin or sulfonylureas. Arch Intern Med 1997;157(15):1681–1686.

46. Matyka K, Evans M, Lomas J, et al. Altered hierarchy of protective responses against severe hypoglycemia in normal aging in healthy men. Diabetes Care 1997;20:135–141.

47. The Diabetes Control and Complications Trial Research Group. Epidemiology of severe hypoglycemia in the diabetes control and complication trial. Am J Med 1991;90(40):450–459.

48. Gabriely I, Shamoon H. Hypoglycemia in diabetes: Common, often unrecognized. Cleve Clin J Med 2004;71(4):335–342.

49. Cryer PE, Childs BP. Negotiating the barrier of hypoglycemia in diabetes. Diabetes Spectrum 2002;15:20–27.

50. Heller SR, Amiel SA, Mansell P. Effect of the fast-acting insulin analog lispro on the risk of nocturnal hypoglycemia during intensified insulin therapy. U. K. lispro study group. Diabetes Care 1999;22(10):1607–1611.

51. Ratner RE, Hirsch IB, Neifing JL, et al. Less hypoglycemia with insulin glargine in intensive insulin therapy for type 1 diabetes. U. S. study group of insulin glargine in type 1 diabetes. Diabetes Care 2000;23(5);639–643.

52. Wright EE. Treat the target: ABCs for the elderly. DOC News 2006;3(4):4.

53. Gross TM, Bode BW, Einhorn D, et al. Performance evaluation of the minimed continuous glucose monitoring system during patient home use. Diabetes Technol Ther 2000;2(1):49–56.

12
Diabetes and Pregnancy

K. W. Hickey
Georgetown University Hospital, Washington, DC, U.S.A.

J. G. Umans
Medstar Research Institute, Hyattsville, Maryland, U.S.A.

M. Miodovnik
Washington Hospital Center, Washington, DC, U.S.A.

BACKGROUND

Currently, diabetes mellitus (DM) afflicts an estimated 171 million people worldwide and 20.8 million in the United States (though only two-thirds of these are diagnosed). Type 1 DM accounts for 5% to 10% of these cases (1). Diabetes prevalence in women 18 to 44 years old is lower than that in the general population, although with an excess of type 1 cases. Importantly, the prevalence of type 2 DM (and of diabetes overall) is increasing dramatically in young women, perhaps due to the epidemic of adolescent obesity.

One to two percent of pregnancies are complicated by pregestational DM, with type 1 more frequent than type 2. An additional 3% to 5% of pregnancies will be complicated by Gestational Diabetes Mellitus (GDM), including a subset (about 9% of cases) that actually has undiagnosed type 2 DM. Women with type 1 DM, characterized by the complete lack of insulin production, have historically been characterized during pregnancy by White's classification system (Table 1) in attempts to predict pregnancy outcomes and complications by the duration, severity, and medical complications associated with the diabetes (2,3). Pregestational type 2 DM is characterized by increasing insulin resistance and subsequently impaired insulin secretion, which worsen during pregnancy. Type 2 DM is strongly associated with obesity, sedentary lifestyle, ethnicity, and family history. Its incidence is growing dramatically (2).

Gestational diabetes is characterized by glucose intolerance leading to diabetes first detected during pregnancy (4). It will affect up to 14% of some high-risk populations including African-Americans, Hispanic-Americans, American-Indians, Asian-Americans, and Native Hawaiian/Pacific Island ethnic groups (5,6).

Since a growing percentage of young women with pregestational glucose intolerance or frank type 2 DM remains undiagnosed and because this population rarely comes to medical attention outside of pregnancy, these women must be identified during prenatal

Table 1 White's Classification of Diabetes Mellitus in Pregnancy

Class	Criteria
Gestational Diabetes	
A1	Diet controlled gestational diabetes
A2	Insulin controlled gestational diabetes
Pregestational Diabetes	
B	Age of onset 20 yr or greater; duration < 10 yr
C	Age of onset 10–19 yr; duration 10–19 yr
D[a]	Age of onset < 10 yr; duration > 20 yr
R	Proliferative retinopathy or vitreous hemorrhage
F	Nephropathy with over 500 mg of protein/day
RF	Criteria for both R and F
G	Many pregnancy failures
H	Evidence of arteriosclerotic heart disease
T	Prior renal transplant

[a]Historic subdivision of class D, not currently used in clinical practice. D1: age of onset < 10 yr; D2: duration > 20 yr; D3: calcification of vessels of the leg (formerly class E); D4: benign retinopathy; D5: hypertension.

care in order to optimize maternal and fetal health (1). The need for pregnancy prevention or preconceptional planning should be discussed during care by the diabetologist with referral to a perinatologist for further preconceptional counseling.

PRECONCEPTIONAL COUNSELING

Overall, more than two-thirds of pregnancies are unplanned (3). Because first trimester hyperglycemia may lead to fetal malformations and pregnancy loss and because untreated target organ damage may worsen during early pregnancy, women contemplating pregnancy should be referred for preconceptional counseling to optimize maternal health, to tighten glycemic control, and to anticipate maternal diabetic, obstetric, and fetal complications. The preconceptional visit should include a thorough history of disease state, comorbidities, and an extensive maternal examination. Not only will women want to discuss how diabetes will affect the pregnancy but also they will wish to know how the pregnancy may impact their diabetes. Discussion of the anticipated risks may further include questions on how to achieve pregnancy.

REPRODUCTIVE FUNCTION

Preconceptional consultation may reveal abnormalities in reproductive function. Women with DM may report delay in menarche, delay in ovulation, and increased incidence of menstrual irregularities (7–9). Individually or collectively, these may contribute to relative infertility.

Longer duration of type 1 DM as well as higher insulin requirements have been associated with inability to conceive although the mechanism impairing fertility is not entirely clear (10). Abnormalities in the hypothalamic–pituitary axis of diabetic women have also been associated with impaired fertility as demonstrated by decreased response of luteinizing hormone to gonadotropin-releasing hormone (11,12), decreased thyrotropin concentrations (14), decreased synthesis of corticosterone (13), and decreased basal levels on luteinizing hormone and follicle-stimulating hormone (8,14).

Pathways involving the direct effects of insulin on ovarian cells have also been postulated to affect reproductive function. In rats with alloxan-induced DM, the ovarian weights are reduced, apparently due to decreased responsiveness to gonadotropins (15,16). Even women with fair control of their diabetes have impaired insulin-stimulated synthesis of progesterone by granulosa cells (17). Improved glycemic control, as evidenced by lower HbA1c correlates with higher rates of conception (18).

Additionally, DM increases rate of spontaneous abortions (SAB). The SAB rate in prospective studies of women with type 1 DM ranges from 15% to 30% compared to 10% to 12% in nondiabetic women (18–22). The increased rate of SAB has been linked to periconceptional glycemic control (32). This increased rate has been attributed to early developmental insults with ensuing degeneration of the fetus and formation of a blighted ovum or the formation of major congenital anomalies incompatible with extrauterine life. Poor glycemic control may also result in abnormal placentation or abnormal vascularization resulting in SAB (33,34). While it remains unclear whether there is a threshold elevation of HbA1c that predicts SAB, it is clear from both mouse and human studies that poor glycemic control leads to progressive increases in SAB (18,21–31).

MATERNAL EVALUATION

Either prior to conception or at the earliest antenatal visit, it is crucial to evaluate maternal health in order to estimate and limit maternal and fetal risks during pregnancy. This first visit should include the following:

1. Evaluation of glycemic control
   - Hemoglobin A1c
   - Self-monitored blood glucose concentrations: fasting, preprandial, postprandial, and nighttime. An additional 2:00 a.m. and 3:00 a.m. blood glucose concentration may be needed to assess for maternal hypoglycemia. See table 2 for target glycemic values.
2. Evaluation of renal function
   - 24-hour urine collection for protein and creatinine
   - Serum creatinine
   - Estimation of creatinine clearance and GFR
3. Evaluation of blood pressure
4. Evaluation for retinopathy—examination by ophthalmologist with follow-up each trimester or more frequently if retinopathy diagnosed
5. Clinical examination for peripheral and autonomic neuropathy
   - Sensory loss
   - Postural hypotension

Table 2 Goals for Self-Monitored Blood Glucose Concentrations

	Capillary whole-blood glucose
Fasting	60–90 mg/dL
Before meals	80–95 mg/dL
1 hr after meals	< 140 mg/dL
2 hr after meals	< 120 mg/dL

- Gastroparesis
- Heat intolerance
6. Clinical evaluation of peripheral vascular disease
7. Evaluation of thyroid status (TSH and free T_4) in patients with type 1 DM
8. EKG
   - For patients older than 35 or those with comorbidities (hypertension, nephropathy, obesity, diabetes > 10 years, hypercholesterolemia).
   - Abnormalities should be further evaluated with a stress test.

Stratifying disease severity and documenting end-organ damage will provide expectations for pregnancy outcomes and complications. Patients can then be made aware of the care anticipated for a successful pregnancy.

GLYCEMIC CONTROL DURING PREGNANCY

The key to successful obstetrical outcomes with optimization of maternal and fetal health can be achieved primarily through aggressive glycemic control. In order to obtain this narrow window of normoglycemia in pregnancy, the patient, perinatologist, diabetologist, diabetic nurse educator, and nutritionist must embark on a multidisciplinary approach to disease management. Active participation by the patient in her care is essential.

Increasing insulin resistance in pregnancy may require continued meetings with the nutritionist and diabetic educator to optimize a diet and medication regimen that works in pregnancy. The patient will need to self-monitor blood glucose concentrations with a glucometer with memory. The capacity to download glucose concentrations with dates and times will aid adjustment to diet, scheduled food intake, and exercise regimens.

Target Glycemic Values

Women will need to be educated regarding the changing goals for blood glucose concentrations in pregnancy (Table 2). As they learn to manage their diabetes in pregnancy, they will learn when adjustments to therapy should be considered based on the number of out of target glycemic values obtained over the course of their monitoring. Providers should inform their patients that if greater than 15% to 20% of values are outside the target range they should call their physician and relay their glucose concentrations. Women with consistently elevated fasting glucose concentrations should be encouraged to obtain a glucose concentration between 2:00 a.m. and 3:00 a.m. to assess for a Somogyi effect that is discovered with maternal hypoglycemia in the early am with maternal hyperglycemia at the am fasting.

MANAGEMENT WITH DIABETES IN PREGNANCY

Patients should understand normal physiology with a basal rate of insulin secreted to prevent excess hepatic production and mobilization of free fatty acids from adipose. Basal insulin is required whether or not food is consumed. Additional insulin is needed with consumption of food. Understanding the normal physiology and that resistance may increase with pregnancy will then help the patient understand the use of diet, medication, and exercise to obtain normoglycemia.

Traditional Insulin Regimens

The mainstay of management in pregestational diabetes in pregnancy has been through the use of regular and NPH insulins. When calculating doses for insulin regimens in type 1 DM, estimate 0.9 U/kg/day in the first trimester, 1.0 U/kg/day in the second trimester, and 1.2 U/kg/day in the third trimester. In insulin regimens for type 2 DM the requirements are increased: 0.9 U/kg/day in the first trimester, 1.2 U/kg/day in the second trimester, and 1.6 U/kg/day in the third trimester (35–37). Insulin requirements for gestational DM are usually biphasic with dosages frequently increasing from 24 weeks up to 30 weeks estimated gestational age (EGA) and then stabilizing after 30 weeks EGA. Dosage can be estimated based on body mass index (BMI). If the BMI $\leq$ 25, then start with 0.8 U/kg/day. If the BMI $\geq$ 25, then start with 1.0 U/kg/day (38). Once the total dose is calculated, then divide the dose into two-thirds in the morning and one-third in the evening. Further, divide the morning dose into a 2:1 ratio of intermediate to rapid acting, and divide the evening dose into a 1:1 ratio of intermediate- to rapid-acting insulin.

Due to the onset and peak of the regular and NPH insulins, it is recommended that a meal with a mixed carbohydrate load should be eaten to coincide with the peak of regular insulin in 30 minutes with duration of 90 minutes. A second meal or snack, with a significant carbohydrate content should be eaten five to seven hours later.

Insulin Analogs

Short-acting insulin analogs, lispro, and aspart have reduced stability with increased absorption after injection. Administration should occur immediately prior or up to 15 minutes after starting meals. While these agents are reported to increase control and decrease maternal hypoglycemia, they have shown conflicting results with improvement in obtaining target glycemic values. Use of these short-acting analogs should be accompanied by carbohydrate counting to improve glycemic control and decrease maternal hypoglycemia. There are short-term studies showing minor benefit; but, until long-term data for safety are available, use with caution is recommended.

Lantus is a long-acting insulin which is generally dosed once daily. It should be combined with a short-acting analog in the highly motivated patient for aggressive control. Concern for maternal hypoglycemia exists with this long-acting agent. Studies report use in pregnancy, but no long-term data are available and so currently it is listed as a category C drug.

MATERNAL DIABETIC COMPLICATIONS

As evidenced by the key factors in the White's classification scheme and by the components of our recommended initial patient evaluation above, key factors in maternal management, pregnancy risks, and long-term outcome include microvascular diabetic complications, macrovascular complications, and hypertension. We therefore now focus on diabetic retinopathy, nephropathy, coronary artery disease, and hypertension.

Retinopathy

Retinopathy will affect the majority of patients diagnosed with type 1 DM and is the leading cause of blindness in the United States. Of patients followed for 20 years who were diagnosed with diabetes before the age of 30, 50% will have proliferative retinopathy, while 100% will have some form of retinopathy (39,40). In the nonpregnant diabetic patient, glycemic control is correlated with the presence and severity of retinopathy (41–43). Strict glycemic control is associated with slower development and progression of retinal disease in both type 1 and type 2 DM.

Effect of Pregnancy

In pregnancy there are additional physiologic and hormonal changes presenting challenges to determining the cause of progressive retinopathy. Trying to untangle the effects of time, glycemic control, and pregnancy with its resulting increased difficulty in glycemic control, development of pregnancy-induced hypertension, and the circulating angiogenic growth factors has been virtually impossible. Pregnancy may be a state in which the convergence of glycemic control, growth factors, and hypertension accelerate retinal changes and cause worsening of the disease. Review of the literature has contradictory findings due to the heterogeneity between studies as seen in differing designs methodology, inconsistent frequency and method of fundoscopic examinations, and inconsistent length of follow-ups. These variations in study design may explain the difficulty in reconciling the findings. The constraints of limited postpartum follow-up further restrict observations to short-term effects of pregnancy on retinal disease. Several studies have addressed these questions and reached these varying conclusions (44–74):

1. The progression of retinopathy is based on the severity of the preexisting disease. Women with no disease or mild retinopathy are less likely to have progression than those with advanced disease (Table 3). However, 10% to 15% of women with no retinal disease may progress to proliferative retinopathy during pregnancy and require photocoagulation. It is unclear whether this reflects the natural course of disease in these women and would have occurred without pregnancy (60,61,64).
2. While tight glycemic control ameliorates retinopathy in nonpregnant diabetics and tight control at conception predicts good pregnancy outcome, a paradoxical literature suggests that rapid attainment of strict glycemic control early during pregnancy may accelerate retinopathy. Taken together, therefore, existing retinopathy should be photocoagulated, if possible, prior to conception and strict glycemic control achieved gradually, also prior to conception rather than rapidly afterwards (44–51).
3. In addition to intensive glycemic control, humoral and paracrine factors such as growth hormone, insulin-like growth factor 1, vascular endothelial growth factor (VEGF), and other angiogenic factors may contribute to the development of retinopathy (52–56). The significance is that the placenta produces several

Table 3 Progression of Retinal Disease in Pregnancy by Prepregnancy Retinal Examination

Author (year)	No. of pregnancies	None	Background	Proliferative
Horvat et al. (1980)	160	13/118 (11)	11/35 (31)	1/7 (14)
Moloney & Drury (1982)	53	8/20 (40)	15/30 (50)	1/3 (33)
Dibble et al. (1982)	55	0/23 (0)	3/19 (16)	7/13 (54)
Ohms (1984)	100	4/50 (8)	15/48 (31)	1/2 (50)
Rosenn et al. (1992)	154	18/78 (23)	28/68 (41)	5/8 (63)

No. (%) with progression based on initial examination.
Source: Modified from Ref. 126.

angiogenic factors that result in vessel proliferation in vivo and in endothelial cell cultures in vitro. Human placental lactogen with growth hormone-like actions, circulates at levels up to 1000 times that of growth hormone, and placental growth factor acts a full agonist at VEGF type 1 receptors. Theoretically, the presence of placental factors could result in new vessel formation during pregnancy although it is unknown whether the systems' concentrations of these factors is high enough to affect distant target organs, such as the eyes (57,58).

4. Progression of retinopathy is more likely to occur in patients with hypertensive disorders. As 10% to 20% of women with diabetes develop pregnancy-induced hypertension, the relation of hypertension to retinopathy may be particularly relevant during pregnancy. The development of pregnancy-induced hypertension or preeclampsia has been linked to progression of retinopathy in 50% to 60% of women during pregnancy (59–61). In women with preproliferative changes, acute retinal hemorrhage may occur with the increased blood pressure associated with the Valsalva of maternal expulsive efforts. Some obstetricians recommend cesarean delivery due to this concern while others contend that the vascular changes are predominantly postarteriolar and are unlikely to be affected by the Valsalva maneuver.

5. The regression of retinal disease is demonstrated in the majority of postpartum patients. These observations suggest that short-term worsening of retinal disease may not predict overall long-term effects of pregnancy on diabetic retinopathy (60,63,66,71).

In summary, retinal disease may progress during pregnancy, and the risk of progression is related to the severity of baseline retinopathy. While progression of retinal disease can be documented, women should also be followed for several years postpartum monitoring for disease regression. The changes observed in pregnancy may be accounted for by the altered hormonal milieu, the rapid normalization of glycemic control, development of hypertensive complications, or the hemodynamic stresses of pregnancy though their relative importance remains uncertain due to limited data. Except for the subset of women who suffer rapid proliferative changes or retinal hemorrhages, the long-term prognosis for most women is not altered by pregnancy.

Management of Diabetic Retinopathy in Pregnancy

1. Preconceptional counseling with referral to ophthalmology for baseline fundoscopic examination.
2. Gradual tight glycemic control prior to conception.
3. Photocoagulation of proliferative retinopathy to stabilize disease prior to conception.
4. Funduscopic examination at least every trimester and 6 to 12 weeks postpartum.
5. Visual changes should be addressed immediately by their ophthalmologist.

Nephropathy

Diabetic nephropathy is the most common cause of end-stage renal disease in the United States affecting up to 40% of diabetics. Clinically, diabetic nephropathy progresses through four distinct clinical phases including renal hypertrophy with scattered glomerular sclerosis and basement membranes widening, subclinical disease with the development of microalbuminuria followed by proteinuria and ultimately resulting in end-stage renal disease (75).

Like many other advanced complications of diabetes, the incidence of diabetic nephropathy is related to the duration of diabetes. Once nephropathy is present, there is progressive decline in renal function with a decrease in glomerular filtration rate of 10 mL/min each year. With this stepwise decrement, the incidence of nephropathy seen in diabetics is approximately 15% in 15 years, 30% in 20 years, and 40% in 30 years with end-stage renal disease occurring in at least 75% of patients within the following 10 years. Within the past decade, it has become evident that development and progression of nephropathy can be modified by meticulous control of blood pressure, preferably with ACE-inhibitors and angiotensin receptor blockers (ARBs), and strict glycemic control (76–81).

Effect of Pregnancy

Nephropathy in pregnancy may mirror retinal disease in pregnancy as a convergence of factors leading to the development of disease. Indeed, glomerular filtration rate, hypertension, protein intake and excretion, and glycemic control have been associated with the development of nephropathy. Three major factors associated with pregnancy may increase the risk of nephropathy.

1. While glomerular filtration rate increases 40% to 60% in pregnancy, it does so without an increase in glomerular capillary pressure and so should not worsen diabetic nephropathy by a hemodynamic mechanism (82) (Table 4).
2. Likewise, there are no data to suggest any benefit of a low protein diet during pregnancy (83–85).
3. The use of ARBs and ACE-inhibitors for tight control of hypertension slows progression of nephropathy. Hod et al. confirmed this theory in a small uncontrolled study, optimizing therapy to reduce proteinuria prior to pregnancy and improving pregnancy outcome. In a retrospective study by Carr, poor obstetrical outcomes were associated with diminished first trimester blood pressure control. Of greater concern was that many patients with diabetic nephropathy in that academic medical center had inadequately or entirely untreated hypertension prior to conception (86,87).

Table 4 Progression of Diabetic Nephropathy in Pregnancy

Accelerated progressed to author (year)	No.	Follow-up (months)	Progression	ESRD (n)
Kitzmiller (1981)	23	9–35	No	3
Dicker (1986)	5	6–12	No	0
Grenfell (1986)	20	6–120	No	2
Reece (1988)	31	1–86	No	6
Reece (1990)	11	10–45	No	0
Bisenbach (1992)	5[a]	13–42	Yes	5
Kimerle (1995)	29	4–108	No	8
Gordon (1996)	34	34 (average)	Yes	3
Purdy (1996)	11[a]	6–138	Yes	7
Mackie (1996)	6[a]	6–96	No	3
Rossing (2002)	26	36–164	No	5
Bagg (2003)	14	12–192	No	5
Irfan (2004)	35[a]	6–57	Yes	22

[a]Creatinine clearance < 75 mL/min at baseline or serum creatinine > 1.4 mg/dL.
Source: Modified from Ref. 126.

4. Hypertension coexists with many renal disorders, and systemic arterial hypertension may be a factor in the rate of nephropathy progression (88,89). Management of hypertension with angiotensin-converting enzyme (ACE) inhibitors or alternative antihypertensive agents appears to slow the progression to overt nephropathy and may also delay the progression from overt nephropathy to end-stage renal disease (90,91). With 10% to 20% of all women with type 1 DM affected by pregnancy-induced hypertension and additional women affected with some variation of nephropathy, pregnancy may be expected to exert a detrimental effect on renal disease significant cohort of women with diabetes.

While ACE-inhibitors and ARBs are contraindicated in late pregnancy due to fatal fetal renal failure, they had been used up to conception or during the first trimester. However, the recent report that first trimester ACE exposures could be associated with the rare occurrence of severe malformations has led to the avoidance of treatment during attempts at conception to avoid this risk (92). While it seems reasonable to use other agents in women with essential hypertension, balancing the potential risks and benefits would still seem to favor use of ACE inhibitors up to time of conception. The strict glycemic control desired in pregnancy may actually benefit renal function and delay disease progression.

Effect of Nephropathy on Pregnancy

The presence of nephropathy may affect pregnancy outcomes due to three main reasons:

1. The presence of nephropathy increases the likelihood of developing hypertensive complications. While many of these women may have preexisting chronic hypertension, even those that do not, preeclampsia is a common complication of pregnancy. While the diagnosis of preeclampsia may be challenging due to preexisting hypertension and proteinuria, the rate of superimposed preeclampsia is estimated at 50% (92–103).
2. In women with nephropathy, due to declining maternal health or fetal compromise, there is an increased risk of fetal prematurity. Approximately 25% to 30% of pregnancies are delivered prior to 34 weeks gestation and almost one-half are delivered prior to 37 weeks gestation (94–103).
3. In women with nephropathy, there is an increased risk of fetal growth restriction and fetal distress occurring in approximately 20% of pregnancies. The presence of chronic hypertension, worsening nephropathy, decreased creatinine clearance, and superimposed preeclampsia are all associated with this increased risk (101–103).

In diabetic women, the worst perinatal outcomes are seen in women with impaired renal function, with increased serum creatinine concentrations and decreased creatinine clearance. The poor obstetric outcomes are due to prematurity as perinatal survival has approached 100% over the last several decades. To continue this trend, aggressive control of maternal hypertension is of paramount importance while the choices of antihypertensive medications remain limited. The use of ACE-inhibitors during pregnancy is contraindicated due to their potential for fetal renal dysplasia resulting in oligohydramnios and pulmonary hypoplasia. The medications most widely used are Methyldopa, Nifedipine, and alpha-adrenergic blockers, for a targeted blood pressure in the range of 130/80.

Management of Diabetic Nephropathy in Pregnancy

1. Preconceptional counseling with referral to nephrology for comanagement of renal disease and hypertension. If preconception serum creatinine is > 1.4 mg/dL or if creatinine clearance is ≤ 75 mL/min, advise the patient that the risk of maternal and fetal complications is high and that pregnancy may accelerate nephropathy towards end-stage renal disease.
2. Baseline assessment of renal function with serum creatinine, creatinine clearance, and 24-hour urine protein. Proteinuria may increase during pregnancy without signifying worsening of the underlying nephropathy.
3. Repeat assessment of renal function at least every trimester or more frequently if concerns for superimposed preeclampsia exist. The clinical diagnosis of superimposed preeclampsia may be extraordinarily difficult in these women due to baseline proteinuria and hypertension.
4. Aggressive management of hypertension to maintain blood pressure under 130/80. Patients should be taken off ACE-inhibitors upon conception and switched to an alternative agent as needed.
5. Acute worsening of renal function should lead to pregnancy termination or early delivery.

Coronary Artery Disease

Atherosclerosis and fatal myocardial infarction occurs three times more frequently in women with diabetes. In women with preexisting cardiovascular disease, the physiologic changes of pregnancy and delivery can result in inadequate myocardial oxygenation resulting in myocardial infarction and heart failure. The physiologic changes associated with pregnancy increased cardiac output, decreased systemic vascular resistance with shunting of blood from the coronary arteries, increased oxygen consumption combined with the intrapartum changes of increased vascular return during contractions followed by the acute blood loss at delivery can combine with decreasing blood flow to the myocardium and failure to meet the heart's demands. Additionally, these women are extremely susceptible to pulmonary edema and myocardial damage in the immediate postpartum period. Immediately after vaginal delivery, there is a 60% to 80% increase in cardiac output due to autotransfusion of uteroplacental blood, release of venocaval obstruction, and rapid mobilization of extravascular fluid which results in increased stroke volume and increased venous return (104).

Coronary artery disease can be further complicated by maternal hypoglycemia. Strict glycemic control in the type 1 diabetic has been associated with increased episodes of hypoglycemia in pregnancy. This phenomenon is seen primarily in the first half of pregnancy. The concern revolves around the activation of the counter-regulatory responses with the release of catecholamines that lead to tachycardia and increased demand on the myocardium. These changes can result in acute myocardial infarction in the patient with underlying coronary artery disease.

Management of Coronary Artery Disease in Pregnancy

1. Preconceptional counseling with referral to cardiology for comanagement. A thorough examination to assess the extent of coronary artery disease and myocardial function.
2. Counseling should include serious maternal risk of death associated with attempting pregnancy.

3. Option of pregnancy termination should be discussed.
4. Limit maternal physical activity.
5. Aggressive glycemic control with frequent self-monitored blood glucose levels and avoidance of maternal hypoglycemia. Targets for blood glucose levels may have to be adjusted to attempt to further avoid maternal hypoglycemia.
6. Delivery at a tertiary care center. Anesthesia consultation should be obtained well before delivery. Maternal effort should be kept to a minimum.
7. Permanent sterilization should be discussed in advance so that the procedure can be performed at the time of delivery.
8. Close postpartum monitoring due to risk of hemodynamic decompensation.

Neuropathy

Little is known about the effects of diabetic neuropathy on pregnancy or the possible effects of pregnancy on neuropathy. Pregnancy may increase the incidence of polyneuropathy but in the long-term, pregnancy has not increased the prevalence of neuropathy.

Of interest, the presence of gastroparesis may affect pregnancies leading to worsening of nausea and emesis. The results of this gastrointestinal dysfunction are inadequate nutrition, irregular absorption of nutrients, and aberrant glucose control.

FETAL COMPLICATIONS

Congenital Malformations

Congenital Malformations (CM) is the single most important factor impacting perinatal mortality in the diabetic patient. CM in the pregestational diabetic patient accounts for 50% of perinatal mortality compared to the 20% to 30% in nondiabetic women (105–110). The hypothesis is that a hyperglycemic environment, as seen in the poorly controlled pregestational diabetic, is the underlying factor for congenital malformations during embryogenesis. This is underscored by the increased risk of CM seen in women with fasting hyperglycemia first diagnosed in pregnancy. These women likely represent the undiagnosed pregestational diabetic (111,112).

While maternal and fetal management and surveillance have continued to improve with technological advances, the incidence of CM remains the same 4.9% to 9.2%, which is a sevenfold increase in risk over the general population (113–116). Indeed, prevention of congenital malformations can only be achieved with preconceptional and early postconceptional glycemic control. In addition to the obvious benefits of such an approach in terms of clinical outcome, an analysis of the cost–benefit ratio for preconceptional care demonstrates that intensive medical care before conception results in significant cost savings compared with prenatal care only (117,118).

ABNORMAL FETAL GROWTH

Macrosomia

Macrosomia is most commonly defined as a birth weight greater than 4000 g. Normal infants who are constitutionally large will obviously also be labeled macrosomic, but the macrosomia characteristic of the diabetic pregnancy is associated with altered body composition with increased body fat is therefore considered abnormal. In diabetic women, 15% to 45% of pregnancies will be complicated by macrosomia (119).

In understanding intrauterine fetal growth, a biphasic intrauterine growth pattern has been observed with an initial phase of early fetal growth delay in the first half of pregnancy, affecting both head and abdominal growth, followed by the typical accelerated abnormal fetal growth in the third trimester. The accelerated growth in the third trimester is further characterized by abnormal adipose deposition and distribution, visceral organ hypertrophy and hyperplasia, and acceleration of skeletal growth (120–123). The excessive fetal size and asymmetric macrosomia are the principal factors contributing to the increased risk of birth trauma in infants of mothers with DM, with such complications as shoulder dystocia, asphyxia, brachial plexus injuries, and facial nerve palsies (124). Macrosomia is also a major factor in the increased rate of cesarean delivery among women with DM (125).

Fetal Growth Restriction

At the opposite end of the spectrum of disturbances in fetal growth among infants of mothers with DM, infants born to mothers with microvascular disease are at increased risk of fetal growth restriction. Fetal growth restriction can be defined as estimated fetal weight below the 10th centile for a reference population or abdominal circumference less than fifth centile. This risk of growth restriction confounds the fact that these infants are at increased risk of low birth weight because of the increased risk of prematurity among mothers with microvascular disease (94). It appears that the microvascular process in these women may affect placentation and uterine blood flow, possibly leading to compromised fetal nutrition and fetal growth restriction. Indeed, the rate of fetal growth restriction among these infants, defined as birth weight less than the 10th percentile for gestational age, is 11% to 21% (92,94,101,102).

CONCLUSIONS

In summary, pregnancy in the woman with type 1 DM remains challenging. Surprisingly, despite an increase in the tools available for diabetes management and monitoring, the outcomes during and after pregnancy have not dramatically improved. Much of this may still be connected to the fact that there is not enough prepregnancy planning in those women with type 1 DM. Clearly this needs to be addressed by endocrinologists and care providers in communities where those with type 1 DM receive their day-to-day care. Until this reality changes, clearly the risks will remain greater in this population, requiring more aggressive monitoring and greater potential for poor outcomes for both mother and child.

REFERENCES

1. Wild S, Sicree R, Gojka R, et al. Global prevalence of diabetes: Estimates for the year 2000 and predictions for 2030. Diabetes Care 2004;27:1047–1053.
2. National Diabetes Fact Sheet. Center for Disease Control 2005.
3. American Diabetes Association. Standards of medical care in diabetes (Position statement). Diabetes Care 2005;28:S4–S36.
4. White P. Pregnancy complicating diabetes. Am J Med 1949;7:609.
5. American Diabetes Association. Gestational diabetes mellitus (Position statement). Diabetes Care 2004;27:S88–S90.

6. Green JR, Pawson IG, Schumacher LB, et al. Glucose intolerance in pregnancy: Ethnic variation and influence of body habitus. Am J Obstet Gynecol 1990;163:86.

7. King E. Epidemiology of glucose intolerance and gestational diabetes in women of childbearing age. Diabetes Care 1998;21:B9–B13.

8. Bergqvist N. The gonadal function in female diabetics. Acta Endocrinol Copenh 1954;19:1.

9. Djursing H, Nyholm HC, Hagen C, et al. Clinical and hormonal characteristics in women with anovulation and insulin-treated diabetes mellitus. Am J Obstet Gynecol 1982;143:876.

10. Kjaer K, Hagen C, Sando SH, et al. Infertility and pregnancy outcome in an unselected group of women with insulin-dependent diabetes mellitus. Am J Obstet Gynecol 1992;166:1412.

11. Briese V, Muller H. Diabetes mellitus: An epidemiologic study of fertility, contraception and sterility. Geburtshilfe Frauenheilkd 1995;55:270.

12. Kirchick HJ, Keyes PL, Frye BE. An explanation for anovulation in immature alloxan-diabetic rats treated with pregnant mare's serum gonadotropin: Reduced pituitary response to gonadotropin releasing hormone. Endocrinology 1979;105:1343.

13. Djursing H, Nyholm HC, Hagen C, et al. Depressed prolactin levels in diabetic women with anovulation. Acta Obstet Gynecol Scand 1982;61:403.

14. Valdes CT, Elkind-Hirsch KE, Rogers DG. Diabetes-induced alterations of reproductive and adrenal function in the female rat. Neuroendocrinology 1990;51:406.

15. Djursing H, Hagen C, Nyholm HC, et al. Gonadotropin responses to gonadotropin-releasing hormone and prolactin responses to thyrotropin-releasing hormone and metoclopramide in women with amenorrhea and insulin-treated diabetes mellitus. J Clin Endocrinol Metab 1983;56:1016.

16. Liu TYF, Lin HS, Johnson DC. Serum FSH, LH, and the ovarian response to exogenous gonadotropins in alloxan diabetic immature female rats. Endocrinology 1972;91:1172.

17. Diamond MP, Lavy G, Polan ML. Progesterone production from granulosa cells of individual human follicles derived from diabetic and non-diabetic subjects. Int J Fertil 1989;34:204.

18. Nielsen G, Moller M, Sorensen H. HbA1 C in early diabetic pregnancy and pregnancy outcomes. Diabetes Care 2006;29:2612.

19. Miodovnik M, Skillman C, Holroyde JC, et al. Elevated maternal glycohemoglobin in early pregnancy and spontaneous abortion among insulin-dependent diabetic women. Am J Obstet Gynecol 1985;153:439.

20. Mills JL, Simpson JL, Driscoll SG, et al. Incidence of spontaneous abortion among normal women and insulin-dependent diabetic women whose pregnancies were identified within 21 days of conception. N Engl J Med 1988;319:1617.

21. Miodovnik M, Mimouni F, Tsang RC, et al. Glycemic control and spontaneous abortion in insulin-dependent diabetic women. Obstet Gynecol 1986;68:366.

22. Casson IF, Clarke CA, Howard CV, et al. Outcomes of pregnancy in insulin dependent diabetic women: Results of a five year population cohort study. BMJ 1997;31:275.

23. Lorenzen T, Pociot F, Johannesen J. A populations-based survey of frequencies of self-reported spontaneous and induced abortion is in Danish women with type 1 diabetes mellitus. Danish IDDM Epidemiology and Genetics Group. Diabet Med 1999;16:472.

24. Mills JL, Knopp RH, Simpson JL, et al. Lack of relation of increased malformation rates in infants of diabetic mothers to glycemic control during organogenesis. N Engl J Med 1988;318:671.

25. Greene MF, Hare JW, Cloherty JP, et al. First-trimester hemoglobin A1 and risk for major malformation and spontaneous abortion in diabetic pregnancy. Teratology 1989;39:225.

26. Wright AD, Nicholson HO, Pollock A, et al. Spontaneous abortion and diabetes mellitus. Postgrad Med J 1983;59:295.

27. Mills JL, Simpson JL, Driscoll SG, et al. Incidence of spontaneous abortion among normal women and insulin-dependent diabetic women whose pregnancies were identified within 21 days of conception. N Engl J Med 1988;319:1617.

28. Nielsen GL, Sorensen HT, Nielson PH, et al. Glycosylated hemoglobin as predictor of adverse fetal outcome in type 1 diabetic pregnancies. Acta Diabetol 1997;34:217.

29. Rosenn B, Miodovnik M, Combs CA, et al. Glycemic thresholds for spontaneous abortion and congenital malformations in insulin-dependent diabetes mellitus. Obstet Gynecol 1994;84:515.

30. Mello G, Parretti E, Mecacci F, et al. Glycemic thresholds in spontaneous abortion during the first trimester in pregnant women with insulin dependent diabetes. Minerva Ginecol 1997;49:365.

31. Hanson U, Persson B, Thunell S. Relationship between haemoglobin A1c in early Type 1 (insulin-dependent) diabetic pregnancy and the occurrence of spontaneous abortion and fetal malformation in Sweden. Diabetologia 1990;33:100.

32. Torchinsky A, Toder V, Carp H, et al. In vivo evidence for the existence of a threshold for hyperglycemia-induced major fetal malformations: relevance to the etiology of diabetic teratogenesis. Early Pregnancy 1997;3:27.

33. Mimouni F, Tsang RC. Pregnancy outcome in insulin-dependent diabetes: Temporal relationships with metabolic control during specific pregnancy periods. Am J Perinatol 1988;5:334.

34. Rosenn B, Miodovnik M, Combs CA, et al. Preconception management of insulin-dependent diabetes: Improvement of pregnancy outcome. Obstet Gynecol 1991;77:846.

35. Rayburn W. Changes in insulin therapy during pregnancy. Am J Perinatol 1985;2:271.

36. Weiss P, Hoffman H. Intensified conventional insulin therapy for the pregnant diabetic patient. Obstet Gynecol 1984;64:629.

37. Jovanovic L, Peterson M. Optimal insulin delivery for the pregnant diabetic patients. Diabetes Care 1982;5:24.

38. Langer O, Anyaegbunam A, Brustman L, et al. Gestational diabetes: Insulin requirements in pregnancy. Am J Obstet Gynecol 1987;157:669.

39. Bendon RW, Mimouni F, Khoury J. et al. Histopathology of spontaneous abortion in diabetic pregnancies. Am J Perinatol 1990;7:207.

40. Clinical Practice recommendations 2003: Diabetic Retinopathy Diabetes Care 2003;26(Suppl 1):S99.

41. The DCCT Research Group: Progression of retinopathy with intensive versus conventional treatment in the diabetes control and complications trial. Ophthalmology 1995;102:647.

42. Alvarsson ML, Grill VE. Effect of long term glycemic control on the onset of retinopathy in IDDM subjects: A longitudinal and retrospective study. Diabetes Research 1989;10:75.

43. Klein R, Klein BEK, Moss SE, et al. Glycosylated hemoglobin predicts the incidence and progression of diabetic retinopathy. JAMA 1988;260:2864.

44. Brinchmann-Hansen O, Dahl-Jorgensen K, Sandvik L, et al. Blood glucose concentrations and progression of diabetic retinopathy: The seven year results of the Oslo Study. BMJ 1992;304:19.

45. American College of Obstetricians and Gynecologists. Diabetes and pregnancy. ACOG Technical Bulletin No. 200. American College of Obstetricians and Gynecologists, December 1994, Danvers, MA.

46. Alvarsson ML, Grill VE. Effect of long term glycemic control on the onset of retinopathy in IDDM subjects: A longitudinal and retrospective study. Diabetes Research 1989;10:75.

47. Klein R, Klein BEK, Moss SE, et al. Glycosylated hemoglobin predicts the incidence and progression of diabetic retinopathy. JAMA 1988;260:2864.

48. Brinchmann-Hansen O, Dahl-Jorgensen K, Sandvik L, et al. Blood glucose concentrations and progression of diabetic retinopathy: The seven year results of the Oslo Study. BMJ 1992;304:19.

49. Reichard P, Britz A, Carlsson P, et al. Metabolic control and complications over 3 years in patients with insulin dependent diabetes (IDDM): The Stockholm Diabetes Intervention Study (SDIS). J Intern Med 1990;228:511.

50. Kroc Collaborative Study Group. Blood glucose control and the evolution of diabetic retinopathy and albuminuria. N Engl J Med 1984;311:365.

51. The Diabetes Control and Complications Trial Research Group. The effect of intensive treatment of diabetes on the development and progression of long-term complications in insulin-dependent diabetes mellitus. N Engl J Med 1993;329:977.

52. Dahl-Jorgensen K, Brinchmann-Hansen O, Hanssen KF, et al. Rapid tightening of blood glucose leads to transient deterioration of retinopathy in insulin-dependent diabetes mellitus: The Oslo Study. BMJ 1985;290:811.

53. Sevin R. The correlation between human growth hormone (HGH) concentration in blood plasma and the evolution of diabetic retinopathy. Ophthalmologica 1972;165:71.

54. Arner P, Sjoberg S, Gjotterberg M, et al. Circulating insulin-like growth factor I in type 1 (insulin-dependent) diabetic patients with retinopathy. Diabetologia 1989;32:753.

55. Hyer SL, Sharp PS, Sleightholm M, et al. Progression of diabetic retinopathy and changes in serum insulin-like growth factor I (IGFI) during continuous subcutaneous insulin infusion (CSII). Horm Metab Res 1989;21:18.

56. Hill CR, Kissun RD, Garner A. Angiogenic factor in vitreous from diabetic retinopathy. Experientia 1983;39:583.

57. Castellon R, Hamdi HK, Sacerio I, et al. Effects of angiogenic growth factor combinations on retinal endothelial cells. Exp Eye Res 2002;74:523.

58. Presta M, Mignatti P, Mullins DE, et al. Human placental tissue stimulates bovine capillary endothelial cell growth, migration and protease production. Biosci Rep 1985;5:783.

59. Hill DJ, Flyvbjerg A, Arany E, et al. Increased levels of serum fibroblast growth factor-2 in diabetic pregnant women with retinopathy. J Clin Endocrinol Metab 1997;82:1452.

60. Cousins L. Pregnancy complications among diabetic women: Review 1965–1985. Obstet Gynecol Surv 1987;42:140.

61. Rosenn B, Miodovnik M, Kranias G, et al. Progression of diabetic retinopathy in pregnancy: Association with hypertension in pregnancy. Am J Obstet Gynecol 1992;166:1214.

62. Lovestam-Adrian M, Agardh CD, Aberg A, et al. Preeclampsia is a potent risk factor for deterioration of retinopathy during pregnancy in type 1 diabetic patients. Diabet Med 1997;14:1059.

63. Horvat M, Maclean H, Goldberg L, et al. Diabetic retinopathy in pregnancy: A 12-year prospective survey. Br J Ophthalmol 1980;64:398.

64. Moloney JBM, Drury MI. The effect of pregnancy on the natural course of diabetic retinopathy. Am J Ophthalmol 1982;93:745.

65. Dibble CM, Kochenour NK, Worley RJ, et al. Effect of pregnancy on diabetic retinopathy. Obstet Gynecol 1982;59:699.

66. Price JH, Hadden DR, Archer DB, et al. Diabetic retinopathy in pregnancy. Br J Obstet Gynaecol 1984;91:11.

67. Ohrt V. The influence of pregnancy on diabetic retinopathy with special regard to the reversible changes shown in 100 pregnancies. Acta Ophthalmol 1984;62:603.

68. Jovanovic R, Jovanovic L. Obstetric management when normoglycemia is maintained in diabetic pregnant women with vascular compromise. Am J Obstet Gynecol 1984;149:617.

69. Phelps RL, Sakol P, Metzger BE, et al. Changes in diabetic retinopathy during pregnancy. Arch Ophthalmol 1986;104:1806.

70. Serup L. Influence of pregnancy on diabetic retinopathy. Acta Endocrinol (Copenhagen) 1986;277(Suppl):122.

71. Chew EY, Mills JL, Metzger BE, et al. Metabolic control and progression of retinopathy: The Diabetes in Early Pregnancy Study. National Institute of Child Health and Human Development Diabetes in Early Pregnancy Study. Diabetes Care 1995;18:631.

72. Axer-Siegel R, Hod M, Fink-Cohen S, et al. Diabetic retinopathy during pregnancy. Ophthalmology 1996;103:1815.

73. Lapolla A, Cardone C, Negrin P, et al. Pregnancy does not induce or worsen retinal and peripheral nerve dysfunction in insulin-dependent diabetic women. J Diabetes Complications 1998;12:74.

74. Temple RC, Aldridge VA, Sampson MJ, et al. Impact of pregnancy on the progression of diabetic retinopathy in Type 1 diabetes. Diabet Med 2001;18:573.

75. Selby JV, FitzSimmons SC, Newman JM, et al. The natural history and epidemiology of diabetic nephropathy. Implications for prevention and control. JAMA 1990;263:1954.

76. Reichard P, Britz A, Carlsson P, et al. Metabolic control and complications over 3 years in patients with insulin dependent diabetes (IDDM): The Stockholm Diabetes Intervention Study (SDIS). J Intern Med 1990;228:511.

77. The Diabetes Control and complications Trial Research group. The effect of intensive treatment of diabetes on the development and progression of long-term complications in insulin-dependent diabetes mellitus. N Engl J Med 1993;329:977.

78. McCance DR, Hadden DR. Atkinson AB, et al. The relationship between long-term glycemic control and diabetic nephropathy. QJM 1992;82:53.

79. Reichard P, Rosenqvist U. Nephropathy is delayed by intensified insulin treatment in patients with insulin-dependent diabetes mellitus and retinopathy. J Intern Med 1989;226:81.

80. Parving H-H. Impact of blood pressure and antihypertensive treatment on incipient and overt nephropathy, retinopathy, and endothelial permeability in diabetes mellitus. Diabetes Care 1991;14:260.

81. Jerums G, Allen TJ, Tsalamandris C, et al. The Melbourne Diabetic Nephropathy Study Group: Angiotensin converting enzyme inhibition and calcium channel blockade in incipient diabetic nephropathy. Kidney Int 1992;41:904.

82. Hostetter TH. Pathogenesis of diabetic glomerulopathy: Hemodynamic considerations. Semin Nephrol 1990;10:219.

83. Bank N. Mechanisms of diabetic hyperfiltration. Kidney Int 1991;40:792.

84. Zeller KR. Low-protein diets in renal disease. Diabetes Care 1991;14:856.

85. Dodds RA, Keen H. Low protein diet and conservation of renal function in diabetic nephropathy. Diabetes Metab 1990;16:464.

86. Hod M, van Dijk DJ, Karp M, et al. Diabetic nephropathy and pregnancy: The effect of ACE inhibitors prior to pregnancy and fetomaternal outcome. Nephrol Dial Transplant 1995;10:2328.

87. Carr D, Koontz GL, Gardella C, et al. Diabetic Nephropathy in Pregnancy: Suboptimal Hypertensive Control Associated With Preterm Delivery. Am J Hypertens 2006;19:513.

88. Mauer SM, Sutherland DER, Steffes MW. Relationship of systemic blood pressure to nephropathology in insulin-dependent diabetes mellitus. Kidney Int 1992;41:736.

89. Mogensen CE, Hansen KW, Osterby R, et al. Blood pressure elevation versus abnormal albuminuria in the genesis and prediction of renal disease in diabetes. Diabetes Care 1992;15:1192.

90. Parving H-H. Impact of blood pressure and antihypertensive treatment on incipient and overt nephropathy, retinopathy, and endothelial permeability in diabetes mellitus. Diabetes Care 1991;14:260.

91. Jerums G, Allen TJ, Tsalamandris C, et al. The Melbourne Diabetic Nephropathy Study Group: Angiotensin converting enzyme inhibition and calcium channel blockade in incipient diabetic nephropathy. Kidney Int 1992;41:904.

92. Cooper WO, Hernandez-Diaz S, Arbogast PG, et al. Major congenital malformations after first-trimester exposure to ACE inhibitors. N Engl J Med 2006;354:2443.

93. Reece EA, Coustan DR, Hayslett JP, et al. Diabetic nephropathy: Pregnancy performance and fetomaternal outcome. Am J Obstet Gynecol 1988;159:56.

94. Reece EA, Winn HN, Hayslett JP, et al. Does pregnancy alter the rate of progression of diabetic nephropathy? Am J Perinatol 1990;7:193.

95. Gordon M, Landon MB, Samuels P, et al. Perinatal outcome and long-term follow-up associated with modern management of diabetic nephropathy. Obstet Gynecol 1996;87:401.

96. Rosenn BM, Miodovnik M, Khoury JC, et al. Outcome of pregnancy in women with diabetic nephropathy. Am J Obstet Gynecol 1997;176:S179.

97. Dunne FP, Chowdhury TA, Hartland A, et al. Pregnancy outcome in women with insulin-dependent diabetes mellitus complicated by nephropathy. QJM 1999;92:451.

98. Khoury JC, Miodovnik M, LeMasters G, et al. Pregnancy outcome and progression of diabetic nephropathy. What's next? J Matern Fetal Neonatal Med 2002;11:238.

99. Bar J, Ben-Rafael Z, Padoa A, et al. Prediction of pregnancy outcome in subgroups of women with renal disease. Clinical Nephrology 2002;53:437.

100. Ekbom P, Damm P, Feldt-Rasmussen B., et al. Pregnancy Outcome in Type I diabetic Women with Microalbuminuria. Diabetes Care 2001;24:1739.

101. Kitzmiller JL, Brown ER, Phillippe M. et al. Diabetic nephropathy and perinatal outcome. Am J Obstet Gynecol 1981;141:741.

102. Grenfell A, Brudenell JM, Doddridge MC, et al. Pregnancy in diabetic women who have proteinuria. QJM 1986;59:379.

103. Kimmerle R, Zass RP, Cupisti S, et al. Pregnancies in women with diabetic nephropathy: Long-term outcome for mother and child. Diabetologia 1995;38:27.

104. Kalter H. Perinatal mortality and congenital malformations in infants born to women with insulin-dependent diabetes mellitus: United States, Canada and Europe, 1940–1988. Morb Mortal Wkly Rep 1990;39:363.

105. Kucera J. Rate and type of congenital anomalies among offspring of diabetic women. J Reprod Med 1971;7:61.
106. Becerra JE, Khoury MJ, Cordero JF, et al. Diabetes mellitus during pregnancy and the risks for specific birth defects: A populations-based case-control study. Pediatrics 1990;85:1.
107. Cousins L. Congenital anomalies among infants of diabetic mothers: Etiology, prevention, prenatal diagnosis. Am J Obstet Gynecol 1983;147:333.
108. Schaefer-Graf UM,Buchanan TA, Xiang A, et al. Patterns of congenital anomalies and relationship to initial internal fasting glucose levels in pregnancies complicated by type 2 and gestational diabetes. Am J Obstet Gynecol 2000;182:313.
109. Towner D, Kjos SL, Leung B, et al. Congenital Malformations in Pregnancies Complicated by NIDDM. Diabetes Care 1995;18:1446.
110. Rosenn BM, Miodovnik M, Khoury JC, et al. Pregnancy outcome in women with Type 2 diabetes mellitus. Am J Obstet Gynecol 1996;147:394.
111. Schaefer UM, Songster G, Xiang A., et al. Congenital malformations in offspring of women with hyperglycemia first detected during pregnancy. Am J Obstet Gynecol 1997;177:1165.
112. Sheffield JS, Butler-Koster EL, Casey BM, et al. Maternal Diabetes Mellitus and Infant Malformations. Am J Obstet Gynecol 2002;100:925.
113. Casson IF, Clarke CA, Howard CV, et al. Outcomes of pregnancy in insulin dependent diabetic women: Results of a five year population cohort study. BMJ 1997;31:275.
114. Hawthorne G, Robson S, Ryall EA, et al. Prospective population bases survey of outcome of pregnancy in diabetic women: Results of the Northern Diabetic Pregnancy Audit, 1994. BMJ 1997;315:279.
115. Nordstrom L, Spetz E, Wallstrom K, et al. Metabolic control and pregnancy outcome among women with insulin-dependent diabetes mellitus: A twelve-year follow-up in the country of Jamtland, Sweden. Acta Obstet Gynecol Scand 1998;77:284.
116. The DCCT Research Group. Pregnancy outcomes in the Diabetes Control and Complications Trial. Am J Obstet Gynecol 1996;174:1343.
117. Elixhauser A, Weschler JM, Kitzmiller JL, et al. Cost-benefit analysis of preconception care for women with established diabetes mellitus. Diabetes Care 1993;16:1146.
118. Herman WH, Janz NK, Becker MP, et al. Diabetes and pregnancy: Preconception care, pregnancy outcomes, resource utlization and costs. J Reprod Med 1999;44:33.
119. Moore TR. Diabetes in pregnancy. In: Creasy RK, Resnik R, eds. Maternal-Fetal Medicine: Principles and Practice, 4th edn. Philadelphia: WB Saunders, 1999:967.
120. Siddiqi TA, Miodovnik M, Mimouni F, et al. Biphasic fetal intrauterine growth in insulin-dependent diabetic pregnancies. J Am Coll Nutr 1989;8:225.
121. Eriksson UJ, Lewis NJ, Freinkel N. Growth retardation during early organogenesis in embryos of experimental diabetic rats. Diabetes 1984;33:281.
122. Pedersen JF, Molsted-Pedersen L. Early growth retardation in diabetic pregnancy. BMJ 1979;1:18.
123. Ogata ES, Sabbagha R, Metzger BE, et al. Serial ultrasonography to assess evolving fetal macrosomia: Studies in 23 pregnant diabetic women. JAMA 1980;243:2405.
124. Tsang RC, Ballard JL, Braun C. The infant of the diabetic mother: Today and tomorrow. Clin Obstet Gynecol 1981;24:125.
125. Cousins L. Pregnancy complications among diabetic women: Review 1965–1985. Obstet Gynecol Surv 1987;43:10.
126. Langer O, ed. The Diabetes in Pregnancy Dilemma, 1st edn. Lanham: University Press of America, 2006.

13

Psychological Aspects of Type 1 Diabetes in Adults

B. A. Boyer
Institute for Graduate Clinical Psychology, Widener University, Chester, Pennsylvania, U.S.A.

V. Myers
Pennington Biomedical Research Center, Louisiana State University, Louisiana, U.S.A.

D. Lehman
Institute for Graduate Clinical Psychology, Widener University, Chester, Pennsylvania, U.S.A.

INTRODUCTION

When considered from an experiential perspective, type 1 diabetes (DM1) represents a significant stressor for individuals and their families. A comprehensive understanding of psychological factors related to DM1 requires investigation of (*i*) the impact of DM1 upon psychological adjustment and (*ii*) the impact of psychological adjustment upon medical outcomes for DM1. Both of these directions of influence are reviewed below regarding each of the most prevalent and/or problematic psychological adjustment problems for adults with DM1.

When comparing with other chronic health conditions, from an experiential perspective, it is important to consider:

- *disease factors*, including disease onset, disease progression;
- *regimen factors*, including the complexity, the intrusiveness, the cost and the accessibility, and the side-effects that affect regimen adherence;
- *individual factors*, including health beliefs and coping; and
- *comorbid psychopathology* (1).

Disease, regimen, and individual factors specific to DM1, although reviewed more comprehensively elsewhere (2), will be reviewed briefly in this chapter. Several psychological problems that are prevalent and problematic among individuals with DM1, depression, anxiety, and dysregulated eating, will each be reviewed in detail in the chapter.

The disease onset of DM1 may vary in several ways. Some individuals may experience the vague and mildly distressing symptoms of increased thirst and urination, hunger, fatigue, and weight loss, and subsequently seek medical attention at which time they receive the diagnosis of DM1. In such cases, the symptoms are not extreme or greatly distressing, and the individual may perceive the news of the diagnosis and demand for ongoing treatment to be more distressing than the symptoms. In contrast, other individuals may develop diabetic ketoacidosis (DKA) (e.g., a serious and dangerous condition of high levels of ketones, which can result in coma and/or death) prior to diagnosis, and therefore experience the disease onset as more distressing and fear inducing. Additionally, many adults with DM1 have been diagnosed as children or adolescents, and time since diagnosis is an important consideration. The regimen factors are likely to be more important than the disease factors regarding both coping and self-management success among individuals with DM1. The DM1 self-management regimens, as described in more detail in other chapters, are reviewed here with respect to the specific demands they place on patients. Regardless of which exact regimen an individual uses, the DM1 treatment is complex, multifactorial, and requires ongoing consistency (2). The exact regimen, in turn, poses particular challenges and offers particular benefits. In Table 1, the typical current DM1 regimens are compared and contrasted regarding the factors involved in patient self-care.

Table 1 Specific Self-Management Activities and Lifestyle Factors Relevant to Current Insulin Regimen

Type of regimen	Injection therapy with intermediate insulin and rapid insulin (but not at every meal) (e.g., Twice daily NPH [morning and dinnertime, possibly bedtime] with Regular, Aspart or Lispro injections prior to breakfast and dinner)	MDI regimen; basal/bolus therapy by injections, with bolus taken at every meal (e.g., Glargine with Aspart or Lispro injections each time you eat)	CSII; pump therapy
Frequency of injection (or needle insertion)	Fewer, 2–3/day	More injections	Only infusion set changes, 1/every third day
Need for consistency in mealtimes	High	Low	Low
Flexibility in mealtimes	Low	Moderate	High
Flexibility regarding amounts of food eaten/meal	Low	High	High
Need for carbohydrate counting	Varied, but can accomplish control without carbohydrate counting	High	High
Demand to execute arithmetic for meal insulin-to-carbohydrate ratios	Varied, but low if patient is not carbohydrate counting	High	High, but low with newer pump models, in which ratios can be entered into pump.
Ability to dose with insulin for effects of dietary Fats upon BG	Low, very difficult	Low, very difficult	High, ease with use of temporary basal rates.
Ability to achieve euglycemia with exercise/sports activity	Low	Moderate	High

Within the literature addressing DM1 treatment among adolescents and children, an important distinction has been made between *adherence* and *self-management* with accompanying activities and goals relevant to blood glucose (BG) management (3). *Adherence* represents the patient's following of treatment instructions by medical providers, and *self-management* involves an active self-directed process, with elements divisible into *process* to execute the *activities* to reach self-management *goals*. This distinction emphasizes that, although self-management is a process collaborative with medical providers, it truly requires the patients and families to understand the factors that affect BG [e.g., food intake (carbohydrates, fats), insulin dosage, timing of food intake and insulin dosage, BG monitoring, exercise, stress], factors that affect prevention of complications (foot care, ophthalmologic screening), and actively manage these activities in their ongoing life. As highlighted in Table 1, the evolution of regimen, development of newer preparations of insulin (e.g., Glargine), and application of newer delivery methods (e.g., continuous subcutaneous insulin infusion [CSII] pumps) over the past 10 to 15 years, has greatly affected the self-management behaviors required for patients. As a result, many of the old stereotypes among the public, such as DM1 management requiring the elimination of simple carbohydrates and/or severe restriction of carbohydrates, has become an obsolete assumption. For example, those using basal/bolus multiple daily injections (MDI) or CSII pumps, who are accurate in their carbohydrate counting and appropriate use of insulin-to-grams of carbohydrate bolus ratios, may not need to limit carbohydrate intake at all (4). Although regimen such as MDI and CSII pumps have reprieved some patients from requirements of older regimen, successful management continues to require the consistent process of active BG monitoring, use of insulin boli to correct high BG, counting of carbohydrates and use of insulin-to-gram of carbohydrate ratio boli, and other demanding activities to maintain optimal BG.

The individual factors, such as intelligence, knowledge, culture, patient's trust in medical profession, health beliefs, and coping, constitute the variables that interact with the disease and regimen factors overviewed above. For a full review of these issues, the reader is referred to Boyer (2). Here, a brief review of diabetes-specific knowledge and coping are provided.

Diabetes-Specific Knowledge

Since the treatment for DM1 involves a complex regimen of self-management, the amount and accuracy of knowledge is imperative for patients' adherence to treatment (5) and glycemic control (6). The literature on knowledge among the pediatric DM1 population becomes relevant, since those diagnosed as children or adolescents may receive most of their self-management training at diagnosis. Data indicates, however, that individuals show decrease in their maintenance and application of diabetes-specific knowledge over time, and reeducation becomes important (7). Although knowledge is related to self-management (8) and glycemic control (9), it has also been found not to predict management outcome (7,10), as other factors interfere with the application of this knowledge over time (11). Some of these factors are discussed throughout the remainder of this chapter.

Coping

Due to the demand for active and strategic self-management of BG among all treatments for DM1, the coping dispositions of patients and their families are of crucial importance. Empirical investigations regarding coping among those with DM1, and the relationship of coping to medical outcomes, have generally implied that active, approach-oriented coping dispositions show a better match with DM1 self-management demands than passive, avoidant coping. Active coping corresponds with better quality of life among adults with diabetes (12), and better metabolic control among adolescents with DM1 (13). Although much of the research investigating samples of patients with DM1 are adolescent samples, these data are relevant to our discussion, as most adults with DM1 have had the condition across their adolescent years, and may have developed coping dispositions that persist into adulthood. While some studies have shown that coping training interventions for adolescents produced reductions in diabetes-specific stress but not improvements in glycemic control (14), others have produced improvements in self-efficacy as well as metabolic control that maintained for 6 months following therapy (15). Simply put, it appears that individuals who manage stress by approaching the stressful condition, attempting to control the condition, and find the process of exerting strategic control to be distress-reducing are likely to be more easily successful managing DM1 than those who reduce stress by avoiding the stressful condition, employing avoidant strategies to reduce the sense of threat and distress, and experience greater distress when approaching the stress-inducing context.

While the factors reviewed above, knowledge, coping, and self-management difficulties are relevant to any and all individuals with DM1, several psychological disorders have been shown to be more prevalent in those with DM1, and particularly problematic for self-management and glycemic control.

DEPRESSION

A well-developed literature has investigated the comorbidity between DM1 and depression, and the relationship of depression to medical outcomes among those with DM1. It has been shown that individuals with DM have a disproportionately higher rate of psychiatric disorders (16), with affective and anxiety disorders being more commonly diagnosed than in the general population (17,18). In one study of DM1 and type 2 (DM2) inpatients, 52% presented with at least one lifetime psychiatric disorder, and 41.3% presented with a diagnosis within the past 6 months (17). In this sample, affective and anxiety disorders represented 83% of the psychiatric diagnoses. Another study of DM1 outpatients showed rates of anxiety and depressive disorders at 44% and 41.5%, respectively (18).

Some individual studies have found that depression among those diagnosed with diabetes was vastly elevated, compared to the individuals without diabetes, with depression as high as six times higher for those with DM (19). In an epidemiological study of depression in individuals with DM1 and DM2, findings revealed that depression was three to four times more prevalent in this population than in the general population (20). These results suggest that 15% to 20%, or approximately one in five individuals with either DM1 or DM2 are afflicted with depression. Furthermore, approximately 40% of individuals with DM have significantly elevated levels of depressive symptomatology, but are not clinically depressed.

The literature has developed enough to permit meta-analytic studies. Taken together, the evidence from 42 studies regarding rates of depression among those with DM1 or DM2 indicates a 2.0 odds ratio for depression among those with diabetes (21). While these studies include both DM1 and DM2 populations, the data did not suggest a difference between DM1 and DM2. For those with DM1, there appeared to be twice the rate of depression as among those without diabetes. There were, however, differences related to gender. Rates of depression were 28% among women with diabetes, and 18% among men with diabetes, but due to different base rates for depression among men and women without diabetes, the 2.0 odds ratio was consistent for both genders (21). A more recent review, investigating depression among only samples with DM1, and including five additional studies since the Anderson and colleagues study (21), reported that 12% of those with DM1 exhibited comorbid depression, compared with only 3.2% of the comparison group without diabetes (22). These data suggest that, among individuals with DM1, the rates of depression may be above three times the rate as those without DM. Indeed, 27% of children and adolescents diagnosed with DM1 developed a major depressive episode during the 10 years after the diagnosis of DM1 (23). These series of studies and the resulting meta-analytic reviews demonstrate that regardless of the exact degree of increased risk and prevalence, depression appears elevated in prevalence among those with DM1.

Given the elevated prevalence of depression among individuals with DM, a few studies have attempted to characterize the disorder further. In a study by Peyrot and Rubin (24), elevated depressive symptoms varied according to two factors: (*i*) nondiabetes specific (generic) factors and (*ii*) diabetes-related factors. The researchers found higher rates of depression among women, individuals who were unmarried, and those with less education. Higher rates of depression were also found in individuals with three or more medical complications secondary to their diabetes (i.e., retinopathy, neuropathy, kidney disease, etc). Other studies have examined the relationship between social problems and depression in individuals with DM (25,26). Roy (25) found that social problems are reported more often among individuals with DM1. Wilkinson and colleagues (26) found that individuals reporting major social problems had significantly higher levels of psychiatric morbidity.

Relationship of Depression to Medical Outcomes

Of further concern is the relationship between comorbid depression and medical outcomes among those with DM1. Several studies have investigated the influence of depression on glycemic control and other adherence measures. Studies have found that individuals with DM and a history of depression showed significantly worse glycemic control as measured by glycosylated hemoglobin (18,27,28). Additionally, a few meta-analytic studies now exist and have shown a significant relationship between depression and poorer metabolic control among those with both DM1 and DM2 (29,30). Not surprisingly, depression has also shown a relationship to greater complications of persistent hyperglycemia (31). Inquiry continues regarding the exact nature of this relationship between depression and hyperglycemia. One study sought to determine whether depression induced a decrease in diabetes self-care and whether changes in self-management mediated the relationship between depression and hyperglycemia. Although the inclusion of the score from the summary of diabetes self-care activities in regression analyses attenuated the relationship between depression and glycosylated hemoglobin among individuals with DM1, it did not account for a significant mediation of the depression → hyperglycemia relationship (30). As such, continued investigation of this relationship is necessary, to determine the strength of the depression → reduced self-management → hyperglycemia mechanism, or evaluate other psychological and psychophysiological mechanisms for this relationship (30).

The course of depression in the DM population is chronic and severe (16,32,33), and the presence of depression in individuals with DM may significantly worsen the course of both disorders (34). There is sufficient data in the literature demonstrating the (*i*) increased prevalence of depression in the DM1 population, (*ii*) deleterious impact of depression on medical outcomes, and (*iii*) evidence that effective treatments exist. However, depression continues to be underdiagnosed and undertreated (35). In a study of nine primary care practices, 49% of patients with a diagnosis of either DM1 or DM2, reporting clinically significant depression in a systematic screening, were not diagnosed or treated. Only 43% of those patients who were appropriately diagnosed with depression were receiving antidepressant pharmacotherapy, and only 6.7% received four or more psychotherapy sessions during the previous year (36). This suggests that not only were many patients with depression not initially diagnosed, but those who were diagnosed were not adequately treated.

Treatment for Comorbid Depression and Diabetes

A few studies have examined the influence of psychopharmacology and psychotherapy on the treatment of depression in this population; however data remain scarce. Although the prevalence of major depression and diabetes is well established, there are no large-scale, randomized controlled clinical trials. Both antidepressant medications and cognitive behavioral therapy have demonstrated short-term effectiveness in the treatment of depression among DM individuals. The results seem promising with improvement towards a reduction in depressive symptoms, as well as improved glycemic control (16,37–40). As previously stated, data is available showing that depression has been shown to worsen medical outcomes for those with diabetes. Many of the treatment data for depression and diabetes show improvements in medical outcomes (i.e., improved metabolic control); however, depression treatment for those with comorbid depression and diabetes have not consistently shown improvement in patients' self-management (41) or glycemic control (42).

Pharmacological management of depression may be necessary for long-term or resistant depressive symptoms. Monoamine oxidize inhibitors (MAOIs) and tricyclic antidepressants (TCAs) are not commonly used to treat depression in persons with diabetes due to potential adverse side effects (e.g., short-term hyperglycemia, hypoglycemic unawareness, postural hypotension). Notably, a randomized clinical trial of nortriptyline revealed significant reductions in depression; however, there was an adverse effect on glucose control (39). Selective serotonin reuptake inhibitors (SSRIs) appear to be the preferred antidepressant of choice for those with DM. However, SSRIs are not without side effects. This class of drugs may alter the metabolism of certain oral hypoglycemics and certain drugs can be associated with weight gain (43). Effectiveness data suggest that SSRIs are associated with both improved depressive symptoms and metabolic control. The SSRI, fluoxetine, has been evaluated for its efficacy on reducing depressive symptoms in both DM1 and DM2 patients (44). An 8-week, randomized clinical trial found that fluoxetine significantly reduced depressive symptoms compared to placebo and trended towards better glycemic control.

Lack of statistical power is an important note of caution in interpreting the data on antidepressants on depressive symptoms in persons with diabetes. Most of the pharmacotherapy studies have too few participants to robustly measure symptom reduction and symptom burden from diabetes, and no long-term data are available (43).

Cognitive behavioral treatment has been shown useful in the treatment of depression in persons with diabetes; however, data is scant. This therapeutic approach modifies dysfunctional thinking, reduces negative emotions, trains stress reduction, and provides skill building in areas of deficit. Improvements in mood, quality of life, and coping were demonstrated in the only large-scale randomized clinical trial to date in DM2 adults (45). However, other data from less statistically robust studies exists. Cognitive behavioral therapy has shown effects through improved glycemic control and quality of life (15,46), and evidence suggests that CBT techniques may prove beneficial in improving compliance to diabetes regimen (45).

Combined treatment of pharmacotherapy and psychotherapy has been found to be significantly more efficacious in reducing depressive symptoms than placebo alone (47).

Overall, with the limited data available, it appears that both psychopharmacological and psychotherapeutic approaches have beneficial effects on depression reduction in persons with diabetes, and may promote improvement in medical outcomes.

ANXIETY

A significant literature has addressed the prevalence of anxiety comorbid to DM1. A meta-analysis of 2584 individuals with either DM1 or DM2, found that 14% of the sample showed symptoms of generalized anxiety disorder, and 40% of the sample reported elevated symptoms of anxiety (48). Although these studies included participants with both types of diabetes, the rates of anxiety were similar for DM1 and DM2. Thirteen percent of young individuals developed an anxiety disorder during the 10 years following their diagnosis of DM1 (23).

Additionally, some individuals experience anxiety directly related to DM1 and self-management. Although most diabetic complications arise from persistent hyperglycemia, the immediate symptoms of hypoglycemia are much more perceptible subjectively and indeed frightening and uncomfortable. Fear of hypoglycemia (FH) has been observed among individuals with DM1. FH has been found to be related to higher trait anxiety (49) and greater perceived stress (50), past experiences with hypoglycemia (49,50), more daily variability in BG (50), and poorer metabolic control (51). A self-report instrument, the hypoglycemic fear survey, has been developed to measure this phenomenon (51), and has demonstrated good internal consistency and temporal stability (51). FH appears to have two components, each measured by the hypoglycemic fear survey, a cognitive worry component and a behavioral avoidance component. Patients may become persistently worried and fearful of hypoglycemia, and mistake the symptoms of anxiety for the similar symptoms of hypoglycemia, often experiencing persistent difficulty distinguishing whether these symptoms are due to low BG or anxiety (49). In addition, this persistent fear induces some individuals to engage in avoidance behaviors such as overeating in response to early symptoms of low BG (51), intentionally maintaining higher levels of BG to create the perception of safety from hypoglycemia by underdosing their insulin relative to BG levels or food intake (52).

This fact that FH is related to previous frequency and experiences with hypoglycemic episodes hypoglycemia (49,50) and the pattern of persistent and intrusive worry about low BG hypoglycemia (50), the anxious hyperarousal that accompanies this fearful cognition, and the resulting maladaptive behavioral attempts to avoid risk of hypoglycemia (51,52), has led some investigators to question whether this responding may constitute the symptom triad of posttraumatic stress.

In the only study to date, in which the full symptom triad of intrusive ideation, anxious hyperarousal, and avoidance, along with the criterion that these symptoms pose clinically significant interference with functioning, reported that 25% of individuals using basal/bolus insulin regimen (i.e., MDI and CSII pumps) indicated symptoms consistent with current posttraumatic stress disorder (53) related to hypoglycemia.

Relationship of Anxiety to Medical Outcomes

Furthermore, a meta-analysis assessing evidence of a relationship between anxiety and metabolic control found that, while overall results did not support a significant relationship, in studies using interviews to evaluate anxiety, anxiety did show significant relationship to glycemic control (54). It appears that when more rigorous assessment was utilized, a relationship between anxiety and hyperglycemia was detectable, although not supported by studies employing questionnaire assessment of anxiety (54).

Treatment for Comorbid Anxiety and Diabetes

While very few empirical studies have evaluated efficacy of treatment for anxiety among adults with DM1, one case study has demonstrated that cognitive-behavioral therapies (CBT) may be useful, suggesting that CBT may be as effective for this population as for others (55). Since anxiety greatly affects quality of life, since studies utilizing interview assessment of anxiety indicate that it interferes with medical outcomes for those with DM1 (54), and since diabetes-specific anxiety and hypoglycemic fear may interfere with glycemic control, interventions to treat anxiety among those with DM1 are greatly needed (50,51).

Despite the fewer studies regarding treatment of anxiety among those with DM1 compared to the literature addressing depression, the existing evidence suggests that clinicians should have a high suspicion for anxiety among adults with DM1. In addition, the potential detriment regarding metabolic outcomes suggests that therapies to ameliorate anxiety are imperative.

DYSREGULATED EATING

Approximately 5% of women and 1% of men suffer from anorexia nervosa, bulimia nervosa, or binge eating disorder. An estimated 1 in 100 American women binges and purges to lose weight and 15% of young women have significantly disordered eating attitudes and behavior (56). Although eating disorders can strike anyone, the most common demographic affected is adolescent, Caucasian females, of middle to upper middle class socioeconomic status. At particular risk, however, may be people who modify their diet because of an illness such as diabetes or celiac disease (57) When considering the development, prevalence, and medical risks of dysregulated eating among adults with DM1, it is important to remember that most adults with DM1 are diagnosed as children or adolescents (58). For both women and men in the United States, adolescence constitutes the developmental period during which dieting, dysregulated eating, and eating disorders are most likely to develop (59,60). Therefore, a discussion of adolescent eating patterns becomes imperative. Given the physiological and hormonal changes that occur during adolescence, many youth become self-conscious and hyperaware of their body, and may begin to diet. Dieting is often the first step to developing an eating disorder. Although eating disorders are most commonly found in individuals during adolescence and early adulthood, disordered eating patterns are extremely difficult to overcome and often persist throughout life. Relapse rates after treatment among individuals with eating disorders appears as high as 30% to 40% within 3 years posttreatment (61–65), indicating that disordered eating often persists even after treatment.

For adolescents with DM1, diabetes self-care requires an unremitting focus on the balance among food, exercise, and insulin. Therefore, it is reasonable to speculate that people with DM1 may often become more preoccupied with food and their own bodies than the average person. In general, adolescents with a chronic illness, such as DM1, generally report higher body dissatisfaction, and engage in more dangerous weight loss measures than those without a chronic illness (66).

Although intensive insulin therapy represents the most effective current regimen (67), it tends to cause a modest weight gain, and increases the risk for hypoglycemia (low blood sugar). When an individual has a hypoglycemic episode they must eat something to raise their blood sugar, thereby increasing their calorie consumption for the day. These side effects are generally mild and thought to be worth the health benefits that come with intensive insulin therapy. However, the increase in weight that can be caused both by an increase in caloric consumption due to hypoglycemia and the improvement in glycemic control can be upsetting and problematic for some people and, therefore, seems likely to be a risk factor for the development of disordered eating (68).

As a result of this need for hyperawareness about one's body, combined with a higher base weight than average, it is not surprising that the rate of eating disorders among people with DM1 is higher than among the general population. Current estimates suggest that approximately 16% of people with DM1 suffer from a co-occurring eating disorder (69), and many more will suffer from subclinical levels of disordered eating. Research suggests that DM1 may trigger the development of an eating disorder, as DM1 may exacerbate body dissatisfaction following DM1 diagnosis and treatment, in part to their higher-than-average base weight (70).

The diagnostic and statistic manual, (DSM-IV) (71) identifies three forms of eating disorders: anorexia nervosa, bulimia nervosa, and eating disorder not otherwise specified. There is currently a debate about adding a fourth disorder, binge eating disorder, to the next revision of the DSM. A section below is devoted to each.

Anorexia

Anorexia is often the easiest of the eating disorders to diagnose because the physical symptoms are difficult to keep hidden. The symptoms, refusal to maintain a minimally normal body weight (characterized as less than 85% of what is appropriate for an individual's height), an intense fear of gaining weight, severe disturbances and perceptions about the shape of the body, amenorrhea, preoccupation with food, the hoarding of food, concerns about eating in public, cooking for others but refusing to eat, and rigid thinking (71), may readily become apparent to family, friends, or medical professionals.

A meta-analysis that reviewed five controlled studies, found that individuals with DM1 are at no greater risk for developing anorexia than the general population (72). However, an estimated 1% of all females develop anorexia at some point in their lives, and approximately 10% of people with anorexia will die from complications such as starvations, suicide, or an electrolyte imbalance, constituting the highest death rate of any mental illness (71). Therefore, observation and screening for those with DM1 is imperative, even if the rates are not higher than among those without DM.

Anorexia can cause infertility, osteoporosis, and irritable bowel syndrome; however, for those with anorexia and DM1 the risks are even greater. Women with diabetes and anorexia have a mortality rate of 34.6 per 1000 person-years, whereas those with anorexia without diabetes have only a 2.2 per 1000 person-years (73). This staggering difference highlights the essential need for physicians to screen for this disorder, regardless of its prevalence. In addition, people with diabetes face a slew of other potential complications. Skipping meals can put people with diabetes at risk for hypoglycemia, which can result in a variety of symptoms including mental confusion, impaired judgment, mood changes, seizures, coma, and possibly death (4).

Bulimia

Bulimia nervosa is characterized by episodes of binge eating, followed by a variety of compensatory methods to negate the increase in calories consumed (e.g., purging through vomiting, excessive exercise, using laxatives or enemas, starvation). A binge is defined as occurring during a discrete period of time, involves eating an amount of food that is significantly larger than what most people would eat during similar circumstances, and a sense of being out of control during the episode (71). Other symptoms that may become evident in the clinical setting include dehydration, abdominal pain, and the emergence of dental problems (as continuous vomiting wears away the tooth enamel) (74).

Bulimia is diagnosed in approximately 1% to 3% of the population, with males displaying one-tenth the rate for females (71). Since individuals with bulimia often appear physically healthy and are not grossly underweight, prevalence may, in fact, be much higher. In addition, 30% of those with bulimia show a lifetime diagnosis of comorbid disorders, such as substance abuse or dependence disorder (71).

A meta-analysis of controlled studies composed of 748 persons with diabetes and 1587 female participants found that patients with DM1 are significantly more likely to develop bulimia when compared to those without diabetes (75). In addition, it is also estimated that 60% to 80% of people with DM1 engage in episodes of binging at a subclinical rate (76). This binging and purging behavior makes it incredibly difficult to keep BG levels stable. This is because the activity of binging and purging makes it difficult to accurately gauge the amount of food a person is ingesting, and it becomes impossible to accurately assess the amount of insulin that is necessary. In addition, binges often include foods that are high in fats, which may have no immediate impact on blood sugar levels, but may cause them to rise hours later. The results of this can be disastrous. The inability of people with bulimia to keep their BG levels stable can result in BG levels that are perpetually too high, or too low. In turn, this leads to higher HbA1c levels and poorer overall glycemic control.

A recent study compared patients with DM1 and bulimia, to those with DM1 and binge eating disorder. Although both of these are serious forms of disordered eating, the study found that the presence of bulimia nervosa was highly associated with severe disturbances related to depression, anxiety, and eating disorders. In addition, the group with bulimia nervosa showed an overall higher rate or co-occurring mental disorders, psychosocial dysfunction and poorer overall glycemic control (77).

Eating Disorder Not Otherwise Specified

Some eating disorders have unique features that cause them to not fit one of the generally accepted categories of eating disorders (e.g., anorexia, bulimia). To address this problem, DSM-IV identifies a diagnosis known as eating disorder not otherwise specified (ED-NOS). Examples of eating disturbances that would fit this diagnostic profile include a person who purges after eating only a small amount of food or a person who has lost a significant amount of weight by starving themselves but their weight still technically falls in a healthy range.

The most common ED-NOS seen in people with DM1 is the reduction of insulin dosage to lose weight. Studies have found that up to 30% of adolescents with DM1 have intentionally reduced or omitted their insulin doses to control weight in adolescence or young adulthood (69). We have observed several variations of this in the clinical setting: (*i*) episodically omitting insulin administration; (*ii*) consistently under dosing for meals and snacks; or (*iii*) the omission of a bolus for meals albeit maintenance of basal doses by those using insulin pumps or basal/bolus formats of injection regimen (with Glargine basal doses and "per-meal" bolus injections with analogue insulin).

When this happens, blood glucose becomes hyperglycemic and ketones appear in the urine as body fat is broken-down for energy, placing individuals at greater risk for ketoacidosis, nephropathy, and other diabetic complications. Of tremendous clinical difficulty is that, despite the negative impact of insulin omission on glycemic control and risk for potentially irreversible complications, this tactic does successfully result in weight loss. For individuals with DM1 who are rigidly fixated upon weight loss, to the exclusion of long-term DM1-related health concerns, diagnosis and treatment of the eating disorder become imperative.

Relationship of Dysregulated Eating to Medical Outcomes

An eating disorder can be a life-threatening illness for anyone, but for a person with diabetes it is even more dangerous. Eating disorders greatly increase the mortality and morbidity rate among people with DM1. The majority of research has found that having an eating disorder is linked to increased medical complications for people with diabetes (78). As a result, screening for eating disorders should be implemented as part of routine care for people with diabetes in order to prevent the development or exacerbation of diabetes related complications secondary to dysregulated eating patterns. Multiple self-report measures that are reliable and valid are available to assist with screening and diagnosis of dysregulated eating; however, most are not specific to those with diabetes (79).

Treatment for Comorbid Diabetes and Dysregulated Eating

Once an eating disorder or any pattern of disordered eating is diagnosed, treatment should begin immediately. Patients may require inpatient treatment in either a medical or psychiatric hospital, if their eating disorder is particularly severe, or their health is at immediate risk. An example of this circumstance, which is most relevant to people with diabetes, is a person who has intentionally omitted so much insulin from their regimen that they have entered a state of ketosis and require an intravenous insulin drip in order to normalize their blood sugar.

After immediate physical danger has been eliminated or ruled out, long-term treatment can begin. Because of the increased risks associated with having both DM1 and an eating disorder, an interdisciplinary team should be utilized in order to address the complex nature of the problem. Ideally, the team should include a psychotherapist, diabetes educator, endocrinologist, and nutritionist. These professionals should be in regular communication with each other in order to ensure that treatment is progressing; and the physical, emotional and psychological needs of the patient are all being addressed. Depending on the age and circumstances of the patient, family, group, and/or couples therapy may be appropriate as well.

One small study compared 9 young women with bulimia nervosa who were receiving in-patient treatment to 10 young women with bulimia nervosa who were not. These patients were reassessed 3 years after treatment by examining their body mass index, HbA1c results, and psychological test scores. Patients who had received inpatient treatment had lower HbA1c results and demonstrated lower scores on measures assessing depression, anxiety, and binge eating and purging behaviors (80). Although the small sample size of this study makes it difficult to discern how generalizable the results are, these preliminary findings do suggest that inpatient treatment may be a more helpful form of treatment for women with diabetes who are suffering from bulimia nervosa.

CONCLUSION

DM1 is a complicated disease, which can represent a significant stressor for the individual and his/her family. A comprehensive understanding of how this disease impacts psychological factors, and the impact of psychological factors on medical outcomes is crucial in understanding and managing this disease. A well-developed literature has investigated the comorbidity between DM1 and several psychiatric diseases, and has shown that individuals with DM have a disproportionately higher rate of psychiatric disorders. Depression, anxiety, and dysregulated eating appear more prevalent among those with DM1, interfere with important outcomes such as quality of life, self-management, and glycemic control. In addition, psychological factors interact with adjustment to DM1, self-management, and metabolic control, even at subdiagnostic levels of symptomatology. Indeed, it appears nearly impossible to optimize medical outcomes without addressing the role of knowledge, coping, anxiety and mood, and dysregulated eating in the adult DM1 population. Diabetes treatment teams must maintain a high suspicion for these factors among adults with DM1, screen carefully, and treat aggressively, so as to prevent these nonpathophysiological factors from rendering treatment ineffective.

REFERENCES

1. Boyer BA. Theoretical models of health psychology and the model for integrating medicine and psychology. In: Boyer BA, Paharia MI, eds. Comprehensive Handbook of Clinical Health Psychology. Hoboken, NJ: Wiley, in press.
2. Boyer BA. Diabetes mellitus. In: Boyer BA, Paharia MI, eds. Comprehensive Handbook of Clinical Health Psychology. Hoboken, NJ: Wiley, in press.
3. Schilling LS, Grey M, Knafl KA. The concept of self-management of type 1 diabetes in children and adolescents: An evolutionary concept analysis. J Adv Nurs 2002;37(1):87–99.
4. Scheiner G, Goldstein B. Think Like a Pancreas: A Practical Guide to Managing Diabetes with Insulin. New York: Marlowe & Company, 2004.
5. Hanson CL, Henggeler SW, Burghen GA. Social competence and parental support as mediators of the link between stress and metabolic control in adolescents with insulin-dependent diabetes mellitus. J Consult Clin Psychol 1987;55(4):529–533.
6. Grey DL, Marrero DG, Godfrey C, et al. Chronic poor metabolic control in the pediatric population. Diabetes Educ 1988:14:516–520.
7. Johnson SB. Insulin-dependent diabetes mellitus in childhood. In: Roberts MC, ed. Handbook of Pediatric Psychology, 2nd edn. New York: Guilford Press, 1995, pp. 263–285.
8. Christensen K. Self-management in diabetic children. Diabetes Care 1983;6:552–555.
9. Harkavy J, Johnson SB, Silverstein J, et al. Who learns what at diabetes summer camp. J Pediatr Psychol 1983;8(2):143–153.
10. Anderson BJ, Miller JP, Auslander WF, et al. Family characteristics of diabetic adolescents: Relationship to metabolic control. Diabetes Care 1981;4(6):586–594.
11. Wysocki T, Greco P, Buckloh LM. Childhood diabetes in psychological context. In: Roberts MC, ed. Handbook of Pediatric Psychology, 3rd edn. New York: Guilford Press, 2003, pp. 304–320.
12. Coelho R, Amorim I, Prata J. Coping styles and quality of life in patients with non-insulin-dependent diabetes mellitus. Psychosomatics 2003;44(4);312–318.
13. Seiffge-Krenke I, Stemmler M. Coping with everyday stress and links to medical and psychosocial adaptation in diabetic adolescents. J Adolesc Health 2003;33(3):180–188.
14. Boardway RH, Delamater AM, Tomakowsky J, et al. Stress management training for adolescents with diabetes. J Pediatr Psychol 1993;1:29–45.
15. Grey M, Boland EA, Davidson M, et al. Coping skills training for youth with diabetes mellitus has long-lasting effects on metabolic control and quality of life. J Pediatr 2000;137:107–113.
16. Rubin RR, Peyrot M. Psychological issues and treatments for people with diabetes. J Clin Psychol 2001;57(4):457–478.
17. De Mont-Marin F, Hardy P, Lepine JP, et al. Six-month and lifetime prevalences of psychiatric disorders in inpatients with diabetes mellitus. Eur Psychiatry 1995;10:245–249.

18. Friedman S, Vila G, Timsit J, et al. Anxiety and depression disorders in an adult insulin-dependent diabetes mellitus (IDDM) population: Relationships with glycemic control and somatic complications. Eur Psychiatry 1998;13:295–302.
19. Lustman PJ, Griffith LS, Clouse RE, et al. Psychiatric illness in diabetes mellitus: Relationship to symptoms and glucose control. J Nerv Ment Dis 1986;174(12):736–742.
20. Gavard JA, Lustman PJ, Clouse RE. Prevalence of depression in adults with diabetes: An epidemiological evaluation. Diabetes Care 1993;16:1167–1178.
21. Anderson RJ, Freedland KE, Clouse RE, et al. The prevalence of comorbid depression in adults with diabetes: A meta-analysis. Diabetes Care 2001;24(6):1069–1078.
22. Barnard KD, Skinner TC, Peveler R. The prevalence of co-morbid depression in adults with type 1 diabetes: Systematic literature review. Diabet Med 2006;23:445–448.
23. Kovacs M, Goldston D, Obrosky DS, et al. Psychiatric disorders in youths with IDDM: Rates and risk factors. Diabetes Care 1997;20:36–44.
24. Peyrot M, Rubin RR. Levels and risks of depression and anxiety symptomatology among diabetic adults. Diabetes Care 1997;20:585–590.
25. Roy M, Collier B, Roy A. Excess of depressive symptoms and life events among diabetics. Compr Psychiatry 1994;35(2):129–131.
26. Wilkinson G, Borsey DQ, Leslie P, et al. Psychiatric morbidity and social problems in patients with insulin-dependent diabetes mellitus. Br J Psychiatry 1988;153:38–43.
27. Ciechanowski PS, Katon WJ, Russo JE. Depression and diabetes: Impact of depressive symptoms on adherence, function, and costs. Arch Intern Med 2000;160:3278–3285.
28. de Groot M, Jacobson AM, Samson JA, et al. Glycemic control and major depression in patients with type 1 and type 2 diabetes mellitus. J Psychosom Res 1999;46(5):425–435.
29. Lustman PJ, Anderson RJ, Freedland KE, et al. Depression and poor glycemic control: A meta-analytic review of the literature. Diabetes Care 2000;23:934–942.
30. Lustman PJ, Clouse RE, Ciechanowski PS, et al. Depression-related hyperglycemia in type 1 diabetes: A mediational approach. Psychosom Med 2005;67(2):195–199.
31. de Groot M, Anderson RJ, Freedland KE, et al. Association of depression and diabetes complications: A meta-analysis. Psychosom Med 2001;63:619–630.
32. Lustman PJ, Griffith LS, Freedland KE, et al. The course of major depression in diabetes. Gen Hosp Psychiatry 1997;19:138–143.
33. Peyrot M, Rubin RR. Persistence of depressive symptoms in diabetic adults. Diabetes Care 1999;22(3):448–452.
34. Goodnick PJ. Diabetes mellitus and depression: Issues in theory and treatment. Psychiatr Ann 1997;27(5):353–359.
35. Steed L, Cooke D, Newman S. A systematic review of psychosocial outcomes following education, self-management and psychological interventions in diabetes mellitus. Patient Educ Couns 2003;51(1):5–15.
36. Katon WJ, Simon G, Russo J, et al. Quality of depression care in a population-based sample of patients with diabetes and major depression. Med Care 2004;42(12):1222–1229.
37. Goodnick PJ, Henry JH, Buki VMV. Treatment of depression in patients with diabetes mellitus. J Clin Psychiatry 1995;56(4):128–135.
38. Lustman PJ, Freedland KE, Griffith LS, et al. Predicting response to cognitive behavior therapy of depression in type 2 diabetes. Gen Hosp Psychiatry 1998;20:302–306.
39. Lustman PJ, Griffith LS, Clouse RE, et al. Effects of nortriptyline of depression and glycemic control in diabetes: Results of a double-blind, placebo-controlled trial. Psychosom Med 1997;59: 241–250.
40. Harris MD. Psychosocial aspects of diabetes with an emphasis on depression. Curr Diab Rep 2003;3:49–55.
41. Lin EH, Katon W, Rutter C, et al. Effects of enhanced depression treatment on diabetes self-care. Ann Fam Med 2006;4(1):46–53.
42. Katon WJ, Von Korff M, Lin EH, et al. The Pathways Study: A randomized trial of collaborative care in patients with diabetes and depression. Arch Gen Psychiatry 2004;61(10): 1042–1049.

43. Musselman DL, Betan E, Larsen H, et al. Relationship of depression to diabetes types 1 and 2: Epidemiology, biology, and treatment. Biol Psychiatry 2003;54(3):317–329.
44. Lustman PJ, Freedland KE, Griffith LS, et al. Fluoxetine for depression in diabetes: A randomized double-blind placebo-controlled trial. Diabetes Care 2000;23(5):618–623.
45. Lustman PJ, Griffith LS, Freedland KE, et al. Cognitive behavior therapy for depression in type 2 diabetes mellitus. A randomized, controlled trial. Ann Intern Med 1998;129(8):613–621.
46. van der Ven NC, Lubach CH, Hogenelst MH, et al. Cognitive behavioural group training (CBGT) for patients with type 1 diabetes in persistent poor glycaemic control: Who do we reach? Patient Educ Couns 2005;56(3):313–322.
47. Keller MB, McCullough JP, Klein DN, et al. A comparison of nefazodone, the cognitive behavioral-analysis system of psychotherapy, and their combination for the treatment of chronic depression. N Engl J Med 2000;342(20):1462–1470.
48. Grigsby AB, Anderson RJ, Freedland KE, et al. Prevalence of anxiety in adults with diabetes: A systematic review. J Psychosom Res 2002;53:1053–1060.
49. Polonsky WH, Davis CL, Jacobson AM, et al. Correlates of hypoglycemic fear in type I and type II diabetes mellitus. Health Psychol 1992;11(3):199–202.
50. Irvine AA, Cox D, Gonder-Frederick L. Fear of hypoglycemia: Relationship to physical and psychological symptoms in patients with insulin-dependent diabetes mellitus. Health Psychol 1992;11(2):135–138.
51. Cox DJ, Irvine A, Gonder-Frederick LA, et al. Fear of hypoglycemia: Quantification, validation, and utilization. Diabetes Care 1987;10(5):617–621.
52. Surwit RS, Scovern AW, Feinglos MN. The role of behavior in diabetes care. Diabetes Care 1982;5:337–342.
53. Myers VH, Boyer BA, Herbert JD, et al. Adults with insulin-dependent diabetes mellitus: Post-traumatic stress related to hypoglycemia using intensive management regimens. J Clin Psychol Med Settings 2007;14(1):11–21.
54. Anderson RJ, Grigsby AB, Freedland KE, et al. Anxiety and poor glycemic control: A meta-analytic review of the literature. Int J Psychiatry Med 2002;32:235–247.
55. Boyle S, Allan C, Millar K. Cognitive-behavioural interventions in a patient with an anxiety disorder related to diabetes. Behav Res Ther 2004;42(3):357–366.
56. Collins RL, Ricciardelli LA. Assessment of eating disorders and obesity. In: Donovan DM, Marlatt GA, eds. Assessment of Addictive Behaviors. 2nd edn. New York: Guilford Press, 2005:305–333.
57. Khan Y, Montgomery AMJ. Eating attitudes in young females with diabetes: Insulin omission identifies a vulnerable subgroup. Br J Med Psychol 1996;69(4):343–353.
58. http://diabetes.niddk.nih.gov/dm/pubs/statistics/index.htm (2006).
59. Haas HL, Clopton JR. Psychology of an eating disorder. In: Robert-McComb JJ, ed. Eating Disorders in Women and Children: Prevention, Stress Management, and Treatment. New York: CRC Press, 2001:39–48.
60. De Castro JM, Goldstein SJ. Eating attitudes and behaviors of pre-and post-pubertal females: Clues to the etiology of eating disorders. Physiol Behav 1995;58(1):15–23.
61. Freeman RJ, Beach B, Davis R, et al. The prediction of relapse in bulimia nervosa. J Psychiatr Res 1985;19:349–353.
62. Keller MB, Herzog DB, Lavori PW, et al. The naturalistic history of bulimia nervosa: Extraordinarily high rates of chronicity, relapse, recurrence, and psychosocial morbidity. Int J Eat Disord 1992;12:1–9.
63. Mitchell JE, Davis L, Goff G. The process of relapse in patients with bulimia nervosa. Int J Eat Disord 1985;4:457–463.
64. Pyle RL, Mitchell JE, Eckert ED, et al. Maintenance treatment and 6-month outcome for bulimic patients who respond to initial treatment. Am J Psychiatry 1990;147:871–875.
65. Richard M, Bauer S, Kordy H. Relapse in anorexia and bulimia nervosa: A 2.5-year follow-up. Eur Eat Disord Rev 2005;13:180–190.
66. Neumark-Sztainer D, Story M, Falkner NH, et al. Disordered eating among adolescents with chronic illness and disability. Arch Pediatr Adolesc Med 1998;152:871–878.

67. Diabetes Control and Complications Trial Research Group (DCCT). The effect of intensive treatment of diabetes on the development and progression of long-term complications in insulin-dependent diabetes mellitus. N Engl J Med 1993;329:977–986.

68. Daneman D, Olmsted M, Rydall A, et al. Eating disorders in young women with type 1 diabetes. Horm Res 1988;50(1):79–86.

69. Kelly SD, Howe SJ, Hendler JP, et al. Disordered eating behaviors in youth with type 1 diabetes. Diabetes Educ 2005;34(4):572–583.

70. Colton PA. Eating disturbances in young women with diabetes mellitus: Mechanics and consequences. Psychiatr Ann 1999;29(4):213–218.

71. American Psychiatric Association. Diagnostic and Statistical Manual of Mental Health Disorders, 4th edn. Washington, DC: American Psychiatric Society, 2000.

72. Nielsen S. Eating disorders in females with type 1 diabetes: An update of a meta-analysis. Eur Eat Disord Rev 2002;10(4):241–254.

73. Nielsen S, Emborg C, Molback AG. Mortality in concurrent type 1 diabetes and anorexia nervosa. Diabetes Care 2002;25:309–312.

74. Garfinkel PE. Classification and diagnosis of eating disorders. In: Brownell KD, Fairburn CG, eds. Eating Disorders and Obesity: A Comprehensive Handbook. New York: Guilford Press, 1995:125–134.

75. Mannucci E, Rotella F, Ricca V, et al. Eating disorders in patients with type 1 diabetes: A meta-analysis. J Endocrinol Invest 2005;28(5):417–419.

76. La Greca AM, Schwarz LT, Satin W. Eating patterns in young women with IDDM: Another look. Diabetes Care 1987;10(5):659–660.

77. Takii M, Komaki G, Uchigata Y, et al. Differences between bulimia nervosa and binge-eating disorder in females with type 1 diabetes: The important role of insulin omission. J Psychosom Res 1999;47(3):221–231.

78. Rydall AC, Rodin GM, Olmsted MP, et al. Disordered eating behavior and microvascular complications in young women with insulin-dependent diabetes mellitus N Engl J Med 1997;336(26):1849–1854.

79. Kelly SD, Howe CJ, Hendler JP, et al. Disordered eating behaviors in youth with type 1 diabetes. Diabetes Educ 2005;31(4):572–583.

80. Takii M, Uchigata Y, Komaki G, et al. An integrated inpatient therapy for type 1 diabetic females with bulimia nervosa: A 3-year follow-up study. J Psychosom Res 2003;55(4):349–356.

14

Beta-Cell Replacement: Pancreas and Islet Transplantation

R. Paul Robertson
Pacific Northwest Research Institute, University of Washington, Seattle, Washington, U.S.A.

CLINICAL INDICATIONS FOR BETA-CELL REPLACEMENT

Given the very limited availability of donated pancreas, which has been estimated to be roughly 4000 to 6000 a year in the United States of America, relatively few patients with diabetes should be considered for beta-cell replacement. There are three general clinical situations that justify this approach. The first is recurrent hypoglycemia with poor symptom recognition despite optimal medical care. This is a complex area to consider. Recurrent hypoglycemia in diabetic patients is a direct consequence of administration of exogenous insulin. In circumstances where too much insulin has been given, patients inevitably become hypoglycemic. When patients become recurrently hypoglycemic, they develop a decrease in the perception of symptoms related to hypoglycemia. Normally, hypoglycemia causes warmth, hunger, sweating, and rapid heart rate. When hypoglycemia becomes very severe, additional symptoms such as visual loss, lethargy, coma, and even death can occur. With recurrent hypoglycemia, patients become desensitized so that the symptoms begin to occur at lower and lower glucose levels. Usually, humans experience symptoms of hypoglycemia when the blood glucose level drops below 55 to 57 mg/dL. When symptoms begin at glucose levels in this range, ample time is available to remedy the situation by ingesting substances containing sucrose. However, if the symptoms do not begin to develop until the blood glucose level is as low as 30 mg/dL, it continues to decrease, and not much time is left to stop this process before extremely dangerous levels of hypoglycemia are reached.

Patients who have lost symptom recognition of hypoglycemia can fully regain it if hyperglycemia is avoided for several weeks. This intervention may result in somewhat higher levels of hemoglobin A1c, but this need not necessarily be the case. On the other hand, there remains a subcategory of recurrently hypoglycemic patients who have a great deal of difficulty maintaining acceptable levels of hemoglobin A1c when they decrease exogenous insulin dosage to a degree sufficient to avoid hypoglycemia. This is especially frequent in patients with autonomic dysfunction that can result in gastroparesis and diabetic diarrhea. In these cases, the pathophysiology of recurrent hypoglycemia is related to the variation in gastrointestinal transit time of ingested food. This variability in food transit time makes it extremely difficult if not impossible to effectively match insulin dosage to dietary intake and absorption. Beta-cell replacement can be considered the optimal therapy for such patients because the replaced beta cells will be exquisitely sensitive to circulating glucose levels and thereby very quickly and appropriately alter the amount of insulin being released into the blood. This obviously is not the case when insulin is injected exogenously in subcutaneous tissue. Following pancreas and islet transplantation, patients with recurrent hypoglycemia and symptom unawareness report a marked decrease in the frequency of hypoglycemia and a return of symptoms initiated by hypoglycemia.

The second general indication for beta-cell replacement is an unrelenting march of secondary complications of diabetes. This is most often observed in patients who have developed kidney failure and are candidates for kidney transplantation. The most common clinical scenario in which the pancreas is transplanted is the one in which patients are scheduled for kidney transplantation. The rationale for performing simultaneous pancreas and kidney transplantation is that since the recipient will be immunosuppressed for kidney transplantation, no independent justification for immunosuppression for pancreas transplantation is needed. In addition, just as the native kidney of the recipient was harmed by hyperglycemia, the transplanted kidney will be at-risk for developing diabetic nephropathy if the recipient is allowed to remain hyperglycemic. Inclusion of a transplanted pancreas with the transplanted kidney, therefore, serves to protect the transplanted kidney from hyperglycemia.

The third and most difficult clinical indication for beta-cell replacement is psychiatric or emotional disability that prevents patients from cooperating with insulin-based therapy. When such patients begin to develop secondary complications, the ethical and medical decision must be made whether or not to offer them beta-cell replacement. Clearly, such a decision must be preceded by careful evaluation of the patient to be sure they are cooperating to the best of their ability to maintain normoglycemia by conventional measures. Concern has been raised that patients with psychiatric or emotional disabilities will be incapable of maintaining immunosuppressive drug treatment if they are not able to cooperate with exogenous insulin therapy. Experience has demonstrated that this is not necessarily the case because the personal burden of ingesting immunosuppressive drugs is not nearly as great as maintaining rigorous insulin-based regimens.

CLINICAL BURDEN OF IMMUNOSUPPRESSION

Recipients must be systemically immunosuppressed to maintain function of transplanted beta cells, otherwise they will undergo allorejection. Immunosuppression regimens have been vastly improved over the past half century so that now the worldwide pancreas rejection rate 3 years posttransplant is generally less than 30%, and in some centers as low as less than 10%. Nonetheless, immunosuppression carries with it the problems of increased susceptibility to infections, particularly cytomegalic inclusion viral disease. Typically, the difficulties patients have with viral infections are worse during the first year posttransplant, and thereafter become much less intense. Immunosuppressed patients are also at increased risk for developing cancer, although this appears to be a frequent problem only in the case of skin cancer such as basal cell carcinoma and melanoma. There are also drug-specific problems. Most notable among these is a decrease in glomerular function when calcineurin inhibitors, such as cyclosporin and tacrolimus, are used. MMF or mycophenolate can be associated with severe gastrointestinal distress. Rapamycin or sirolimus, can be associated with severe oral ulcers. Long-term use of steroids for immunosuppression can cause severe osteopenia. Currently, transplant centers have demonstrated that with the newer immunosuppressive regimens, steroids can be avoided so that metabolic bone disease will become less of a problem in future years. The clinical burden of immunosuppressive drugs also includes a financial cost. These drugs must be taken continually for as long as the transplanted organ is functional, otherwise the organ will undergo allorejection. This cost has been variously estimated to run $10,000 to $15,000 annually. However, it has also been estimated that this cost is much less than the alternative cost, for example, of forgoing kidney transplantation and maintaining patients on dialysis programs for the indeterminate future.

PANCREAS TRANSPLANTATION

The most common scenario in which a pancreas is transplanted is simultaneous pancreas and kidney (SPK) transplantation as described above. Another variation is pancreas after kidney (PAK) transplantation. In other situations, clinical complications other than kidney failure may indicate the need for pancreas transplantation alone (PTA). In 2001, of 1297 pancreas transplants reported, the distribution by procedure was 70% SPK, 22% PAK, 8% PTA in the United States (1).

Organ and Patient Survival Rates

Pancreas transplantation was first performed in 1966 (2). Since then organ survival rates have improved dramatically. Currently, pancreas survival rates at 1 year posttransplant are 92%, 88%, and 91% and at 5 years are 70%, 45%, and 45%, respectively, for the procedures of SPK, PTA, and PKA (1) (Fig. 1) The most common cause for organ failure in the first year following transplantation is the technical failure of the transplant itself. Great vigilance and efforts are expended during the initial transplant period to detect threatened rejection

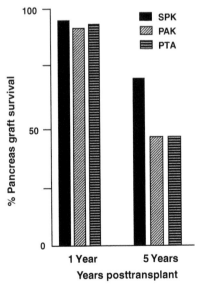

Figure 1 Pancreas graft survival rates following SPK, PAK, and PTA. The data at 3-years posttransplantation indicate an approximately 90% graft survival rate for all three categories. The 5-year data indicate a fall off to 70% for SPK and to 45% for PAK and PTA (1). *Abbreviations*: SPK, simultaneous pancreas and kidney transplantation; PAK, pancreas after kidney transplantation; PTA, pancreas transplantation alone.

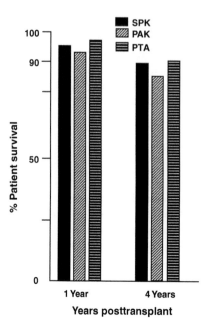

Figure 2   Patient survival rates after undergoing the SPK, PAK, and PTA procedures. At 1 year, the patient survival rate is approximately 95% for all three procedures. At 4-years posttransplant, the survival rates are 90%, 85%, and 90% for SPK, PAK, and PTA, respectively (1). *Abbreviations*: SPK, simultaneous pancreas and kidney transplantation; PAK, pancreas after kidney transplantation; PTA, pancreas transplantation alone.

of the organ. During these times, immunosuppressive therapy is intensified until the blood glucose level returns to normal. In the most common instance where both the pancreas and kidney are transplanted simultaneously, blood creatinine levels also serve as a sentinel for impending allorejection; immunosuppression is intensified until the blood creatinine returns to prerejection levels. These levels will not necessarily be normal because of the use of calcineurin inhibitors. Typically, creatinine levels are 1.5 to 1.9 mg/dL in patients immunosuppressed by calcineurin inhibitors. Another indicator for impending rejection is an increase in urinary amylase in instances where the exocrine drainage of the transplanted pancreas is diverted into the urinary bladder. The predictive benefits of urinary amylase are not available when the exocrine drainage is diverted into the duodenum—a commonly used alternative site.

Patient survival rates for pancreas transplantation at 1 year posttransplant are 95%, 94%, and 98% and at 4 years are 90%, 85%, and 90% for SPK, PAK, and PTA, respectively (1) (Fig. 2). The degree to which patient mortality is related to the transplantation procedure itself as opposed to secondary complications of chronic diabetes has not been established. However, it is unusual for patients to die in the operative or immediate postoperative period. Typically, patients who die experience a cardiovascular death at times 3 months beyond the pancreas transplantation. A recent retrospective study examined whether there is excessive patient mortality following pancreas transplantation (3). The study compared patient mortality in patients on waiting lists for pancreas transplantation compared to patients who received a pancreas transplant. In the most common procedure of SPK, a statistically significant increase in the 3-month posttransplant mortality was reported in patients having undergone pancreas transplantation compared to those who remained on the waiting list. However, mortality in posttransplant time periods thereafter were significantly less in recipients than patients on the waiting list. The degree to which the conclusions of this study are accurate has been called into question (4) because of several concerns. First, no control was in place for individuals on the waiting list who, when given the opportunity to be transplanted, chose to pass up this opportunity and to remain on the waiting list because they did not feel the need to go through with this procedure. This could have enriched the waiting list with healthier patients. Second, 8% of the people on the waiting list left it to undergo kidney transplantation, so would have been among the sickest of the patients waiting. Third, some patients on waiting lists were listed on multiple lists and therefore counted more than once. All three of these factors tend to bias the data toward improved survival in patients on the waiting list compared to those patients who elected to undergo pancreas transplantation.

Clinical Outcomes of Successful Pancreas Transplantation

Glycemic Control

The two most often used measures of glycemic control are the fasting glucose level and the hemoglobin A1c level. Typically, recipients of successful pancreas transplants have average fasting levels of 80 mg/dL, which signals excellent glycemic control (5) (Fig. 3). Similarly, hemoglobin A1c levels are typically in the normal range, usually between 5.5% and 6%. The excellence of these outcomes can be appreciated by comparing hemoglobin A1c levels after pancreas transplantation with those obtained in the Diabetes Control and Complications Trial (DCCT) (5,6) (Fig. 4). Intensive insulin-based management augmented by frequent patient contact with physicians, nurses, and social workers was studied in the DCCT and outcomes were compared to less rigorous insulin-based management. The intensively treated patients were able to achieve average hemoglobin A1c levels of 7%. Attempts to achieve lower levels were met with an increasing incidence of clinical hypoglycemia. In contrast, hypoglycemia following pancreas transplantation is an unusual event. These outcomes clearly illustrate the advantage of beta-cell replacement over exogenous insulin-based management.

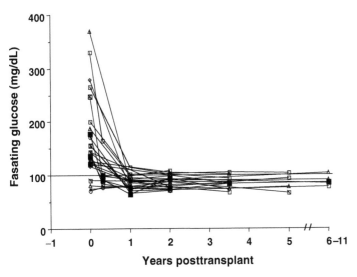

Figure 3 Levels of fasting plasma glucose in recipients before and up to 11-years postpancreas transplantation. By the end of the first posttransplant year, virtually all fasting glucose levels are below 100 mg/dL and average approximately 80 mg/dL (5).

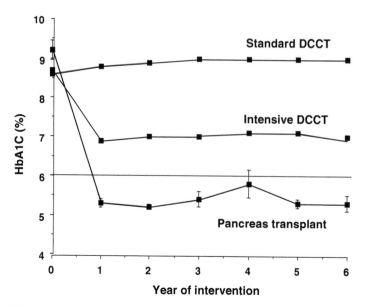

Figure 4   Levels of hemoglobin A1c up to 6-years postintervention with either standard or intensive medical therapy versus pancreas transplantation. The comparison of standard and intensive insulin therapy was the major focus of the DCCT. The data indicated that intensive insulin therapy could provide, at best, levels of hemoglobin A1c in the 7% range. By comparison, successful pancreas transplantation lowers hemoglobin A1c levels into the normal range (5,6). *Abbreviation*: DCCT, diabetes care and complicatioons trial.

Beta-Cell Function

When assessing beta-cell function in humans, plasma levels of insulin and C-peptide are determined from a variety of tests such as the oral glucose tolerance test, the intravenous glucose tolerance test, and the meal tolerance test. Insulin levels are measured most often. C-peptide levels are measured when patients take exogenous insulin as treatment. Injected insulin does not contain C-peptide, whereas C-peptide and insulin molecules are released in a constant molar ratio from the beta cell during endogenous insulin secretion. During the oral glucose tolerance and the meal tolerance tests, enough samples are taken to calculate areas under the curve for hormone secretion. When intravenous glucose tolerance is assessed, sampling times are more frequent so that first phase (the first 5 minutes after the glucose challenge) and the second phase (the subsequent 85 minutes after the intravenous challenge) of insulin secretion can be measured.

The usual recipient of a pancreas transplant has type 1 diabetes mellitus and, therefore, has no living beta cells and no stimulatable insulin secretion. After successful pancreas transplantation, recipients typically have normal-to-supernormal first-phase insulin response to intravenous glucose and elevated second phase (7) (Fig. 5). The reason for the greater than normal insulin levels is that the venous effluent from the transplanted pancreas is drained via a systemic vein (usually the iliac vein) rather than the hepatic portal vein, as is the case for the native pancreas. As the blood passes through the hepatic circulation, 50% to 90% of insulin is degraded during the first pass. When a transplanted pancreas has systemic venous drainage, only 20% of the secreted insulin is delivered to the liver during the first pass. Despite this surgically created state of relative hyperinsulinemia in pancreas recipients, hypoglycemia is not usually a problem in the fasting state and only rarely in the postprandial state (8). Reported results from the oral glucose tolerance test in successful

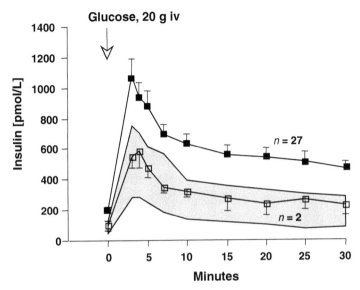

Figure 5 Circulating insulin levels before and after an intravenous injection of glucose, 20 g. Within the first 5 minutes, first phase insulin secretion has reached its peak, which in turn is followed by second phase insulin secretion throughout the ensuing 30 minutes. Shaded area represents the mean ± 95% response for normal controls. The upper line with the closed boxes represents data from 27 recipients of pancreas transplantation. The line describing the responses from the open boxes represent data from two patients with portal venous drainage of the allograft. Basal circulating levels are higher in the pancreas recipients who had systemic venous drainage of the graft, whereas the two patients with portal venous drainage were in the normal range. Recipients with systemic venous drainage also had elevated insulin levels in the basal state prior to the intravenous glucose injection (7).

recipients of pancreas transplantation are varied but most show normal or nearly normal oral glucose tolerance in successful pancreas recipients.

Alpha-Cell Function

The principal product secreted by the alpha cell is glucagon and the primary stimulus for glucagon secretion is hypoglycemia. Glucagon secretion from the native pancreas is released into the hepatic portal vein through which it quickly reaches the liver to stimulate glycogenolysis. The resultant increase in glucose production releases glucose into the hepatic vein and thence the systemic circulation, thereby correcting hypoglycemia. The transplanted pancreas secretes glucagon in sufficient quantities to counterregulate hypoglycemia. Thus, successful pancreas transplantation not only restores beta-cell function but also alpha-cell function. The combination of restored alpha and beta-cell function are the major determinants in the reestablishment of normoglycemia and lack of hypoglycemia that the recipient enjoys posttransplantation. Assessment of glucagon secretion is most accurately made by the hypoglycemic, hyperinsulinemic clamp. This is a test in which insulin is infused at a sufficient rate to lower circulating glucose levels and at the same time glucose is also infused to ensure that glucose levels are not lowered too rapidly or too far. During this study, termed the hypoglycemic clamp, samples of blood are drawn for determination of glucagon and epinephrine levels and the patient's symptoms are carefully monitored. As mentioned earlier, patients with type 1 diabetes typically have no glucagon response and delayed counterregulation of hypoglycemia. In addition, their epinephrine response,

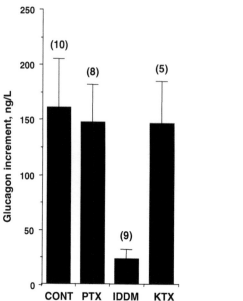
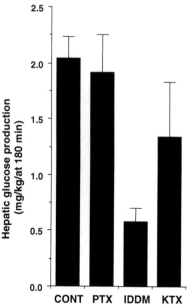

Figure 6 Comparison of the increases in glucagon secretion and in hepatic glucose production during hypoglycemia induced by a hyperinsulinemic, hypoglycemic clamp. Patients with IDDM had markedly diminished glucagon responses compared to CONTs, PTX, and KTX receiving the same immunosuppressive regimens. There were no significant differences between the subjects in the PTX and KTX groups compared to CONT. Similarly, patients in the CONT and PTX groups were not significantly different with regards to hepatic glucose production whereas patients with IDDM had markedly suppressed values. Patients with KTX had intermediate values (7,8). *Abbreviatons*: IDDM, type 1 diabetes; CONT, control subject; PTX, pancreas transplantation recipients; KTX, kidney transplant recipients.

a secondary line of defense against hypoglycemia that also stimulates glycogenolysis, is greatly diminished. After successful pancreas transplantation, glucagon responses and symptom recognition are normal and epinephrine responses are improved during insulin-induced hypoglycemia. This leads to normalization of hepatic glucose production during hypoglycemia (9,10) (Fig. 6).

Nephropathy

Nephropathy associated with chronic diabetes is manifested clinically by elevated serum creatinine, decreased creatinine clearance, and albuminuria as well as structural changes in the glomerulus involving excessive accumulation of mesangium and increased basement membrane thickness. In some instances, PTA has been performed in patients who have progressive renal failure that has not yet required kidney transplantation. Studies comparing recipients of transplanted kidneys versus recipients of both transplanted kidney and pancreas, as well as longitudinal studies of PTA, demonstrate that pancreas recipients have normalization of glycemia and stabilization and even reversal of basement membrane thickness and mesangial accumulation in their native kidneys, whereas kidney alone recipients do not (11,12). This is not necessarily accompanied by an improvement in renal function, however, such patients are generally maintained on calcineurin inhibitors for immunosuppression, which themselves decrease glomerular function. Nonetheless, this positive outcome in terms of renal structure provides the optimistic prediction that patients being

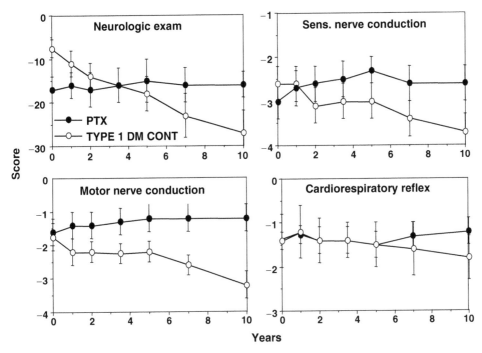

Figure 7 The 10-year posttransplant assessment of neurologic status by physical exam, sensory nerve conduction, motor nerve conduction, and cardiorespiratory reflex. In all instances, successful recipients of pancreas transplantation had stable scores for 10 years after successful pancreas transplant whereas a cohort of type 1 diabetic control subjects who had not undergone pancreas transplant in general had steadily deteriorating values (13).

managed with conventional insulin-based therapy rather than beta-cell replacement can look forward to improved renal structure should they be able to maintain near normal levels of hemoglobin A1c.

Neuropathy

Patients who achieve normal glucose levels after pancreas transplantation often volunteer that they experience stabilization if not improvement in neuropathies. This has been documented in one 10-year study that reported stabilization of neural function as reflected by physical examination as well as by studies of motor and sensory nerve conduction and autonomic nerve function (13) (Fig. 7). More dramatically, patient survival has been reported to be significantly increased by pancreas transplantation in diabetic patients who have the syndrome of autonomic insufficiency (14).

Retinopathy

Early studies of the effects of successful pancreas transplantation on retinopathy failed to detect a statistically significant beneficial effect (15), although the data indicated a trend in that direction. A more recent study reported statistically significant beneficial effects on retinopathy. In this study, patients receiving kidney alone transplantation were compared to patients receiving kidney and pancreas transplants (16) (Fig. 8). The parameters used were fundoscopic changes and the need for additional laser therapy posttransplant. Using both measures, patients receiving pancreas and kidney transplantation had significant

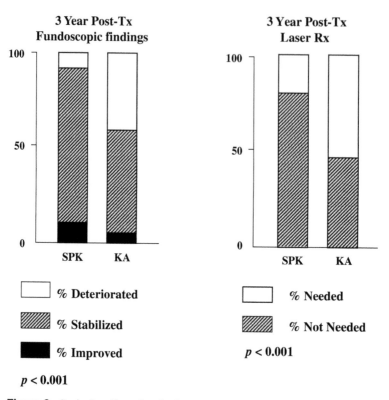

Figure 8   Retinal studies using fundoscopy and the need for laser therapy as measures of successful 3 years after successful transplantation with either pancreas and kidney together or kidney alone. The pancreas transplant recipients established normal circulating glucose levels whereas the kidney transplant recipients did not. By fundoscopic findings, SPK recipients had less deterioration and more stabilization of retinal lesions. Successful pancreas transplant recipients had less need for further laser therapy (16).

improvements in retinal structure and less need for laser treatment compared to the group receiving kidney transplantation alone.

Macrovascular Disease

It has been difficult to detect a statistically significantly improvement in macrovascular outcomes, even in large therapeutic trials comparing conventional versus intensive medical-based management of diabetic patients, (6,17). This has also been true in studies of pancreas transplantation. However, macrovascular benefits were reported in one longitudinal study of patients receiving simultaneous pancreas and kidney transplant (18) (Fig. 9). Coronary atherosclerosis, assessed by quantitative coronary angiography, documented that narrowing of the interior diameter of the coronary arteries continued to increase in patients who lost their pancreatic graft, whereas the group that retained the transplanted pancreas had no mean change in intracoronary artery diameter after a mean follow-up of approximately 4 years.

Quality of Life

Quality of life studies in recipients of simultaneous pancreas and kidney and pancreas alone transplantation have invariably reported improvement in quality of life (19,20). Such studies

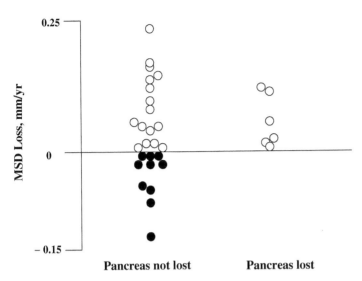

Figure 9 Qualification of coronary atherosclerosis as assessed by quantitative coronary angiography in PTX who had or had not lost the transplanted graft with a mean follow-up of 4-years posttransplantation. Data are expressed as MSD loss. As a group, the successful PTX stabilized with no worsening of MSD, whereas the patients who were successfully transplanted but lost their graft continued to have an increase in MSD loss, indicating further narrowing of coronary arteries (18). *Abbreviations*: PTX, pancreas transplant recipients; MSD, mean segmental diameter.

take into account many outcomes, including the adverse impact of using immunosuppressive drugs and the surgery itself. The issue of longevity of life is more difficult to assess because trials of pancreas transplantation have never been randomized or controlled with a contemporary group of cohorts that is medically managed.

ISLET TRANSPLANTATION

There is great interest in transplanting isolated pancreatic islets instead of transplanting the organ. The rationale for this approach is that it will be less invasive and less costly in terms of morbidity and financial expense. The first successful allogeneic islet transplantation in diabetic animals was published in 1972 (21), and was followed by successful autoislet transplantation in humans in 1980 (22). Between 1980 and 2000 many attempts were made to establish alloislet transplantation in diabetic patients, but the success rate was minimal. In 2000, a study was published from the University of Alberta in Edmonton reporting 100% success in 7 patients who were on average 12-months posttransplant (23). The major differences in this study were the elimination of glucocorticosteroids from the immunosuppression regimen, use of daclizumab, and multiple infusions (usually two) of islets. Over the time, however, this initial success of intrahepatic alloislet transplantation diminished to approximately 80% at 2-years posttransplant and to 8% at 5-years posttransplant (24) (Fig. 10). However, at 5 years, 85% of the recipients still had measurable C-peptide in their blood and were taking roughly half as much insulin as they had pretransplant. The reasons for the fall off in the success rate are not yet clear. Candidates are allorejection, return of autoimmune damage to the new islets, loss of islets due to trauma during the isolation procedure, and toxicity of immunosuppressive drugs. The latter is an important issue because therapeutic concentrations of the drugs tend to be toxic to beta cells in the

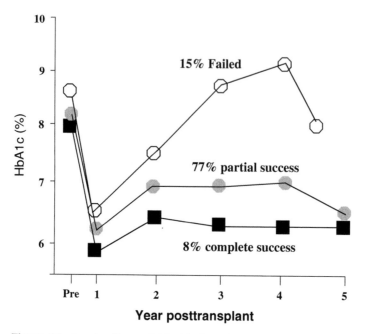

Figure 10 Levels of hemoglobin A1c from the Edmonton patients 5 years after intrahepatic islet transplantation. At this time, 85% of the patients remain C-peptide positive but only 8% were independent of exogenous insulin treatment. 15% of recipients were reported as failures because they had no sign of islet function and returned to full doses of insulin therapy. Seventy-seven percent were deemed partially successful because they were still C-peptide positive, although they returned to using half of their usual dose of daily insulin. Eight percent of patients remain insulin-free and maintained hemoglobin A1c levels in a nearly normal range (24).

native pancreas, and all the more toxic when islets are put into the liver because the drugs are given orally, absorbed via the gastrointestinal tract, and highly concentrated in the liver (25).

The metabolic outcomes of successful alloislet transplantation include normal fasting glucose levels and normal hemoglobin A1c levels, but mildly impaired glucose tolerance (23). In this sense, islet transplantation is not as successful as pancreas transplantation. One drawback in intrahepatic islet transplantation is that it does not provide restored glucagon responses to hypoglycemia (26,27) (Fig. 11), a major benefit of pancreas transplantation. This defect appears to be specifically related to the transplantation site, since islets transplanted into the peritoneum and spleen do have normal glucagon responses to hypoglycemia (28). The mechanism for absent glucagon responses from intrahepatic islets is probably related to glycogen stores and increased hepatic glucose flux during hypoglycemia. This results in high-glucose concentrations in the environment of the alpha cell, which in turn negates the hypoglycemic signal the alpha cell receives from the blood coming to it from the general arterial circulation.

Few studies have been published that report the clinical outcomes of successful islet transplantation in terms of the usual secondary complications of diabetes such as eye, kidney, nerve, and macrovascular disease. One publication has appeared reporting that islet recipients have generally improved cardiovascular measures that are independent of improvement in hemoglobin A1c levels, although C-peptide levels were improved (29). Several studies indicate that successful islet transplantation is associated with improved quality of life, and this is primarily related to decreased incidence of hypoglycemia (30,31).

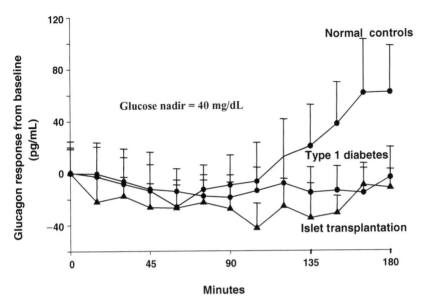

Figure 11 Levels of glucagon before and during induction of hypoglycemia using the hyperinsu-linemic, hypoglycemic clamp in a group of normal control subjects, subjects with type 1 diabetes, and successful recipients of islet transplantation who were normoglycemic and not using insulin. The normal control group had the expected rise in the glucagon counterregulatory response during hypo-glycemia. In contrast, neither the type 1 diabetic patients nor the recipients of islet transplantation had a significant increase in circulating glucagon. This is in contrast to the normal glucagon response experienced by successful recipients of pancreas transplantation, as shown in Fig. 6 (27).

CHOOSING BETWEEN PANCREAS AND ISLET TRANSPLANTATION AS TREATMENTS FOR DIABETES

Since pancreas transplantation has been shown to be very effective in controlling acute and chronic complications of diabetes over long periods of time, and islet transplantation has not, pancreas transplantation must be viewed as the more effective option. However, individual recipients who do not want to undergo the extensive surgery and potentially complicated postoperative course of organ transplantation may logically choose islet transplantation. This should be done, however, with the full knowledge that the majority of islet recipients need to return to insulin-based treatment and that intrahepatic islet transplant recipients do not have restored glucagon secretion during hypoglycemia. The latter is a significant issue given the number of islet transplant recipients who return to insulin treatment and are once again at-risk for hypoglycemia. There are few data that address the impact of islet transplantation on the secondary complications of diabetes mellitus. However, it can be anticipated that those islet transplant patients who are successful in maintaining islet function and normal levels of hemoglobin A1c should have the same beneficial effects on secondary complications of diabetes that has been demonstrated in successful recipients of pancreas transplantation.

REFERENCES

1. Cecka, JM, Terasaki, PI, eds. Clinical Transplants 2002, Vol. 18. Los Angeles: UCLA Immuno-genics Center, 2003:43–52.

2. Kelly WD, Lillehei RC, Merkel FK, et al. Allotransplantation of the pancreas and duodenum along with the kidney in diabetic nephropathy. Surgery 1967;61:827–837.
3. Venstrom JM, McBride MA, Rother KI, et al. Survival after pancreas transplantation in patients with diabetes and preserved kidney function. JAMA 2003;290:2817–2823.
4. Gruessner RW, Sutherland DE, Gruessner AC. Mortality assessment for pancreas transplants. Am J Transplant 2004;4:2018–2026.
5. Robertson RP. Seminars in medicine of the Beth Israel Hospital, Boston: Pancreatic and islet transplantation for diabetes—cures or curiosities. N Engl J Med 1992;327:1861–1868.
6. DCCT RG. The effect of intensive treatment of diabetes on the development and progression of long-term complications in insulin-dependent diabetes mellitus. N Engl J Med 1993;329: 977–985.
7. Diem P, Abid M, Redmon JB, et al. Systemic venous drainage of pancreas allografts as independent cause of hyperinsulinemia in type I diabetic recipients. Diabetes 1990;39:534–540.
8. Redmon JB, Teuscher AU, Robertson RP. Hypoglycemia after pancreas transplantation. Diabetes Care 1998;21:1944–1950.
9. Barrou Z, Seaquist ER, Robertson RP. Pancreas transplantation in diabetic humans normalizes hepatic glucose production during hypoglycemia. Diabetes 1994;43:661–666.
10. Kendall DM, Teuscher AU, Robertson RP. Defective glucagon secretion during sustained hypoglycemia following successful islet allo- and autotransplantation in humans. Diabetes 1997;46:23–27.
11. Bilous RW, Mauer SM, Sutherland DE, et al. The effects of pancreas transplantation on the glomerular structure of renal allografts in patients with insulin-dependent diabetes. N Engl J Med 1989;321:80–85.
12. Fioretto P, Steffes MW, Sutherland DE, et al. Reversal of lesions of diabetic nephropathy after pancreas transplantation. N Engl J Med 1998;339:69–75.
13. Navarro X, Sutherland DE, Kennedy WR. Long-term effects of pancreatic transplantation on diabetic neuropathy. Ann Neuro 1997;42:727–736.
14. Navarro X, Kennedy WR, Loewenson RB, et al. Influence of pancreas transplantation on cardiorespiratory reflexes, nerve conduction, and mortality in diabetes mellitus. Diabetes 1990;39:802–806.
15. Ramsay RC, Goetz FC, Sutherland DE, et al. Progression of diabetic retinopathy after pancreas transplantation for insulin-dependent diabetes mellitus. N Engl J Med 1988;318:208–214.
16. Koznarova R, Saudek F, Sosna T, et al. Beneficial effect of pancreas and kidney transplantation on advanced diabetic retinopathy. Cell Transplant 2000;9:903–908.
17. UKPDS UPDSG. Intensive blood-glucose control with sulphonylureas or insulin compared with conventional treatment and risk of complications in patients with type 2 diabetes (UKPDS 33). Lancet 1998;352:837–853.
18. Jukema JW, Smets YF, van der Pijl JW, et al. Impact of simultaneous pancreas and kidney transplantation on progression of coronary atherosclerosis in patients with end-stage renal failure due to type 1 diabetes. Diabetes Care 2002;25:906–911.
19. Zehrer CL, Gross CR. Quality of life of pancreas transplant recipients. Diabetologia 1991;34(Suppl 1):S145–S149.
20. Piehlmeier W, Bullinger M, Nusser J, et al. Quality of life in type 1 (insulin-dependent) diabetic patients prior to and after pancreas and kidney transplantation in relation to organ function. Diabetologia 1991;34(Suppl 1):S150–S157.
21. Lacy PE, Kostianovsky M. Method for the isolation of intact islets of Langerhans from the rat pancreas. Diabetes 1967;16:35–39.
22. Najarian JS, Sutherland DE, Baumgartner D, et al. Total or near total pancreatectomy and islet autotransplantation for treatment of chronic pancreatitis. Ann Surg 1980;192:526–542.
23. Shapiro AM, Lakey JR, Ryan EA, et al. Islet transplantation in seven patients with type 1 diabetes mellitus using a glucocorticoid-free immunosuppressive regimen. N Engl J Med 2000;343: 230–238.
24. Ryan EA, Paty BW, Senior PA, et al. Five-year follow-up after clinical islet transplantation. Diabetes 2005;54:2060–2069.

25. Robertson RP. Islet transplantation as a treatment for diabetes A work in progress. N Engl J Med 2004;350:694–705.
26. Pyzdrowski KL, Kendall DM, Halter JB, et al. Preserved insulin secretion and insulin independence in recipients of islet autografts. N Engl J Med 1992;327:220–226.
27. Paty BE, Ryan EA, Shapiro AM, et al. Intrahepatic islet transplantation in type 1 diabetic patients does not restore hypoglycemic hormonal counterregulation or symptom recognition after insulin independence. Diabetes 2002;51:3428–3434.
28. Gupta V, Wahoff DC, Rooney DP, et al. The defective glucagon response from transplanted intrahepatic pancreatic islets during hypoglycemia is transplantation site-determined. Diabetes 1997;46:28–33.
29. Fiorina P, Folli F, Bertuzzi F, et al. Long-term beneficial effect of islet transplantation on diabetic macro-/microangiopathy in type 1 diabetic kidney-transplanted patients. Diabetes Care 2003;26:1129–1136.
30. Poggioli R, Faradji RN, Ponte G, et al. Quality of life after islet transplantation. Am J Transplant 2006;6:371–378.
31. Barshes NR, Vanatta JM, Mote A, et al. Health-related quality of life after pancreatic islet transplantation: A longitudinal study. Transplantation 2005;79:1727–1730.

Index

9 780367 388270